Exotics and Wildlife: a manual of veterinary nursing care

For Butterworth-Heinemann:

Commissioning Editor: Mary Seager
Development Editor: Catharine Steers
Project Manager: Morven Dean
Designer: Andy Chapman
Illustration Manager: Bruce Hogarth

Exotics and Wildlife: a manual of veterinary nursing care

Edited by
Caroline Gosden VN
Veterinary Nurse, Animal Care/VN Lecturer, UK

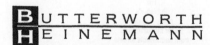

EDINBURGH LONDON NEW YORK OXFORD PHILADELPHIA ST LOUIS SYDNEY TORONTO 2004

BUTTERWORTH-HEINEMANN
An imprint of Elsevier Limited

First edition 2004
  Reprinted 2007

ISBN-13: 978 0 7506 5415 9

British Library Cataloguing in Publication Data
A catalogue record for this book is available from the British Library

Library of Congress Cataloging in Publication Data
A catalog record for this book is available from the Library of Congress

Veterinary knowledge is constantly changing. Standard safety precautions must be followed, but as
new research and clinical experience broaden our knowledge, changes in treatment and drug therapy
may become necessary or appropriate. Readers are advised to check the most current product information
provided by the manufacturer of each drug to be administered to verify the recommended dose, the
method and duration of administration, and contraindications. It is the responsibility of the practitioner,
relying on experience and knowledge of the patient, to determine dosages and the best treatment for
each individual patient. Neither the Publisher nor the author assumes any liability for any injury
and/or damage to persons or property arising from this publication.

The Publisher

Transferred to digital print 2008
Printed and bound by CPI Antony Rowe, Eastbourne

The
Publisher's
policy is to use
paper manufactured
from sustainable forests

Contents

Contributors **vii**

Acknowledgements **ix**

Preface **xi**

SECTION 1 Rodent care

Introduction **3**
1. Rabbits **5**
   Mary Fraser

2. Rodents **23**
   Sara Cowen

SECTION 2 Snakes, lizards and chelonia care

Introduction **47**
3. Snakes and lizards **51**
   Beverly Shingleton

4. Chelonia **87**
   Beverly Shingleton

SECTION 3 Bird care

Introduction **117**
5. Cage birds **119**
   Emma Brooks

6. Birds of prey **141**
   Sara Cowen

7. Wild birds **149**
   Sara Cowen

SECTION 4 Wildlife care

Introduction **167**
8. Bats **171**
   Sara Cowen

9. Foxes **179**
   Sara Cowen

10. Hedgehogs **191**
    Sara Cowen

11. Squirrels **207**
    Sara Cowen

12. Deer **217**
    Sara Cowen

13. Badgers **223**
    Sara Cowen

Appendices

Appendix 1. Rabbits **231**

Appendix 2. Drug dosages **233**

Appendix 3. General information on hand
rearing mammals **237**

Appendix 4. Feeding and caring for baby
birds **241**

Index 245

Contents

Contributors vii

Acknowledgements ix

Preface xi

SECTION 1 Rabbit care

Introduction 3

1. Rabbits 5
Mary Fraser

2. Rodents 25
Sara Cowen

SECTION 2 Snakes, lizards and chelonia care

Introduction 47

3. Snakes and lizards 51
Beverly Shingleton

4. Chelonia 87
Beverly Shingleton

SECTION 3 Bird care

Introduction 119

5. Cage birds 126
Elaine Brooks

6. Budgerigar 141
Sara Cowen

7. Wild birds 156
Sara Cowen

SECTION 4 Wildlife care

Introduction 167

8. bats 171
Sara Cowen

9. foxes 179
Sara Cowen

10. Hedgehogs 191
Sara Cowen

11. squirrels 207
Sara Cowen

12. Deer 219
Sara Cowen

13. Badgers 223
Sara Cowen

Appendices

Appendix 1: Rabbits 251

Appendix 2: Drug dosages 257

Appendix 3: General information on first feeding mammals 242

Appendix 4: feeding and caring for baby birds 241

Index 1245

Contributors

Emma Brooks VN
Veterinary Nurse, Lansdown Veterinary
Surgeons, Stroud, Gloucestershire, UK

Sara Cowen VN BScHONS PGCE
Veterinary Nurse and Education Officer,
Wildlife Aid, Leatherhead, Surrey, UK

Mary Fraser BVMS PhD CertVD CBiol MIBiol MRCVS
Veterinary Surgeon, Strathmore Veterinary
Clinic, Andover, Hampshire, UK

Beverly Shingleton VN Cert Ed
National Diploma in Animal Management,
Programme Leader, Plumpton College,
Nr Lewes, UK

Acknowledgements

The Editor and Publisher would like to thank Wildlife Aid for providing some of the excellent photographs in the Wildlife care section.

Wildlife Aid (reg. charity no. 297610) is dedicated to the rescue, care and rehabilitation of sick, injured and orphaned British wildlife. Over the past 20 years the centre has grown to be one of the largest and most successful wildlife rehabilitation hospitals in the UK, dealing with more than 12 000 wildlife incidents a year. Staffed mostly by volunteers, the charity has a successful rehabilitation rate of over 70%. The aim of the charity is to return every animal that is capable of surviving back into its natural environment. All the animals are treated and rehabilitated completely free of charge.

Education is our future

Wildlife Aid believes that education plays an important part in helping to preserve our heritage. Through school talks, presentations, website and many other means of communication, the charity plays an active role in helping future generations understand and learn about environmental issues that affect us all. Work experience placements are provided for students across the country and Wildlife Aid liaises regularly with agricultural and training establishments on the content of the wildlife section of veterinary courses. Whatever the problem, if it concerns British wildlife, Wildlife Aid will find the answer.

To find out more about the work of the charity, visit their website at: www.wildlifeaid.com.

Wildlife Aid, Randalls Farmhouse, Randalls Road, Leatherhead, Surrey KT22 0AL, UK. Tel: +(0)1372 377332 (admin only); E-mail: wildlife@pncl.co.uk.

Preface

Exotics and wildlife have always featured in the work of a veterinary nurse but the specialist knowledge and training have not always been readily available. However, these topics are now integrated into all levels of veterinary nurse training.

The Exotics and Wildlife manual is written by veterinary nurses and veterinary surgeons experienced in treating these species, in a user-friendly and easy-to-absorb manner. It covers many relevant areas in the veterinary nursing syllabus as well as other aspects and will equip the veterinary nurse with the knowledge and understanding to appropriately house, feed and treat exotic and wildlife patients in practice.

SECTION 1

Rodent care

Introduction

The popularity of rabbits and small furries as pets is on the increase, particularly as more and more adults are appreciating the benefits of keeping these animals. With this, the expectations of owners are ever rising.

So, what role can you as the veterinary nurse play in the care of these animals? Well, in addition to nursing sick animals, education of owners is a vital component of preventative health care.

IDENTIFICATION

This first point may seem rather unusual to say the least, but it is important that you are able to identify the species and breed of the animal that you are presented with as many owners will take this as an indicator of your veterinary knowledge. This knowledge can also make you invaluable to the veterinary surgeon!

HUSBANDRY

Be prepared for the common questions that owners will ask. As many of the problems that these animals are presented with are related to problems in husbandry, this is the main area where owners need to be provided with information. Know the type and size of housing that is appropriate for particular species; whether they should be kept singly or in groups; if male and female should be kept together; whether they should be kept indoors or outdoors; how the animal should be handled; if they need to be groomed and how often; etc.

NUTRITION

This is a major area of importance. Many owners will be aware that guinea pigs require vitamin C in their diet, but how many will know that rats shouldn't be fed a high meat protein diet, or exactly how much fibre should be given to rabbits?

Commercial companies are realising the potential of rabbits and small furries and a whole range of diets are available. Know which diets are available and what you would suggest as best for an individual animal.

VACCINATION

Make sure that owners know that rabbits can be vaccinated against myxomatosis and VHD, and how often these vaccinations should be given.

BREEDING AND NEUTERING

Some owners may not realise how young some small furries can be when they reach sexual maturity. Indeed, I'm sure you have all seen cases where small furries have arrived home from the pet shop already pregnant! Know the ages from which they can breed, the gestation periods and how to tell male from female. Advise owners that if there is any doubt to bring them in to the veterinary surgery soon after they buy them to ensure that they are not keeping male and female animals together.

Neutering of rabbits and other small furries is a routine operation in many practices now and owners should be given information about the advantages of this, such as the prevention of disease in addition to preventing unwanted pregnancies.

DENTAL HEALTH

Although you are all aware how common dental disease is, particularly in rabbits, remember that if the client has never owned a rabbit before then they may not appreciate that there can be a problem. Most owners will bring a pup or a kitten to the practice for a health check soon after purchasing it, but it is just as important to get rabbits and small furries checked for problems. Making sure that owners are aware of the clinical signs of dental disease, such as problems with eating and drooling; teeth grinding allows conditions to be treated early before irreversible problems result. Also, make sure that owners are aware of the importance of correct diet in the prevention of problematic conditions.

COMMON DISEASE CONDITIONS

Make sure that owners are aware of the common problems that may be found in their particular animal, such as fly strike in rabbits. Make sure they know how to prevent it and what to do if they find that their pet has been affected.

Obesity is another problem that is becoming more common in small furries and rabbits. Clinics are held for dogs and cats that are overweight, so why not do the same for rabbits and small furries? This gives you a chance to discuss nutrition and carry out general health checks.

HEALTH AND SAFETY

Ensure that owners are aware of the health risks that all of the animals can pose. Although we are all aware that as long as basic hygiene principles are followed then there is not a problem, many of these animals are looked after by children, so it is important that owners are aware that infections such as *Salmonella*, *E. coli* and *Yersinia pseudotuberculosis* can be carried by them and can affect humans. In addition, ectoparasites such as fleas and *Cheyletiella* can also affect their human handlers.

INSURANCE

More and more insurance companies are now offering insurance for rabbits and other small furries. Although it may seem strange to some owners, it is not unheard of for owners to pay hundreds of pounds for veterinary treatment of small furries that have only cost a fraction of this.

NEW DEVELOPMENTS

Keep up to date with new developments in the veterinary care of these animals. New treatments and diets are coming onto the market all the time. One of the best ways of doing this is to join one of the societies, such as the Rabbit Welfare Association, Rabbit and Rodent Enthusiasts Club or the British Veterinary Zoological Society. These societies organise regular meetings and produce bulletins that contain a lot of valuable material. Advertising in the practice that you are a member of these societies lets owners know that you have a special interest in these species and may even gain you a few clients.

INVALUABLE

So, what can you as the veterinary nurse do in the care of these animals? Well, make yourself a source of knowledge about the care of these species. Make up information packs for owners covering the points mentioned above. Most of all though, show owners that you are enthusiastic about these species and you may become invaluable to the practice.

SOCIETIES

The British Veterinary Zoological Society
www.bvzs.org
  The Rabbit and Rodent Enthusiasts Club
www.therrec.co.uk
  Rabbit Welfare Association
www.rabbitwelfare. co.uk
  The British Rabbit Council, Purefoy House, 7 Kirkgate, Newark, Nottinghamshire. NG24 1AD.

Chapter 1

Rabbits

Mary Fraser

INTRODUCTION

The popularity of rabbits as pets is increasing and veterinary nurses will deal with rabbits on a daily basis.

Historically, rabbits undergoing veterinary procedures did not have a good survival rate, due to the fact that rabbits are a prey species and do not demonstrate clinical signs of illness until they are severely ill. However, as many rabbits are now kept as house rabbits, owners are more aware of small changes in their behaviour and this, combined with the increase in veterinary knowledge and elective surgery, means that the success rate is now much greater.

Veterinary nurses are in the ideal position to liaise with owners, provide information about husbandry and feeding, help prevent problems occurring and deal with them if they do (Fig. 1.1).

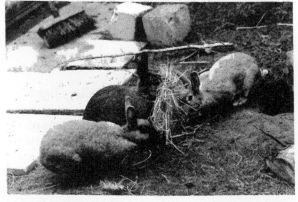

Fig. 1.1 Rabbits in garden.

Rabbits are presented to the surgery for a variety of conditions, some examples of which are given in Table 1.1. It must be remembered that rabbits are a prey species and, therefore, will not demonstrate any clinical signs of illness until the later stages of the disease process. It is important that owners are aware of this and that they do not have unrealistic expectations of veterinary care. However, this does not mean that every case is a lost cause and with dedicated nursing many of these cases will respond to treatment.

Table 1.1 Some examples of first aid situations

1. Owner dropping rabbit	Fractured bones
	Paralysis
	Teeth damage
2. Collapse	Heat stroke
	Shock
	Infection – *E. cuniculi*
	Viral haemorrhagic disease
	Poisoning
	Metabolic diseases, e.g. diabetes, pregnancy toxaemia
3. Respiratory distress	Infection
4. Head tilt/circling	*E. cuniculi*
	Middle/inner ear disease
	Coenuris cyst
	Infection
5. Fly strike	
6. Electrocution (house rabbits)	
7. Fitting	

The role of the veterinary nurse in the first aid case will vary in different practices. If there is a veterinary surgeon available then they may carry out the clinical examination and the nurse will deal with owners, take a history and prepare any equipment. However, there may be times when the veterinary nurse is expected to deal with these cases, carry out a clinical examination and make an initial assessment.

If transporting a rabbit to the practice, owners should be advised to keep the rabbit warm by wrapping it in a towel and providing a heat source such as a hot water bottle.

Tip: The temperature of the rabbit should be just warm to the touch when wrapped in a towel.

If there is any bleeding, owners should stem this as best as possible by applying pressure to the wound.

As many rabbits are owned by children it is better if an adult can come to the practice. This is essential for the completion of consent forms and may help when taking a history.

Once at the practice a history needs to be obtained from the owner. Useful questions to ask are:

1. Is the rabbit a house rabbit or kept outdoors?
2. How long has the rabbit been ill (sudden onset or progressive)?
3. Are there any other rabbits in the house?
4. Are there any other pets in the house?
5. Is the rabbit vaccinated against myxomatosis/viral haemorrhagic disease?
6. Could the rabbit have eaten anything unusual?
7. Has the rabbit suffered any trauma (e.g. being dropped, attacked)?
8. Was the rabbit eating normally/producing faeces?

Finding out whether the rabbit is an outdoor rabbit or a house rabbit will determine the type of things that the rabbit will come into contact with and is particularly important in suspected poisonings.

You may have to give advice to an owner over the telephone and it is helpful to ask the questions given above. You also need to assess if the rabbit is in pain which can be difficult. Any change in normal behaviour could be regarded as a sign of pain. Other signs include immobility, hunching, grinding teeth or possibly even aggression and anorexia. If the rabbit is demonstrating any of these signs it is better if the rabbit is seen at the veterinary practice.

INITIAL ASSESSMENT

The rabbit should be handled as little as possible during any examination to reduce stress.

The initial assessment should take place before handling the rabbit. Things to observe include:

- wounds
- swellings
- haemorrhage
- fractures
- respiratory rate
- respiratory manner.

Tip: If the rabbit shows respiratory problems then give oxygen during examination.

Mouth breathing in the rabbit is not a good clinical sign as they are obligate nose breathers and will only mouth breathe if in severe respiratory distress.

Standard parameters should then be recorded:

- mucous membrane colour
- capillary refill time
- body temperature
- pulse rate
- pulse strength
- pulse regularity
- examination of the eyes – pupillary light response and nystagmus
- examination of the ear canals for signs of infection possibly associated with middle ear disease.

Examination of the nervous system and spinal reflexes can be carried out in rabbits just as for dogs.

Examination of bladder control (present or absent), hindlimb reflexes and deep pain sensation can indicate damage to the spine. Examination of the mammary glands and reproductive system should also take place, observing any swelling, discharge or haemorrhage.

TREATMENT

Obviously the treatment required will depend on the clinical problem. When stressed rabbits can develop shock. In rabbits the shock organ is the lungs where vasodilatation will take place. This means that a rabbit in shock may well present in respiratory distress and collapse. As the circulation is affected, fluid therapy is vitally important for these cases. Placement of an intravenous catheter is essential and will also allow blood to be taken for haematology/biochemistry analysis. Some examples of first aid scenarios and their treatment are given in Table 1.2.

Table 1.2 Common first aid scenarios

Problem	Treatment
Sudden collapse	Provide heat and warmth Clinical assessment Blood sample
Head tilt/circling	Clinical examination – ears, eyes X-ray Blood sample
Fractures	Provide warmth, oxygen, fluids Examine for compound fractures Stabilise fracture if possible and bandage to reduce swelling Provide pain relief
Teeth damage	Examine for bleeding Assess degree of damage Provide pain relief
Respiratory distress	Reduce stress levels as much as possible Provide warmth and oxygen
Fly strike	Fluids for endotoxic shock Antibacterial therapy Pain relief Remove maggots
Heat stress	Measure body temperature IV fluids Cool with wet towels Keep in well-ventilated room

HOSPITAL CAGE SET UP

Siting

The cage should be situated in an area where the rabbit will not feel stressed – ideally, not facing the cats in the hospital! The cage should be big enough for the rabbit to turn round in, but also ensure that it is easy for the nurse to remove the animal from the cage when needed. Ideally, the cages should be near the ground and made of stainless steel, as rabbits will gnaw at their surroundings and bowls.

Food and water

Rabbits need to be provided with water at all times. You will need to ask the owner how the rabbit is usually provided with water, as, although most rabbits will use a water bottle, some may use a bowl. Providing the wrong form of water container can result in the rabbit refusing to drink. Most cages are suitable for attaching a water bottle to, but you must ensure that the height of the bottle suits the rabbit and that it is not too high/low for the rabbit to reach.

The feeding bowls should be easy to clean and impossible to gnaw – either metal or ceramic bowls are best.

Bedding

Bedding is important as rabbits are prone to developing hock lesions if this is not adequate. Newspaper is the ideal substrate. Materials such as sawdust or straw are not ideal in practice as they are messy and can obscure any body fluids that may be needed for examination. If the rabbit uses a litter tray then you should also find out what the owner puts in the litter tray – cat litter, straw or newspaper are usually used. Newspaper is best if the rabbit will use it as any urine or faecal material will be obvious when produced; cat litter can be a problem as some rabbits will eat it; hay or straw are usually well tolerated.

Even rabbits not used to litter trays are generally very clean and will use one corner of the cage as a toilet. Again, this is more likely if the cage is big enough.

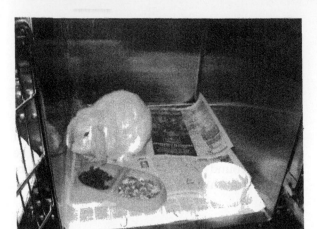

Fig. 1.2 Hospital cage set up.

Temperature

The environmental temperature should be kept below 25°C to prevent heat stress, as rabbits cannot sweat. The room should be well ventilated to reduce the risk of respiratory disease.

If rabbits are only hospitalised for a short time (a few hours) then it is possible to keep them in a carry box inside the cage. This may make them more secure, although this cannot be used for long-term hospitalisation (Fig. 1.2).

FOOD AND FEEDING

Normal diet

When dealing with rabbit nutrition it is important to remember the diet of the wild rabbit in comparison with that of its domestic cousin. Rabbits are naturally herbivorous and in the wild will eat large amounts of fibre. Their gastrointestinal system is designed to deal with this fibre and obtain nutrition from it.

> **Tip:** Ideally, hay should make up 50% of the diet.

Fibre is important for a number of reasons:

- Fibre wears down the continuously growing incisors and molars
- Indigestible fibre induces peristalsis
- Fibre is utilised by the bacteria in the caecum.

Thus, if a rabbit's diet is low in fibre a variety of problems can result:

- Overgrowth of incisors and molars
- Gut stasis
- Inadequate or imbalanced nutrition.

The best source of fibre is hay. Figures vary but, ideally, at least 25% and up to 50% of the diet should be composed of hay. A large amount of fibre in the diet means that the rabbit needs to chew and this will help prevent dental problems such as overgrown teeth and crowns or hyperextended roots. Hay is also useful in that it is a good source of vitamin D, which is required for normal calcium metabolism.

The remainder of the diet can be made up of vegetables and some commercial food.

Rabbits have a very sweet tooth and if given the chance will be selective about what they eat, usually only eating high-calorie cereals and leaving hay and vegetables.

Rabbits produce caecotrophs, which appear different to normal faeces as they are softer, often green coloured and covered in mucous. They are usually consumed directly from the anus, often at night. The mucous covering protects them from the acidic environment of the stomach. Once the mucous layer is dissolved, nutrients including vitamins B and K are absorbed from the caecotrophs' bacterial contents.

As caecotrophs are consumed when they are produced they should not be seen lying around the cage. If the owner does see caecotrophs this could be due to spinal injury, obesity, vestibular disease or dental disease. If caecotrophs are not being produced or consumed then it is important that these rabbits are given vitamin supplements.

Vegetables deteriorate rapidly and so fresh vegetables need to be given twice daily. Useful examples include celery, spinach, kale, dandelion leaves, parsley, carrots or green peppers. Fruits such as apples, pears and melons can also be given. You should find out the normal diet of any rabbit that is coming in to the hospital as changing diet can result in diarrhoea.

In the wild, rabbits will eat mainly at dusk and dawn and it is possible that rabbits may not be observed eating in the practice. However, it is important to record accurately exactly what and how much the rabbit has eaten by counting the number of pieces of individual vegetables that are given to the rabbit and then left.

Calcium

Rabbits will absorb calcium from the diet and if they are fed food containing large amounts of calcium (such as alfalfa) then they will absorb large amounts of calcium. The only way that rabbits can deal with this excess calcium is to excrete it in the urine, which can result in the production of sludgy urine or even urinary calculi. Monitoring urine colour and consistency is important in these cases.

Calcium is also a factor in rabbit dental disease. Nutritional osteodystrophy due to low levels of calcium and vitamin D can result in abnormal tooth growth. It is important, therefore, that rabbits are given sufficient quantities of fresh vegetables in the diet to reduce this problem. As other factors are involved in the production of dental disease, provision of a good diet alone will not prevent dental disease occurring in all cases.

Water

Fresh water should always be available and, as mentioned earlier, you need to find out whether the rabbit is used to using a dropper bottle or a bowl. If using a dropper bottle you need to ensure that it is positioned at the correct height for the rabbit. Rabbits will normally drink between 50 and 100 ml/kg/24 hours, so this should be measured. Water bowls can result in wetting of the dewlap and dermatitis so any rabbit provided with water by this method should be checked for these problems and the dewlap kept dry.

Pre-operative feeding

Rabbits should be fed up until about 30 minutes before an operation. This is because they cannot vomit and, therefore, do not need long periods of fasting to ensure that the stomach is empty prior to an anaesthetic. Also, if food is withdrawn then this can lead to gut stasis, a common problem with rabbits undergoing anaesthesia. Some vets do not withdraw food from rabbits at all prior to surgery, but removing food for around 30 minutes means that it is unlikely that there will be any food material in the mouth when the rabbit is anaesthetised. This makes intubating the rabbit or carrying out a dental examination much more straightforward.

Post-operative feeding

Rabbits should be encouraged to eat as soon as they come round from an anaesthetic. Offering fresh vegetables and food that the rabbit is known to eat is usually sufficient. As mentioned earlier, it is important to ensure that the rabbit is actually eating and to monitor the amounts that are being eaten. Any period of anorexia can result in gut stasis and/or hepatic lipidosis.

Faecal production should also be monitored as the absence of faeces suggests gut hypomotility. The only faeces that should be observed are hard faecal pellets. Softer caecotrophs should not be evident in the cage. Diarrhoea should also be noted.

The rabbit should be kept in the hospital until it is seen to be eating regularly. It should be stressed to owners that it is vitally important that the rabbit continues to eat at home and that any evidence of anorexia should be reported to the veterinary practice right away.

Anorexia

You will deal with anorexic rabbits for a variety of reasons. It is possible that the rabbit was brought to the practice anorexic or that the condition developed following an anaesthetic. The main causes of anorexia include:

- dental disease
- low fibre content in the diet
- any illness and pain.

As mentioned earlier, gut peristalsis is stimulated by the presence of fibre in the gastrointestinal tract. If rabbits are anorexic then gut stasis will develop. This can result in bacterial overgrowth and the absorption of toxins, which result in the development of shock and collapse. If this is not corrected then it can lead to death.

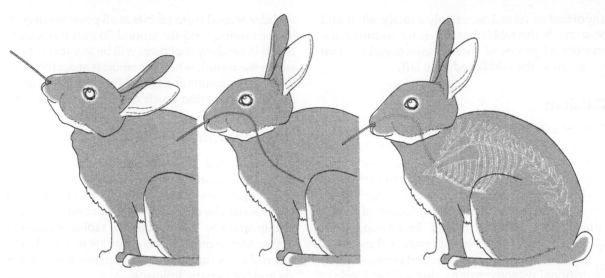

Fig. 1.3 Naso-oesophageal tube.

> **Tip:** Sugar-rich foods can be offered to anorexic individuals to encourage them to eat, as rabbits have a sweet tooth.

Also, anorexic rabbits can develop hepatic lipidosis, which will result in metabolic problems due to liver disease.

Where a rabbit is not eating, syringe feeding or naso-oesophageal feeding should take place.

A naso-oesophageal tube should be placed in the following way (Fig. 1.3):

1. Suitable restraint of the rabbit – usually carried out on the conscious rabbit.
2. Place local anaesthetic into nostril – lignocaine gel or eyedrops.
3. Using a 3 or 4 French naso-oesophageal tube measure from nares to 7th rib and mark tube with marker pen.
4. Insert tube with rabbit's head elevated as this eases insertion and aim medially.
5. Once inserted into the nose flex head so that tube can pass into oesophagus.
6. X-ray the rabbit to ensure correct placement of tube. Passing water into the tube and watching for coughing if the tube is in the trachea does not work in the rabbit.

The simplest method of feeding is to blend a commercial rabbit food, add some water and syringe feed or feed through a naso-oesophageal tube. The volume of water that is required will depend on the consistency of the diet, but you should aim to give the rabbit 3–15 ml four to six times daily (Girling 2001). If making up your own preparation, then adding supplements such as Avipro (VetArk) is beneficial. You can calculate how much to add based on the amount of water that you have added to your preparation, but in general only a very small amount of Avipro will be required.

Specific critical care diets can also be used and may be useful as these are designed to pass through a syringe. There is some controversy over the use of diets that are designed to pass through a syringe as this may mean that the fibre particles are not large enough to stimulate gut motility (Harcourt Brown 2002). However, they are a very useful source of nutrition for the debilitated animal.

Fresh hay should always be offered to these animals to encourage them to feed for themselves and stimulate gut motility.

Medical treatment of anorexia

A variety of drugs may be needed in the treatment of anorexia dependent on the underlying cause.

Often the main problem in an anorexic rabbit is pain, therefore, using analgesics can often encourage the rabbit to eat:

- buprenorphine
- carprofen
- ketoprofen
- meloxicam.

Other drugs such as gut motility stimulants (cisapride or metoclopramide) will prevent gut stasis; appetite stimulants such as nandrolone, anti-ulcer drugs such as ranitidine, and probiotics can all be used in the anorexic rabbit.

It should be remembered that the cascade must be followed when treating rabbits and that many of the drugs used for the treatment of rabbits are not licensed. Prescribing these drugs is the decision of the veterinary surgeon and, although the majority of rabbits will be pets, as they are classified as food-producing animals, data sheet drug withdrawal times must be followed.

Nutrition of the neonatal rabbit

In the wild, neonatal rabbits will only feed for a short period of time once or twice a day. Up until 21 days of age they should only be fed milk replacer. This should be as similar to doe's milk as possible. A suggested formula from Okerman (1994) is one quarter of full-fat cow's milk added to three-quarters condensed milk. To 100 ml of this 6 g of skimmed milk powder is added. Hand rearing neonatal rabbits is very difficult, however, as the gut microflora often does not develop properly and enterotoxaemia can develop.

> **Tip:** In theory, introducing caecotrophs from the adult could help to rectify this problem. However, it is probably best to avoid this due to the risk of introducing pathogenic bacterial parasites.

ANAESTHESIA AND PRE/POST-OPERATIVE CARE

Pre-anaesthetic care

There are a variety of reasons as to why a rabbit may require a general anaesthetic, from emergency surgery through to routine neutering. Wherever possible it is advisable to arrange an appointment for the owner prior to the day of the operation. This will give the owner a chance to find out exactly what is involved in the surgery and anaesthesia and will allow a clinical examination to be carried out to ensure that the rabbit is fit enough to receive an anaesthetic.

Whether the clinical examination is carried out by the vet or the veterinary nurse is at the discretion of the veterinary surgeon. All findings should be reported to the veterinary surgeon, particularly where any abnormalities have been detected. Clinical parameters that should be checked are given below:

- Confirm sex of rabbit.
- Obtain accurate weight for the rabbit.
- Check teeth – incisors and cheek teeth. Look for abnormal growth, presence of dental spurs or ulcers often seen on the cheeks. Any dental disease will need to be rectified prior to carrying out elective surgery as this could lead to anorexia following the anaesthetic.
- Examine ears for mites and any infection. Any pus in the ear could suggest a middle ear infection. If this is a possibility then the rabbit will need an X-ray and treatment prior to anaesthesia.
- Examine for signs of respiratory disease. This includes the presence of a nasal discharge, staining of the inner aspect of the forelimbs.
- Auscultate the lung fields preferably with a paediatric stethoscope.
- Monitor respiratory rate (normal 30–60/min).
- Assess degree of thoracic wall movement – there should only be a little movement in a healthy rabbit.
- Examine eyes for any ocular discharge, which could suggest disease of the nasolacrimal duct (dacryocystitis).
- Examine eyes for nystagmus, which could indicate middle ear disease.
- Measure body temperature (normal 38.5–40°C).
- Measure heart rate and pulse (normal 180–300/min).
- Check for diarrhoea, faecal matting, vaginal discharge in does.
- Check hydration status.

• Observe for signs of head tilt or any circling when moving. Head tilt may not be observed if rabbit is stressed. It can help if rabbit can move around the consulting room.

Owners should be given an information sheet informing them of the procedure that the rabbit is going to undergo and instructions for the day of the operation. Many owners will be used to removing food and water from cats or dogs prior to receiving an anaesthetic and will expect to do the same with their rabbit. They need to be informed and preferably given written instructions not to do this.

> **Tip:** Only withdraw food for a short time prior to anaesthesia.

On the day of the operation the checks listed above should be carried out again as it is possible for rabbits to develop conditions in the time between the initial check and the operation.

Premedication

The choice of premedicant will depend on the procedure that is going to be carried out. It is possible that the procedure may be carried out under deep sedation, as in the case of some dentals, or that a full general anaesthetic may be required.

Premedication should be used when anaesthetising rabbits, as when they are exposed to a gaseous anaesthetic they may breath hold. This is a problem not only because of the lack of oxygen, but also because the stress of breath holding causes the rabbit to release catecholamines from the adrenal glands. These have a direct effect on the lungs and the heart causing a spasm of the smooth muscle of the airways and the pulmonary artery, which results in further breath holding, tachycardia and, if not corrected, right-sided heart failure. This can lead to fatalities during the early stages of an anaesthetic.

The drugs used as premedicants for rabbits are often the same as those given to cats and dogs. The more common drugs include:

• fentanyl/fluanisone combination
• medetomidine

• xylazine
• acepromazine
• diazepam
• midazolam.

These drugs can be given in various combinations and specific anaesthesia texts should be consulted for further information on this topic.

Atropine does not tend to be used in rabbits as it is broken down by the rabbit's metabolism and, therefore, does not have the desired effects. Where an anticholinergic drug is needed then glycopyrrolate should be used.

Fluid therapy

It is helpful to give fluids to most rabbits before they are anaesthetised, as this will reduce the chances of dehydration occurring post-operatively. In the healthy rabbit fluids can usually be given subcutaneously over two or three sites. Up to 30–50 ml can be given over the scruff and the thorax. In more debilitated animals it is better to give fluids intravenously. The best vein to use is the marginal ear vein (Fig. 1.4). The hair can be shaved here and local anaesthetic gel placed over the vein to allow easy access. With an assistant putting pressure over the vein at the base of the ear a butterfly catheter (25 or 27 gauge) can be put into the vein and taped into place. Intraperitoneal administration of fluids can be carried out if intravenous access is difficult, but fluid absorption by this method will be slower.

The choice of fluid will depend on the condition of the rabbit. For example, glucose saline can

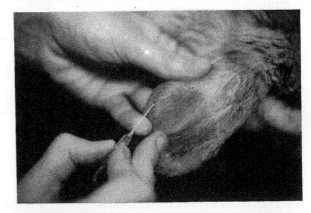

Fig. 1.4 Marginal ear vein.

be used for animals undergoing elective surgery, or if they are anorexic. It should be remembered, however, that the glucose content of these fluids is not sufficient to supply all of the energy requirements of an anorexic rabbit.

Fluids such as Hartmann's can be used where rabbits are suffering from metabolic acidosis or gastrointestinal problems.

Where rabbits lose more than 10% of their body fluids then colloids can be used instead of crystalloids.

Maintenance fluid requirements in rabbits are higher than those in cats and dogs, and 80–100 ml/kg/day should be used when calculating fluid requirements.

Anaesthesia

Anaesthetic induction can be carried out with either injectable or inhalational agents. For minor procedures it is possible that agents such as fentanyl/fluanisone (Hypnorm) may be used alone. Alternatively, medetomidine/ketamine or xylazine/ketamine combinations may be used. Gaseous anaesthetics such as halothane, isoflurane or newer agents such as sevoflurane may also be used.

Gaseous anaesthetics can be given by face mask, endotracheal tube or incubation chamber.

Intubation is the best method as this will allow oxygen to be supplied throughout the procedure and intermittent positive pressure ventilation (IPPV) to be carried out should there be any problems.

As many rabbits have subacute respiratory disease, it is helpful to supply oxygen via an endotracheal tube when using injectable anaesthetics to ensure that they are adequately oxygenated. The main reason for intubation not being commonly used in the rabbit, is that the anatomy makes placement more difficult than in the dog or cat, although many vets are skilled in the procedure.

> **Tip:** Supply oxygen by endotracheal tube to all anaesthetised rabbits, as many have subacute respiratory disease.

If using an anaesthetic chamber then it will need to be quite large for a rabbit and will take some time for gaseous anaesthetics to reach adequate levels. Face masks are not ideal as they can be quite stressful for the rabbit. If the rabbit is stressed at any point during the anaesthetic then this will result in the release of catecholamines (see earlier).

Isoflurane is currently the gaseous agent of choice, but this has a distinctive smell, which can result in the rabbit breath holding. Using a premedicant will reduce this risk. Isoflurane also has the advantage that it makes the heart less sensitive to catecholamines. Newer agents, such as sevoflurane, are likely to be used more in the future.

The use of nitrous is controversial. Based on dogs and cats you would expect nitrous to allow a reduction in the dose of anaesthetic agents. However, rabbits respond differently to nitrous and very high doses of nitrous are needed before any reduction in anaesthetic agent is seen. For this reason it is unlikely that nitrous will be used in rabbit anaesthetics.

The usual circuits used in rabbit anaesthesia are an Ayres T-piece, a Bain or a Mapleson C (Fig. 1.5) as these have a low dead space volume.

Monitoring the depth of anaesthesia is similar to that of dogs and cats. The main checks to make are:

- Monitor respiratory rate, depth, character.
- Monitor mucous membrane colour, capillary refill time.
- Ear pinch reflex – absent in the anaesthetised rabbit.

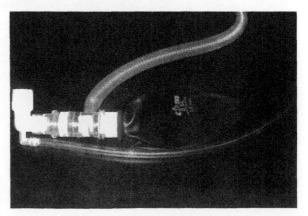

Fig. 1.5 Ayres T-piece, a Bain or a Mapleson C.

- Pedal withdrawal reflex – weakly present in the anaesthetised rabbit.
- If possible use pulse oximeter and electrocardiogram (ECG).

Tip: Protect corneas during surgery with topical ointment.

Preparation of the operating site should involve removing only enough fur to enable sterile access. Rabbits can easily develop hypothermia and heat loss can be minimised by removing as little fur as possible, being careful when scrubbing up the operation site that the rabbit does not become soaked, and don't use spirit as this is cooling.

Throughout any procedure the rabbit should be kept warm either on a heat mat (Fig. 1.6) or wrapped in bubble wrap. It is, however, important that the rabbit's body temperature is monitored to ensure that they do not become too hot, as they cannot lose heat by sweating.

Obviously positioning will depend on the procedure, but it is helpful to keep the abdomen lower than the thorax to reduce the weight of ingesta on the lungs.

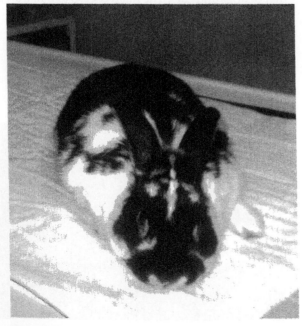

Fig. 1.6 Rabbit on heat mat.

Should the rabbit develop any problems during the anaesthetic then it can be dealt with just as you would for a cat or dog. For example, if respiratory depression occurs then:

- decrease/stop gaseous anaesthetic
- increase oxygen supplementation
- extend neck, ensure airway is patent
- apply doxapram under the tongue
- use artificial respiration – IPPV or chest compressions
- fluids – ensure not bleeding.

Reversal of anaesthesia

This will depend on the agents given. Where the rabbit has received injectable anaesthetics, including medetomidine, xylazine or fentanyl, then it is possible to give a reversal agent.

As for cats and dogs, atipamazole can be given to reverse the effects of medetomidine. This will also reverse the effects of xylazine, although it is not licensed for this use.

Both butorphanol and buprenorphine will reverse the effects of fentanyl and quickly bring the rabbit round.

If using gaseous anaesthesia, then rabbits can be treated in exactly the same way as cats and dogs, leaving them on pure oxygen until they come round from the gaseous anaesthetic agent.

Post-operative care

After surgery the rabbit should be monitored in a warm recovery area. Ideally, it should still be kept on a heat mat until it is up and moving about.

Post-operative antibacterial therapy will depend on the reason for anaesthesia, but in most cases it is desirable to give some form of antibacterial treatment. Analgesics should be given at the beginning of surgery and, if needed again, before the animal is conscious.

The rabbit should be monitored for the signs of pain during the recovery period. These include:

- unwillingness to move
- remaining at the back of the kennel
- teeth grinding
- drawn-in abdomen

- piloerection
- abnormal gait if the rabbit does move
- aggression
- not eating or drinking.

The importance of ensuring that the rabbit begins eating as soon as possible following recovery has already been mentioned.

Being in pain is one of the commonest reasons for anorexia. If the rabbit is demonstrating any of the above signs then pain relief should be given. Some of the more common analgesics given to rabbits include non-steroidal drugs such as meloxicam or carprofen or opioid derivatives such as buprenorphine or butorphanol.

You need to remember that the length of time for which these agents have an effect varies and some can act for as little as 30 minutes. Therefore, the rabbit needs to be monitored to ensure that the treatment is having the desired effect – this can be seen if the rabbit starts to move around the cage and starts to eat – and that the effect is prolonged and the rabbit doesn't return to showing signs of pain.

In cases of elective surgery, fluid therapy will probably have been given prior to operating. As dehydration is an important consideration, the rabbit's hydration status and whether or not it is drinking should be monitored and fluids administered where appropriate.

It is helpful to give them a bed of hay once they have recovered from the anaesthetic to encourage them to eat. Not only can they bury into it and, therefore, feel secure, hay is also the best food to encourage gut motility. They should also be offered fresh vegetables and fruit. If the rabbit is not keen to eat, then it should be hand fed.

Exercise is useful in stimulating gut motility post-operatively – although whether this is feasible or not will depend on the procedure that the rabbit received. Where the rabbit can move about, it can help if there is a safe area that it can move around in rather than sitting in a kennel all day.

Ideally, the rabbit should not be sent home until you are happy that it is eating and is not in pain. Owners should be made aware of the clinical signs of pain and the fact that if the rabbit becomes anorexic then they should contact the surgery right away.

DISEASES

Dental disease

Dental disease is one of the commonest problems seen in veterinary practice. A variety of reasons for the development of dental problems have been put forward and it is fair to say that all of these, either alone or in combination, have a role to play:

- Genetics – some breeds are more prone to dental disease than others, e.g. Dutch and Netherland dwarf.
- Diet – not enough abrasive material in the diet (i.e. hay) to allow for normal wearing of the teeth.
- Calcium imbalance – low levels of calcium in the diet will result in abnormal tooth development.

Dental disease can be very obvious if the incisor teeth are affected. Often the incisors will not meet and do not wear down properly, so the teeth continue to grow with the result that the rabbit appears to have tusks protruding from its mouth – something that the owners will notice (Fig. 1.7). These teeth can easily become damaged or broken and infection of the tooth root can result. The abnormal teeth also make eating very difficult so that the rabbit will probably lose weight.

It is more difficult to observe any abnormality of the cheek teeth. These teeth also grow continuously and are ground down by the food that the rabbit eats. Overgrowth of these teeth leads to pain

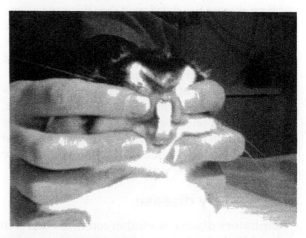

Fig. 1.7 Overgrown incisors.

and ulceration of the cheeks where tooth spurs can develop. Roots can elongate and in severe cases these can be felt as bumps along the mandible. Tooth root extension of the maxillary teeth can also affect the nasolacrimal duct and dacryocystitis can develop, which will often present as an eye problem rather than a dental problem.

The main clinical signs of a rabbit with dental disease are anorexia, salivation, abnormal growth of incisors and obvious oral discomfort or pain.

In order to examine the teeth properly specific equipment is needed (Fig. 1.8):

- laryngoscope or otoscope to visualise the cheek teeth
- a light source
- rabbit tooth gag
- pouch dilator
- possibly sedation
- an assistant to hold the rabbit's head.

Radiography is also very helpful to visualise the tooth roots or observe any abscess formation in the jaw.

Treatment of dental disease is often long term. Immediate relief can be given by reducing the length of overgrown incisors (Fig. 1.9) and removing any spurs on the cheek teeth that are causing pain.

In some cases it may be preferable to remove the incisors as rabbits can manage perfectly well without them as long as they are able to grind food with the cheek teeth.

If an abscess has developed then this can be very difficult to cure. Most cases will require surgery in addition to medical management to debride infected tissue, but the long-term prospects are not good once osteomyelitis has developed.

If rabbits are affected when young then correcting any underlying problems, such as diet, will help, but once the teeth have started to grow abnormally it is very difficult to correct. In most cases, rabbits with dental disease will require regular visits to the veterinary practice.

Respiratory disease

Respiratory disease is another common condition of rabbits. Indeed, many of the rabbits that you see

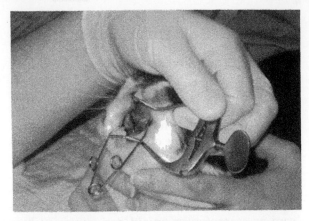

Fig. 1.8 Equipment for examining teeth.

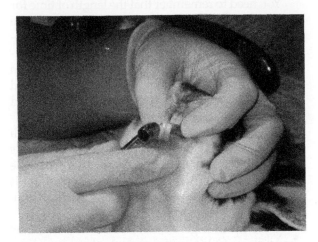

Fig. 1.9 Trimming overgrown incisors.

in practice will have some degree of respiratory disease.

Acute respiratory disease is easy to detect (Fig. 1.10) with clinical signs including:

- nasal discharge
- staining of the forepaws with dried nasal discharge
- increased respiratory rate, depth and pattern
- mouth breathing – a very poor sign
- cyanosis
- eye disease – conjunctivitis
- abnormalities on auscultation (using a paediatric stethoscope).

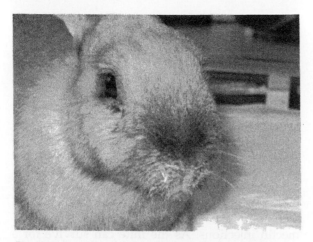

Fig. 1.10 Rabbit with clinical signs of respiratory disease.

Milder respiratory disease may be heard on auscultation but it is possible that no clinical signs will be seen at all. This is a problem when carrying out rabbit anaesthetics as you cannot assume that all of the lung volume is functional. When carrying out anaesthesia with injectable agents rather than gaseous anaesthesia it is advisable to still intubate them and supply oxygen to ensure that they are adequately oxygenated.

Various agents can be responsible for respiratory disease:

- Bacterial – *Pasteurella multocida*, *Bordetella bronchiseptica* and *Pseudomonas aeruginosa*.
- Viral – myxomatosis and viral haemorrhagic disease.
- Other – neoplasia and irritation of the respiratory tract.

Examination of a rabbit with respiratory disease should be carried out with oxygen supplementation and you should stress the rabbit as little as possible.

Treatment of respiratory disease will obviously depend on the underlying cause. General treatment includes: fluid therapy (rabbits with respiratory disease are often dehydrated due to fluid loss in discharge and decreased fluid intake), antibacterial therapy, mucolytics, and steam inhalation to decrease congestion. Rabbits with respiratory disease will often be anorexic, so it is important to ensure that they are eating and if not provide assisted nutrition.

Infectious disease

Encephalitozoon cuniculi

Encephalitozoon cuniculi is a protozoal disease that is surprisingly common in rabbits. Recently, it has been shown that this organism is, indeed, pathogenic (earlier texts state that *E. cuniculi* infection is insignificant) and can be responsible for nervous system disease and renal disease.

E. cuniculi is transmitted between rabbits via infected urine and many animals can carry the infection without demonstrating clinical signs. However, it can cause disease and clinical signs include:

- kidney disease – polyuria, polydypsia
- nervous system disease – head tilt, tremors, convulsions
- muscle weakness.

Examination of a blood sample for antibodies against *E. cuniculi* can confirm that the rabbit has met the infection but does not confirm disease and histology of affected organs is required in order to confirm an infection. Therefore, it is likely that a suspected case will be treated on the basis of clinical signs and a serology result. Treatment relies on the use of anthelmintics such as albendazole, which have some effect against the agent.

Myxomatosis

This condition is caused by a myxoma virus (part of the pox virus group), which is transmitted between rabbits via the rabbit flea (*Psilopsyllus cuniculi*). It is possible for rabbits to die suddenly from the disease without demonstrating any clinical signs. More commonly, though, they will demonstrate signs such as oedema of the periocular region, base of the ears, and genital area; anorexia; lethargy and increased body temperature before dying.

Where rabbits have been vaccinated, but do not have full immunity, then swelling and crusting nodules can be found affecting the skin around the eyes, base of ears and nose (Fig. 1.11) and these animals can make a recovery.

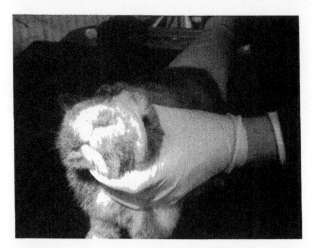

Fig. 1.11 Rabbit suffering from myxomatosis.

Diagnosis is generally made on clinical signs, although it is possible to confirm the condition with a biopsy.

Treatment of myxomatosis is only possible in milder forms of the condition. Nursing includes warmth, intravenous fluids, supported nutrition, cleaning any lesions and antibacterial therapy to prevent secondary infections as these animals are prone to developing respiratory disease.

Ideally, all rabbits should be vaccinated against myxomatosis. Where rabbits live in a high risk area then they can be vaccinated every 6 months rather then once a year. The vaccine does not contain myxomatosis virus but a related virus. Therefore, there is no chance that a rabbit can develop myxomatosis from the vaccine.

Viral haemorrhagic disease

This is a condition caused by a calicivirus, which was first reported in rabbits in the 1980s. Morbidity and mortality are high as the virus is highly contagious.

Clinical signs include:

- sudden death
- haemorrhage
- increased body temperature
- decreased appetite/anorexia
- diarrhoea – often haemorrhagic.

Treatment of infected animals is very difficult due to the short duration of the illness.

Parasites

Cheyletiella

Cheyletiella parasitivorax is a surface living mite which can be asymptomatic when present in small numbers but where the population rises can cause irritation, hair loss and profuse dandruff mainly affecting the dorsum. The mite is zoonotic, with owners often bitten on the forearms and abdomen. The condition is treated with ivermectin injections. As the mite can survive for a short time in the environment any treatment protocol must include thorough disinfection of the environment and disposal of bedding materials.

Psoroptes

Psoroptes cuniculi is the rabbit ear mite. Infestations cause severe otitis externa with crusting and exudate. Treatment includes soaking the ear to remove excess crusting, ivermectin to kill the parasite and antibacterial therapy as these rabbits are prone to secondary bacterial infections.

Fly strike

Fly strike or myiasis is surprisingly common in rabbits kept outdoors. Any problem that results in faecal matting will allow flies to lay their eggs around the rabbit's rump:

- infectious diarrhoea (bacterial or parasitic)
- obesity – cannot carry out copraphagy
- wrong diet – diarrhoea
- dental problems – diarrhoea
- rabbit kept in unsanitary conditions
- matting of the coat in longer coated breeds (poor grooming).

Blowflies lay their eggs in faeces, which quickly hatch into maggots. These maggots then bury into the flesh of the rabbit and feed on this, causing physical damage to skin and muscles, infection, gangrene and release of toxins into the rabbit's bloodstream. It is surprising how quickly these problems can develop and owners need to monitor their animals daily for this condition, as affected animals can quickly die.

Prevention is better than cure and all outdoor rabbits should be treated with Rear Guard (Novartis) to prevent this occurring. If a rabbit is presented with fly strike, then the maggots need to be physically removed, and the damaged tissue treated like any other infected wound. These rabbits are often ill when presented and can die during treatment.

CASE HISTORY 1

Patient

Adult Dutch rabbit, 1 year old, weighing 2.5 kg.

Reason for hospitalisation

The owner had dropped the rabbit and, on examination, the rabbit was found to have a separated mandibular symphysis. The rabbit was admitted for surgery.

Type of accommodation and bedding material used and relevant environmental factors

The rabbit was placed in a metal kennel (dimensions: 40 cm width; 60 cm depth; 50 cm height) in a ward reserved for small mammals/exotics. The bedding material consisted of newspaper and hay. The rabbit was house trained, so a litter tray containing straw was placed towards the back of the kennel. A water bottle was attached at a suitable height on the front of the kennel. The environmental temperature is kept at 15–20°C and the room is well ventilated.

Accommodation cleaning protocol

The litter tray was checked regularly throughout the day and waste material emptied into clinical waste. The tray was cleaned with standard disinfectant, dried and returned to the kennel with fresh straw. Newspaper was changed daily or

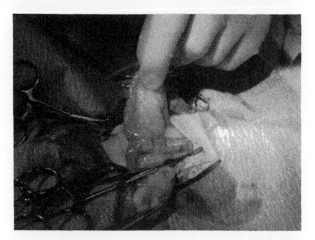

Fig. 1.12 Rabbit spay.

more frequently if soiled (particularly as the newspaper often became wet underneath the water bottle). Newspaper was disposed of in clinical waste. At this time the kennel was cleaned with standard disinfectant, dried and fresh newspaper placed in the kennel.

Feeding regime

As the rabbit had a separated mandibular symphysis it was unwilling to eat prior to surgery. This was not a problem as surgery was carried out soon after the injury. Following surgery, assisted feeding via a naso-oesophageal tube was performed (the tube was placed whilst the rabbit was still anaesthetised and X-rayed to ensure correct placement).

Rabbit pellets were crushed and mixed into a runny paste with some water. The rabbit was restrained by another member of staff and a little water was passed down the tube to ensure that it was patent. The food mixture was then passed slowly down the tube. A little water was then passed down the tube to ensure that there were no blockages and that the rabbit had received all of the food. This feeding regime was carried out four times a day until the rabbit was discharged.

On the day after surgery fresh greens and hay were offered to the rabbit as the surgical repair had been carried out in such a way that the rabbit was able to take some food orally.

Nursing care and monitoring of the animal

The rabbit's temperature, pulse and respiration were monitored twice daily following the operation – these were found to be within normal parameters (see Appendix 1). The skin wounds on either side of the wire that had been placed to repair the damaged mandible were checked throughout the day and any crusting of blood that was present was cleaned with dilute chlorhexidine.

The rabbit was salivating more than normal and excess saliva was cleaned from around the mouth, dewlap and forelimbs. These areas were also kept dry.

Gut motility was monitored – the rabbit was found to be producing normal faeces and no faecal matting was observed. There was concern that the rabbit would not be able to carry out coprophagy but this was not the case – probably due to pain relief given to the rabbit.

Grooming was carried out daily, but as the rabbit was short coated this was not a major problem.

The rabbit was used to being handled and appeared quite bright the day following surgery. Therefore, it was allowed to exercise in the kennel room while a nurse was present. The owner also visited the rabbit during the hospitalisation period.

Medication administered

At the time of surgery:

- Meloxicam (metacam) 0.2 mg/kg intramuscularly (IM)
- Enrofloxacin (baytril) 5 mg/kg subcutaneously (SC)

Daily post-operatively:

- Meloxicam (metacam) 0.2 mg/kg IM once daily – anti-inflammatory and pain relief
- Enrofloxacin (baytril) 5 mg/kg SC twice per day – antibacterial
- Cisapride 0.2 mg/kg orally (PO) twice per day – gut motility stimulant.

Comments

This was a very unusual case. The rabbit responded very well to treatment and was able to eat with the fixation wire in place. However, placement of the naso-oesophageal tube ensured that the rabbit did not have a break in feeding, thus reducing the risk of gut stasis developing.

CASE HISTORY 2
Presentation

A 1-year-old Dutch rabbit was presented with overgrown incisors and anorexia.

Clinical examination

The incisor teeth were obviously overgrown with the lower incisors protruding from the mouth due to the abnormal angle that they were growing. On examination of the mouth both upper and lower molars were found to be overgrown and ulceration of the tongue was present. The rabbit was not considered underweight at 2.5 kg. A full physical examination of the rabbit was carried out and body temperature, heart rate and respiratory rate were within normal parameters. There was no evidence of respiratory disease.

Pre-op

Food was withheld for 30 minutes prior to carrying out a dental. The rabbit was given fentanyl/ fluanisone (Hypnorm) intramuscularly followed by midazolam intravenously. Fluids (40 ml of glucose saline) were given subcutaneously over both flanks. Pain relief was provided with carprofen intramuscularly.

During operation

The rabbit was placed on disposable paper bedding which sat on top of a heat mat. Throughout the procedure the respiratory rate, heart rate, pulse and level of anaesthesia were monitored.

Post-op

The rabbit was revived with intravenous butorphanol. Once the rabbit could sit in sternal recumbency it was returned to a recovery cage. Fresh vegetables were given along with some Milupa in a bowl. The rabbit was monitored to ensure that it began eating. Within an hour of recovery the rabbit was seen eating some vegetables and had passed faeces. As the rabbit was bright and eating it was discharged that evening.

CASE HISTORY 3

Presentation

A 6-month-old female entire Netherland Dwarf rabbit was presented for spaying.

Clinical examination

A full physical examination of this rabbit revealed harsh lung sounds probably due to an underlying respiratory infection. It was therefore decided not to operate on the rabbit at this time. The rabbit was prescribed 10 days of antibiotic therapy to which it responded very well. On examination 2 weeks after the initial presentation, the lung sounds had improved and it was felt that the rabbit could undergo surgery. No other abnormalities were detected.

Pre-op

Food was withheld for 30 minutes prior to anaesthesia. Premedication with fentanyl/fluanisone (Hypnorm) was given intramuscularly. Fluids were given (40 ml subcutaneously). Carprofen was also given at this time for pain relief.

During operation

Once sedated the rabbit was induced with isoflurane given by face mask. Initially a low concentration of isoflurane (0.5%) was given with oxygen and the isoflurane concentration gradually increased to 2.5% ensuring that the rabbit was breathing at all times during induction. The rabbit was then intubated and maintained on isoflurane anaesthesia.

The rabbit was placed in dorsal recumbency in a cradle and the abdomen clipped from just proximal to the umbilicus to the pubis and laterally to the flank. The skin was then surgically prepared with chlorhexidine taking care not to soak the rabbit. During the operation the level of anaesthesia was monitored by observing the pedal reflex and ear pinch reflex in addition to heart rate, respiratory rate and pulse.

Post-op

The rabbit continued to be monitored following reversal of anaesthesia with butorphanol. Once the endotracheal tube was removed and the rabbit could sit in sternal recumbency it was returned to a recovery cage and provided with warmth, fresh vegetables and Milupa. The rabbit did not show any interest in food and was fed 10 ml Milupa with a syringe. After taking this the rabbit was returned to its kennel and did show some interest in the vegetables. It was decided that the rabbit should remain in the surgery overnight to ensure that it was eating. The wound was checked hourly for any discharge or interference by the rabbit. The following morning the rabbit had eaten and passed faeces and was sent home with instructions that the owners should ensure that it continued to eat.

Acknowledgements

The author is grateful to Mrs Hare, Edinburgh for providing Figure 1.1.

REFERENCES

Girling S 2001 City & Guilds Certificate in Veterinary Nursing of Exotic Species. Edinburgh's Telford College, Edinburgh

Harcourt Brown F 2002 Anorexia in rabbits 2: diagnosis and treatment. In: Practice 24(8): 450–467

Okerman L 1994 Breeding problems. In: Okerman L (ed) Diseases of domestic rabbits, 2nd edn. Blackwell Scientific Publications, Oxford, pp. 113–120

FURTHER INFORMATION

Rabbit Welfare Association, PO Box 603, Horsham, West Sussex RH13 5WL, UK
www.rabbitwelfare.co.uk

Chapter 2

Rodents

Sara Cowen

INTRODUCTION

Rodents are increasing in popularity as pets and as such are more frequently being presented at surgeries for treatment and procedures. All rodents have a variety of common conditions that appear. The surgery can become a very stressful and frightening place for all animals; with the appropriate care and nursing the stress levels can be minimised. This is vital to ensure a speedy recovery and allow treatment to be successful. It may often be that secondary problems can occur due to increase in stress (see Tables 2.1 & 2.2 for classification and biological data).

GUINEA PIGS

Guinea pigs are extremely popular with young children and make ideal pets. They are easy to handle and are communicative. Also known as cavies (*Cavia porcellus*) they originate from South America. In the UK there are three main breeds kept as pets:

- Abyssinian (coarse haired, with rosettes)
- English (smooth, short haired) and
- Peruvian (long haired).

Within these breeds numerous colour variations are observed.

GERBILS

Gerbils (*Meriones unguiculatus*) are ideal pets for older children. They are active and entertaining; however, their speed and agility make them unsuitable for small children to handle. They are fairly robust health-wise and require minimal care.

The Mongolian gerbil is normally agouti in colour, although numerous varieties are now being bred. They have a furred tail, ears and feet unlike rats and mice.

HAMSTERS

Hamsters are popularly kept as pets, the most common varieties being the Syrian or Golden hamster (*Mesocricetus auratus*) and dwarf varieties such as the Chinese hamster (*Cricetulus griseus*).

Hamsters are nocturnal in activity and require consideration regarding their normal patterns of activity, such as feeding and preferring to be handled at night.

They have specialised cheek pouches for food storage, as in the wild they would travel up to 8 miles a night searching for food.

> **Tip:** Never feed soft sticky foods as these can cause impaction of the cheek pouches.

RATS AND MICE

Rats (*Rattus norvegicus*) and mice (*Mus musculus*) are increasing in popularity with children and make ideal pets. They have normal activity patterns throughout the day, and are active, inquisitive and intelligent. They come in a range of coat patterns and markings. In the rat, the hooded variety appears to be the most common pet variety.

Table 2.1 Classification of small animals

	Class	Order	Family	Genus	Species	Common name
Rabbit	Mammalia	Lagomorpha	Leporidae	*Oryctolagus*	*cuniculus*	Domesticated rabbit
Chinchilla	Mammalia	Rodentia	Chinchillidae	*Chinchilla*	*lanigera*	Long-tailed chinchilla/small chinchilla
Degu	Mammalia	Rodentia	Octodontidae	*Octodon*	*degus*	Degu
Guinea pig	Mammalia	Rodentia	Caviidae	*Cavia*	*porcellus*	Guinea pig
Hamster	Mammalia	Rodentia	Cricetidae	*Mesocricetus*	*auratus*	Golden/Syrian hamster
Hamster	Mammalia	Rodentia	Cricetidae	*Cricetulus*	*griseus*	Chinese hamster
Hamster	Mammalia	Rodentia	Cricetidae	*Phodopus*	*sungorus*	Dwarf Campbell's Russian hamster (Dzungarian)
Hamster	Mammalia	Rodentia	Cricetidae	*Phodopus*	*sungorus*	Dwarf winter white Russian hamster
Hamster	Mammalia	Rodentia	Cricetidae	*Phodopus*	*roborovskii*	Roborovski hamster
Jird	Mammalia	Rodentia	Cricetidae	*Meriones*	*shawi*	Shaw's Jird
Gerbil	Mammalia	Rodentia	Cricetidae	*Meriones*	*unguiculatus*	Mongolian gerbil
Gerbil	Mammalia	Rodentia	Cricetidae	*Gerbillus*	*syrticus*	Pygmy gerbil
Gerbil	Mammalia	Rodentia	Cricetidae	*Gerbillus*	*perpallidus*	Pallid gerbil
Gerbil	Mammalia	Rodentia	Cricetidae	*Gerbillus*	*pyramidum*	Large Egyptian gerbil
Gerbil	Mammalia	Rodentia	Cricetidae	*Gerbillus*	*gerbillus*	Small Egyptian gerbil
Gerbil	Mammalia	Rodentia	Cricetidae	*Meriones*	*crassus*	Jerusalem gerbil
Gerbil	Mammalia	Rodentia	Cricetidae	*Meriones*	*sacramenti*	Negev gerbil
Gerbil	Mammalia	Rodentia	Cricetidae	*Pachyuromys*	*duprasi*	Duprasi's/fat-tailed gerbil
Rat	Mammalia	Rodentia	Muridae	*Rattus*	*norvegicus*	Brown rat
Mouse	Mammalia	Rodentia	Muridae	*Mus*	*musculus*	Mouse

Mice are now bred in numerous coat colours and include fancy mice species and the more unusual species such as spiny mice.

They are sociable animals, but care must be taken to have single sexed pairs or groups, as they have an exceptionally high breeding capacity, and mixing the sexes will soon result in numerous unwanted individuals.

CHINCHILLAS

Chinchillas (*Chinchilla lanigera*) are rodents similar in relation to guinea pigs and are found native in the Andes and Peru, South America.

They are very friendly and active, and can live for up to 20 years. They were originally bred for their fur due to the thick soft coat and lack of guard hairs. They are born fully developed like guinea pigs and are generally nocturnal in activity.

HANDLING

Tip: Before attempting to handle any small rodent first place a closed fist near the animal and allow it to sniff. Once accepting of the hand you can then proceed with the relevant technique.

Never grab them from above as this represents a claw from a predator and will usually result in attack.

Guinea pigs

Handling of guinea pigs is easy and straightforward, and will hardly ever result in aggression. Always use both hands to restrain and handle

Table 2.2 Biological data of rodents

	Chinchilla	Guinea pig	Hamster	Rat	Mouse	Gerbil
Physiological data						
Lifespan (average)	10 years	4–5 years	18–24 months	2–3 years	1+ years	3–5 years
Lifespan (max)	20 years	8 years	36 months	4 years	3 years	5 years
Adult body weight (male)	400–500 g	750–1000 g	85–130 g	400–800 g	20–40 g	60 g
Adult body weight (female)	400–600 g	750–1000 g	95–150 g	400–800 g	20–40 g	50 g
Respiratory rate (bpm)	40–80	90–150	33–127	80–150	150–250	90–140
Heart rate (bpm)	100–150	130–190	280–412	260–350	500–600	250–500
Rectal temperature (°C)	38.0–39.0	37.2–39.5	36.8–38.3	38	37.5	37.4–39.0
Reproductive data						
Sexual maturity	4–12 months	45–70 days	6–8 weeks	6–10 weeks	5–8 weeks	10–12 weeks
Fertility limit	15 years	3 years	10–18 months	12–16 months	12–18 months	15–20 months
Oestrus season	Nov–May	Polyoestrus	All year round	Polyoestrus	Polyoestrus	Polyoestrus
Oestrus cycle	28–60 days	16 days	4 days	4–5 days	4 days	4–6 days
Length of oestrus	2 days	50 hours	4 days	12 hours	12 hours	12 hours
Post-partum oestrus	12 hours	2–15 hours	18–21 days	24 hours	24 hours	24 hours
Gestation period	108–115 days	59–72 days	15–18 days	20–22 days	19–21 days	24–26 days
Birth weight	30–40 g	70–100 g	2–3 g	5–7 g	1.5 g	1–3 g
Litter size	1–2 kits	1–6 piglets	4–12 pups	6–16 pups	8–12 pups	3–10 pups
Litters per year	2	2	numerous	numerous	numerous	numerous
Number of mammae	4	2	14–22	6 pairs	5 pairs	6
Eyes open	at birth	at birth	12–14 days	10–16 days	12–14 days	17 days
Weaning age	8–10 weeks	3 weeks	3 weeks	3–4 weeks	3–4 weeks	21–24 days

guinea pigs. Place one hand over the shoulders and support the body by placing the other hand over the rump.

Rats and mice

For examination purposes mice can be cupped in the hands and rats can be gently held by grasping around the shoulders and supporting the rump. Then allow the animal's feet to rest on something solid.

Gently holding the base of the tail can assist in controlling movement during procedures. It is possible to restrain by taking the scruff of the neck and holding in the palm of the hand; keep the tail out of the way by placing under your fourth and fifth digits.

Tip: Be careful not to scruff too tight as this can result in bulging or prolapsed eyes and choking.

Gerbils

Gerbils are very quick and agile, but are generally easy to handle. Approach the animal and present an open palm; they may well choose to crawl onto your hand or be gently scooped up. Never grab at the tail, as the skin may slough, an escape mechanism in response to capture. The tail can be gently held at the base to assist restraint.

Chinchillas

Always handle gently and calmly as rough handling can cause them to shed patches of their fur, known as 'fur slip'.

Never lift or handle them using their ears.

Secure by gently catching the base of the tail and lift by supporting the rest of the body in your other hand. For more secure restraint place hands around the shoulders.

> **Tip:** Be wary of chinchillas when handling; if they become stressed or aggressive they may spray urine over you.

Hamsters

When handling hamsters it is important to remember that they do not see well, especially in bright lights. During the day they are sleeping and will often resent being woken to be handled. So approach calmly and slowly, and allow them to wake fully before handling to prevent being bitten.

Place your hand near the animal palm upwards and gently scoop the animal onto the hand.

It is inadvisable to scruff hamsters as this can cause prolapse of the eye.

HOUSING

The majority of small animals are prey species rather than predators. They have poor vision, an acute sense of hearing and smell, and require visual security in their environment.

The surgery represents possibly one of the most stress-inducing environments possible to these species. Humans and other animals represent a threat; a human is 3000 times bigger than a hamster, and can be frightening, especially if unfamiliar.

The housing for these pets is important in terms of both what is provided and where it is located. Consider being a guinea pig placed opposite a dog while its natural instincts are to run and hide. The smell and noises of the kennel area can increase the stress levels of prey species making recovery that much harder.

Try to locate them somewhere quiet and secluded; use an isolated area if available. If an isolated area is not possible, place a towel over the front of the cage for privacy.

Some animals may pine if taken from their mates; it may be necessary to place a well animal (their usual cage mate) with them during the recovery period. Where possible, send them home for treatment, there is nothing better than being with their owner and in their home environment to assist the recovery process and limit stress.

Try to consider the normal patterns of behaviour and replicate this, such as maintaining daylight hours, or allowing nocturnal animals, such as hamsters, to sleep during the day and feed at night.

Provide adequate and appropriate bedding, e.g. woodshavings or a paper pulp bedding, to ensure the animal is warm, or following surgery place on a heat mat to prevent hypothermia.

Give the animal something to hide under or behind, such as logs or branches, for additional security and to create a more realistic environment. A dust bath should be given to desert species, such as chinchillas, hamsters and gerbils, to encourage them to clean themselves. This is especially important if being hospitalised.

Many small animals are neophobic and will avoid new objects in their unknown environment, such as water bottles and bowls that are not familiar to them. Try to get the owner to bring in the animal's own accessories and current diet to ensure they feel settled in the housing and to prevent dietary upset.

When hospitalised they may not require the same living space as they do on a daily basis. Most cages will be suitable in size and structure but ensure they are completely escape proof.

NUTRITION

There are a number of frequently presenting conditions in rodents that often have one thing in common, poor or inappropriate nutrition.

Whilst vets need to be able to treat life-threatening conditions through surgery and drug intervention, providing the owner with sound nutritional advice and tips on feeding at routine check ups can prevent many conditions from arising in the first place. Nutritional support can also be just as important, in promoting the recovery of a convalescing animal.

Small animals are often lumped into the same nutritional groups, but following extensive studies it is now observed that each has a different nutritional requirement and, as such, it is important to provide a species-specific diet.

All animals are sensitive to any form of dietary introduction or change and these may often be the predisposing factor for illness. It is vitally important that the owner brings in a sample of the food they are currently feeding and to ensure this is all that is fed during the animal's stay.

In some cases, where animals are not eating, syringe feeding may be necessary. Try to provide appetising food such as fresh herbs, vegetables and fruit in very small quantities to see if any of these entice them. Failing that, with the herbivores, there is a complete syringeable food available called Science – Recovery, a lifesaving diet that provides the appropriate levels of nutrition, rehydrates the animal and replaces friendly gut bacteria.

Dietary changeovers for small animals

Small animals have very complex and sensitive guts, and many situations and conditions can lead to dietary upset, such as stress, antibiotics and dietary change.

Rodents on the whole are unable to tolerate dramatic changes in their daily diet and may suffer from loosening of faeces or, at worst, diarrhoea. This may then lead to inappetance, dehydration and weight loss.

Dietary upset often occurs due to the purchase, or introduction, of new foods.

Table 2.3 Dietary changeover guidelines

Day 0	100% Original diet		0% New diet	
Days 1–4	75%	" "	25%	" "
Days 5–8	50%	" "	50%	" "
Days 9–12	25%	" "	75%	" "
Days 13–14	0%	" "	100%	" "

Tip: Always check first with owners presenting animals with acute diarrhoea that it is not due to a rapid alteration in the animal's diet.

Changes in an animal's diet should be introduced gradually in order to avoid physiological stress upon the digestive system.

Table 2.3 gives a recommended changeover period for a diet, but obviously this will require some prior planning. The animal should be gradually weaned onto the new food by altering the percentages of original diet to the new recipe. Calculate beforehand the quantity of existing food required and check there is sufficient for adequate acclimatisation.

Introduction of any new forms of food to pets may affect their gut motility and flora, so it is useful to introduce treats and titbits in small amounts initially to allow the gut to acclimatise. This also gives you the opportunity to observe the response.

FIRST AID

When treating and caring for small animals, such as rodents, it is important that you consider and provide all the factors that are conducive to treatment and recovery. Small furries suffer from stress very easily and that can cause the animal to withdraw and prevent treatment being successful.

The essential requirements of sick animals are:

- warmth, environmental or an additional heat source
- fluids, drinking on own or provided subcutaneously or c.p.

- appropriate nutrition, avoid unnecessary dietary change
- environmental security, safe and natural
- good ventilation or if necessary oxygen.

> **Tip:** Know your patient:
>
> - Type of animal – prey or predator.
> - Habits and lifestyle – nocturnal, diurnal, activity patterns.
> - Diet – herbivore, omnivore, grazer, current diet, vegetables, etc.
> - Environment – desert living, forest, grassland, over- or underground.
> - Lifestyle – group, solitary, companions.
> - Biological data – temperature, pulse, respiration, urine and blood values, etc.
> - Common ailments – wet tail, pasturella, malocclusion, torticollis, etc.

PRE- AND POST-OPERATIVE CARE

Until recently, only simple surgery was performed on small animals, e.g. neutering, lumpectomy and dental care, as surgery costs were often in excess of the animal's value. With pet insurance, more complicated procedures are now being performed, e.g. cystotomy.

A physical examination of every animal should be carried out prior to any form of anaesthesia as any health concerns may lead to complications and even death. In all small animals good surgical preparation and intensive post-operative nursing are essential, as they are generally not good candidates for anaesthesia:

Cautions:

- If analgesia is incomplete, increasing the anaesthetic may result in overdose.
- Evaluation of depth of anaesthesia may be difficult – vital signs are often a poor indicator and heart rate may be immeasurable.
- Absence of pedal reflex and ear pinch are useful indicators of sufficient depth.
- Response is extremely variable, especially in guinea pigs.
- Recovery can be prolonged.

Pre-operative checks

Successful surgery relies greatly upon effective preparation. Consider the following:

- Minimise stress due to pre-operative handling by giving a sedative, e.g. ketamine.
- Look for oculonasal discharge; this may indicate the presence of respiratory congestion leading to further complications during anaesthesia.
- Listen to the lungs; impairment or damage may result in respiratory failure during surgery; rats commonly suffer respiratory congestion.
- Fasting is not recommended prior to surgery (rodents do not have a vomit reflex and, therefore, there is minimal threat of choking during anaesthesia, and recovery may be delayed).
- If the animal has not been drinking, pre-operative fluids can be given subcutaneously, e.g. Hartmann's or Ringer's lactate.

> **Tip:** A rough guideline for maintaining fluid levels is 75–100 ml/kg.

> **Tip:** Small animals suffer from hypothermia and circulatory shock very easily. During anaesthesia and recovery, the body temperature should be maintained (heated mat), and the surgical area kept to a minimum, as this will be a source of heat loss.

Intensive post-operative nursing

Recovery depends heavily on the appropriate care given after surgery. The following procedures should be followed:

- Place the animal on a heated mat. Removal of the heat source can result in rapid heat loss.
- Heat lamps can be used but avoid overheating; ensure that the animal can move away from the heat if it needs to – excessive heat can cause dehydration.
- Administer oxygen and respiratory stimulants where necessary.

- Warm to body temperature any fluids given to or used upon the animal before use.
- Ensure all urine is cleaned up and the animal is dried to prevent hypothermia.
- Encourage the animal's appetite and eating (to stimulate gut motility) by providing a few small pieces of fresh herbs, carrot, lettuce, etc. as soon as awake.
- If appetite is poor administer subcutaneous fluids instead.
- Use liquid feeds (e.g. Science – Recovery) to syringe feed if not eating within 6–12 hours.
- Administration of a probiotic may assist in maintaining gut flora and stimulate appetite for a week following anaesthetic and may assist in preventing enterotoxaemia.
- Administer vitamin C – stress depletes the stores of vitamin C that assist in promoting the recovery of the animal and tissue healing. It can also assist in binding toxins in the gut.
- Administer TLC – encouraging and stimulating the animals will be rewarded.
- Keep the animal at a constant environmental temperature following recovery (do not just place back in a cold outdoor hutch) and encourage movement and exercise.

ANAESTHESIA

> **Tip:** Every anaesthetic carries a risk; small furries are even more susceptible – don't forget that a 1-year-old hamster carries the equivalent risk of a 13-year-old cat, so always pre-warn owners of the risks with these patients.

Induction is usually carried out by placing the animal in an induction chamber. This provides less stress to the patient. There are now masks available for the smaller species and these are designed to minimise environmental contamination with a sealed nozzle.

Isoflurane is the most suitable for the smaller species.

During treatment or surgery you should monitor the animal's hydration levels observing capillary refill time, colour of mucous membranes, skin tension, urine production and concentration, etc.

In smaller animals it may be useful to administer the fluid orally or intra-peritoneally, rather than subcutaneously, as there is a high absorption rate from the gut (see Table 2.4 for clinical data).

Small animals have a high surface area to body weight ratio. This results in rapid hypothermia with subsequent hypoxia (reduced blood oxygen) and hypoglycaemia (low blood sugar) especially during surgical operations.

They have a short lifespan, longevity ranging from 1 to 10 years depending on species; operating on a 5-year-old guinea pig represents possibly the senior stage of its life, a geriatric patient, with all the complications that come along with it.

Many small animals will also have pre-existing conditions or subclinical infections, such as *Pasteurella* or respiratory disease. This may not be a problem until anaesthesia or hospitalisation, where the subclinical condition manifests as a complication to the treated illness. Enterotoxaemia (disruption of normal flora, resulting in production of toxins that affect the gut) may follow anaesthesia and can be induced by inappropriate use of antibiotics. The disruption causes multiplication of pathogenic bacteria, which results in rapid dehydration, collapse and death. Avoid using penicillins and use the parenteral rather than the oral route.

> **Tip:** Oral administration introduces the antibiotics directly into the gut where they will break down the gut microflora, often resulting in an imbalance causing growth of pathogenic bacteria. Consider administration of probiotics to counterbalance the effect.

COMMON ILLNESSES
Enteritis

Enteritis is defined as inflammation of the intestines. Whilst diarrhoea can be a symptom of enteritis, chronic soft stools also indicate caecal dysbiosis. Inactivity, inappetence and abdominal distension often accompany enteritis. The main causes are rapid fermentation of diets containing too little fibre, sudden dietary change, and parasitism.

Table 2.4 Small animal clinical data table

	Chinchilla	Guinea pig	Hamster	Rat	Mouse	Gerbil
Haematological values						
RBC ($\times 10^6$ mm^3)	5.2–10.3	4.3–6.6	5.5–8.9	6–10.0	8.7–12.5	8.1–8.6
PCV (%)	25–54	35–49	44.1–53.9	39–55	42–44.0	47.5–45.8
Haemoglobin (g)/dl	8–15.4	12–16.0	14.5–18	11–19.5	10.2–16.2	14.1–14.8
WBC ($\times 10^3$ mm^3)	4.6–19.5	6.2–16.5	6.3–10.1	6–15.0	5–12.0	9.7–12.0
Neutrophils (%)	11–59.0	26–42.0	18.6–32.1	9–34.0	7–40.0	20–26.0
Eosinophils (%)	0–5.0	1–5.0	0.46–1.22	0–6.0	0–40.0	1
Basophils (%)	0–5.0	0–3.0	0–3.0	0–1.5	0–1.5	1
Lymphocytes (%)	35–87.0	39–74.0	59.4–81.9	65–85.0	55–95.0	73–78
Monocytes (%)	0–12.0	39–74.0	1.4–2.4	0–5.0	0.1–3.5	0.9–1.0
Platelets ($\times 10^3$ mm^3)	45–740.0	250–850	339–485	500–1300	100–1000	400–600
Blood volume (ml/kg)	65	60–75	0.078 ml/g	6 ml/100 g	5–6 ml/100 g	78
Clinical chemistry values						
Calcium (mg/dl)	10.0–25.0	5.3–12.0	9.8–13.2	5.3–13.0	3.2–10.0	3.7–6.2
Phosphorus (mg/dl)	4–8.0	3.0–7.6	3.0–9.9	5.3–8.3	2.3–9.2	3.7–8.2
Sodium (mEq/l)	149–157.8	120–152	106–146	140–150	132–162	141–171
Chloride (mEq/l)	98.9–107.0	90–115	86–112	100–113	92–106	93–118
Potassium (mEq/l)	3.4–4.2	3.8–8.9	2.3–9.8	4.3–5.6	5.0–7.6	3.3–6.3
Glucose (mg/dl)	106.9–144.0	60–180	37–198	50–135	60–228	40–140.7
BUN (mg/dl)	negative	9–32.0	12–26.0	6–23.0	17–28.0	16.8–31.3
Creatinine (mg/dl)	–	0.6–2.2	0.4–1.0	0.2–0.8	0.3–1.0	0.5–1.4
Bilirubin (mg/dl)	negative	0.3–0.9	0.1–0.9	0.2–0.55	0.1–0.9	0.2–0.6
Protein (g/dl)	5–6.0	4.7–6.4	5.2–7.0	5.6–7.6	3.5–7.2	4.8–16.8
Albumin (g/dl)	3–3.2	2.1–3.9	3.5–4.9	3.8–4.8	2.5–2.8	1.8–5.8
Cholesterol (mg/dl)	40–100	16–43.0	55–181	40–130	26–82.0	90–130
Alkaline phosphatase (iu/l)	3–12.0	55–108	86–187	16–90.0	47–85.0	12–37.0
SGOT (iu/l)	–	27–68.0	28–122	–	74–232	–
SGPT (iu/l)	–	25–59.0	22–128	20–90.0	26–54.0	–
LDH (iu/l)	405–636	–	140–412	–	–	–
Globulin (g/100 ml)	2–2.6	1.7–2.6	2.7–4.2	1.8–3.0	0.6	0.6–14.3

Gastrointestinal disorders

The digestive system of rodents is not quite as complex and sensitive as that of rabbits, but is still susceptible to disorders. Guinea pigs are herbivorous, hindgut fermenters, existing in the wild on a range of grasses, seeds, weeds and fruits. Fermentation occurs in both the caecum and the colon and, although they practise coprophagy, they do not produce different faeces, i.e. caecotrophs as a rabbit would. Fibre is important for the maintenance of the gut flora, and so an inability to chew fibrous food, or a diet lacking in fibre can cause gastrointestinal disorders in guinea pigs, just as in rabbits.

Clinical signs

The clinical signs to watch out for include:

- faeces – absence, abnormal type, size, condition, colour, quantity
- behaviour and demeanour – altered, depressed, reluctance to move or be handled
- appetite – reduced or totally suppressed, acute or chronic weight loss
- abdominal distension – bloated, gastric tympany, tucked appearance
- indication of pain – teeth grinding, rate and regularity of nose twitching
- gut sounds – absence, reduced, borborygmus.

There are a number of gastrointestinal disorders, including:

- gastric stasis/intestinal ileus
- gastric/intestinal obstruction
- chronic soft stools
- enteritis
- bacteria and viral infections – salmonellosis, E. coli
- diarrhoea
- Tyzzer's disease
- enterotoxaemia
- parasites – coccidiosis, flagellates, flukes, worms, etc
- mucoid enteropathy
- trichobezoars (fur balls).

Some of the factors that can affect gastrointestinal function include:

- dietary – low fibre, high starch, protein, fat, sudden change
- reduced food intake
- inadequate water intake
- inactivity/immobility
- stress (injury, weaning, transportation, predation)
- disease/parasites
- genetic predisposition
- inappropriate antibiotic use.

Treatment

Treatment involves a number of approaches. Analgesia is used to enhance patients' comfort – useful in dental, skeletal and intestinal disorders.

GI motility agents are given to promote gut peristalsis. These should not be used for obstructions. Commonly used agents are metoclopramide for upper tract and cisapride for hindgut problems.

Histamine blockers are given, and aggressive fluid therapy is used to rehydrate gut contents and stimulate peristalsis.

The carers should endeavour to keep animals' interest for food – offer small quantities of a wide variety of suitable foodstuffs. Vitamin supplementation is important until normal feeding is established. Pre- and probiotics may assist re-colonisation of gut.

Treatment for specific disorders

Enterotoxaemia. This condition is extremely difficult to treat, so prevention is the best method through healthy diet, low stress and avoidance of certain antibiotics, including lincomycin, clindamycin, and those from the penicillin group, particularly ampicillin and macrolides. Well-tolerated antibiotics are chloramphenicol preparations and tetracyclines.

Trichobezoars. This condition usually requires medical not surgical treatment, including aggressive fluid therapy, force feeding (syringe or nasogastric tube) and a high-fibre diet. Surgery may need to be considered if treatment is ineffective.

Caecal impaction. Aggressive fluid therapy, but may require immediate surgery.

> **Tip:** Syringing fresh pineapple juice is believed to break up the fur ball, rehydrate the gut and assist in removal naturally. It is often that the gut is dehydrated causing a blockage rather than the fur ball being the actual problem.

Scurvy – vitamin C deficiency

Vitamin C or ascorbic acid is a white crystalline water-soluble carbohydrate, an antioxidant and an essential nutrient. It is reported to have anti-inflammatory and analgesic properties, and is viewed as a useful prophylactic.

Most animals are able to manufacture their own vitamin C. However, guinea pigs (like humans) are unable to do so.

Vitamin C is retained in the tissues for a maximum of 4 days. If not replenished, tissue stores quickly become depleted, and these processes are impaired. Vitamin C deficiency is more commonly known as scurvy.

Scurvy is an unpleasant condition and if not addressed may progress to convulsions and/or death within 3–4 weeks.

> **Tip:** Deficiency is easily preventable by ensuring that an adequate supply of vitamin C is available, by feeding fresh fruit and vegetables daily or a diet complete with added vitamin C.

Factors that can affect vitamin C stasis include:

1. lifestage, e.g. pregnancy
2. activity and environment, e.g. temperature, humidity
3. stress, e.g. handling, transportation
4. disease/intestinal parasites
5. dietary vitamin C, e.g. type and concentration
6. reduced food and water intake
7. absorption, e.g. age of animal.

The symptoms of scurvy are as follows:

1. behaviour – depressed, weak and lethargic
2. appetite – reduced, weight loss
3. mouth – anaemia, loose or broken teeth, bleeding gums, gingivitis
4. lowered disease resistance – susceptibility to secondary infections
5. skin condition – poor, hair loss, re-opening of healed wounds
6. indications of pain – reluctance to move or be handled, lameness and joint swelling
7. faeces – abnormal size, quantity, consistency.

> **Tip:** Water supplementation of vitamin C is not advisable – may affect taste, water intake is extremely variable and there is rapid loss of potency on exposure to water, light and metal.

Treatment for vitamin C deficiency is 100 mg/kg/day until symptoms disappear. Under normal circumstances, a daily rate of 10 mg/kg/day is all that is required, increasing to 30 mg/kg/day during pregnancy and general illness.

Dental overgrowth

Rodents have open-rooted, continuously growing teeth. The incisors and molars are kept in trim, by the surfaces meeting in an appropriate eating action. However, there are times when things go wrong, and, just as in rabbits, there are several factors that can contribute to overgrowth. These are:

- genetic
- traumatic
- dietary.

Grinding and abrasion from fibrous material encourages wear. Fewer instances of dental overgrowth tend to be seen in guinea pigs, as they seem to relish hay and dried grass, the ideal substrates for keeping teeth in trim. The nutrient balance of the overall diet may also have an impact.

Obesity in small animals

Obesity occurs when energy intake is greater than requirement. The animal stores excess energy in adipose tissue and gains weight.

Causes

The causes are poor or inappropriate nutrition, overfeeding and lack of exercise. The consequences are a reduced life expectancy, animals that may be predisposed to disease and disorders and increased anaesthetic and surgical risks should an operation ever be required.

The common signs are a generally overweight appearance, gastrointestinal disturbances, a reduction in activity, e.g. grooming, general movement and behavioural changes.

Treatment

This involves getting a detailed history of the animal's life and environment to assess level of care. The animal should be weighed and the results should be compared to the average adult weight for species (see Table 2.2). Give the owners specific target weights for the species and a weekly weight loss that they can aim for. Provide guidelines as to the quantities that should be fed for an animal at that weight. Most small animals are massively overfed often enabling the animal to selectively feed. Reduce the energy dense diet instead by encouraging the animal to eat more vegetables, hay or grass (if appropriate to nutritional needs). Don't reduce the amount of food, just alter the type, i.e. a small amount of concentrated food and plenty of hay. Replace starchy, sugary treats with healthier ones, e.g. vegetables. Encourage the owner to exercise the animal either indoors or outdoors. Monitor weight reduction weekly; gradual weight reduction is the key – aim for 1% per week.

Alopecia

Alopecia is a condition that often occurs in small animals. The animal loses hair from either specific areas or all over. Alternatively, it can be the total absence of hair.

Alopecia can happen at any stage of life. There are a variety of types:

- alopecia totalis, which is a complete hair loss/baldness
- alopecia areata, which is banded or loss of hair in patches
- temporary alopecia, which happens in older and frequently bred animals or after a short period of poor nutrition
- senile alopecia, which happens in old age and often affects hamsters
- barbarism, through self-mutilation or by cage mate, both due to boredom or poor diet.

Causes

Alopecia may be the result of:

- hormonal imbalance
- poor nutrition
- poisoning
- illness or disease
- genetics and age
- ectoparasites such as mange, ringworm and lice infestation.

Treatment

Before treatment can begin it is important to differentiate between loss of hair due to irritation (ectoparasites) or some other skin condition that may require drug intervention.

In guinea pigs, alopecia during gestation is thought to be caused by the extra nutritional demands upon the sow's body by the litter of piglets, and so the diet should be supplemented with vitamins B and C, zinc, EFAs and EAA.

If boredom is thought to be the cause then increasing the level of fibre within the diet may help; the animal will need to eat more, thereby increasing their time eating and reducing boredom time.

Mites

Mites are permanent ectoparasites, i.e. they live and spend their entire lifecycle on the outside of the host animal.

Clinical signs

These include:

- small patches of non-itchy dandruff within the fur
- dry flaky skin, fur loss and lesions
- weight loss due to intense irritation making the animal so restless that it does not feed properly
- sores and wounds from scratching
- pain and discomfort.

Diagnosis

This involves identifying the type of mite using microscopy. Surface mites and eggs may be obtained from coat brushings. Burrowing (sub-surface) mites' scrapings must be taken from the skin using a scalpel blade.

Treatment

Treatment comprises an injection of ivermectin subcutaneously, normally three injections 1 week apart. It may be necessary to use it in combination with a shampoo or other product. A thorough clean of the animal's environment is essential. Although mites do not live very long off the host, all bedding will require to be disposed of and intense cleaning and disinfection of cage and all accessories is essential.

> **Tip:** Place the entire cage and accessories in a hot bath of disinfectant to allow penetration of every part of the housing to ensure fully treated and prevent re-infection. Rinse thoroughly and dry before replacing the animal.

Urolithiasis in small animals

Rodents presenting at surgery show signs of urolithiasis, similar to those in other species:

- dysuria
- polyuria
- polydipsia
- haematuria
- perineal irritation due to urine scalding
- straining to urinate
- depressed and anorectic
- dehydrated.

A physical examination of the animal is necessary, although palpation of the abdomen may be difficult if the patient is in pain. Urinalysis and radiography (Fig. 2.1) are essential to aid diagnosis. Cystotomy to remove the urolith may be necessary (Fig. 2.2). Although the majority are calcium carbonate, other calcium salts may also be present.

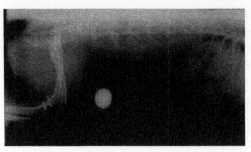

Fig. 2.1 Diagnostic radiograph of rabbit, visualising a large urolith.

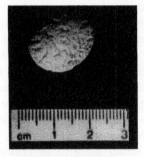

Fig. 2.2 Urolith removed by cystotomy.

Pre-disposing factors for urolithiasis may include:

- high dietary levels of digestible calcium
- dietary factors, which influence urine pH
- chronic underlying cystitis
- low water intake
- obesity, limited exercise, neutering and breed are also suspected to contribute.

Management

Management involves minimising the level of dietary digestible calcium by dietary alteration and aiding diuresis. Assess the animal's diet to determine the level of calcium present in the foods it has been eating, but also the form in which it exists (as dietary calcium varies in digestibility).

Fresh vegetables are an essential part of the management of the condition, and should be introduced into the diet gradually. Not only do they contain calcium oxalate as opposed to calcium carbonate but they also aid diuresis.

Certain vegetables should not be fed as they can exacerbate the condition, e.g. kale, spinach, and other dark, leafy greens, which are exceptionally high in calcium. Useful fresh foods are carrots, celery, lettuce (in moderation), cucumber, sweetcorn, apple and grass.

Restrict access to dry food, especially if there are any uncertainties over the calcium level.

> **Tip:** It is advisable to supplement with additional vitamin C as this acts as a urine acidifier, and is reported to aid dissolution of uroliths in guinea pigs.

Torticollis

Commonly known as head tilt or wry neck, this is spasm of the cervical muscle resulting in the head being twisted to one side. The condition is usually due to otitis media and otitis externa often accompanying *Pasteurella* infection; however it may be indicative of a different disorder or trauma.

Individuals suffering from torticollis may gradually improve over several months and they may learn to live a fairly normal life by compensating for the condition, although symptoms rarely disappear completely.

Clinical signs

These include:

- head tilted to one side
- unbalanced gait or movement
- nystagmus
- circling
- inappetant or unable to eat
- pus in the ear canal.

Treatment

Treatment should include long-term antibiotics, intensive nursing and supportive care, e.g. syringe feeding. For infections, the recommended treatment is enrofloxacin orally for 4–6 weeks, but can be for longer. Alternatively, trimethoprim-sulpha, tetracycline, chloramphenicol and glucocorticoids may assist.

Treatment may not make symptoms disappear, but can reduce their severity enabling the animal to cope. In severe cases a 'bulla osteotomy' may need to be performed to allow permanent drainage.

Animals may develop corneal ulcers if the head is rubbing on the floor and protection may need to be applied to the area.

In all cases the animal will require constant reassessment, but it should learn to compensate and should improve with time if it is able to eat and drink, although it may require some support.

Handling of the animal should be avoided unless necessary as this can cause it to spin. If handling is necessary then hold close to the body and make movements very slow.

Wet tail in small animals

Wet tail (proliferative ileitis) is a very common, highly infectious, condition usually seen around the age of 8 weeks following weaning and separation. The condition is usually fatal and animals are often in poor condition on presentation.

Clinical signs

These include:

- lethargy
- diarrhoea
- huddled appearance due to abdominal pain
- wet soiling around the rear end
- inappetence and weight loss.

Treatment

Treatment will require a course of enrofloxacin (baytril) orally. Fluids are vitally important to prevent acute dehydration and death. Administer lectade to replace the electrolytes lost through diarrhoea.

> **Tip:** Feed little and often; place in bottle if still able to drink on their own or use a small paintbrush dipped in the solution and placed on the animal's mouth. It will suck the fluids off the brush.

If the animal is unable to eat provide it with a suitable liquid feed such as milupa or complan.

Place the animal on a hot water bottle wrapped in a towel. Heat assists recovery and helps to alleviate the abdominal pain. Ensure the animal has room in the cage to move away from the heat source if it wants to.

This disease is highly infectious and so it is vitally important that the animal is isolated and barrier nursing is carried out.

Diabetes mellitus

Diabetes mellitus is a condition that often arises spontaneously. In diabetes, insufficient insulin is produced, which results in elevated glucose levels. Diabetes has been reported in guinea pigs and hamsters with a possible genetic disposition. Degus are highly susceptible to diabetes as they are unable to metabolise any sugar in the diet.

Clinical signs

These include:

- weight loss even though it is still eating well
- polydipsia
- development of cataracts in some animals
- glucosuria, can predispose the animal to cystitis.

Diagnosis

This is made by a urine dipstick test which will show elevated levels of glucose within the urine. The specific gravity may also be reduced, as greater quantities tend to be produced. Alternatively blood glucose can be determined.

Treatment

With regard to treatment, in most cases involving small animals it is unlikely that insulin will be administered as it is not seen to be essential (and also the dose would be so minute). The condition appears to be self-limiting in many cases. Nutritional management can improve the regulation of blood sugar levels without the need for insulin therapy.

Many small animals are provided with a large bowl of food and fed infrequently. It is recommended that quantity given is reduced and frequency of feeding is increased. This encourages the animals to eat more regularly – little and often. It is also recommended that the owner reduce the levels of simple sugars and lipids in the diet, and avoid sugary treats and dried foods sprayed with molasses; in the wild these animals do not consume simple sugars in quantity. The amount of foods rich in fats, e.g. nuts, should also be reduced. If drastically reducing the fat content of a diet for say a gerbil or hamster, diet should be supplemented with fat-soluble vitamins and some essential fatty acids. In herbivores increasing the levels of fibre helps to decrease blood lipid and glucose levels. Dried grass, hay, and small additions of bran to the dried food may help.

Diabetes insipidus

Diabetes insipidus is a condition resulting from a deficiency of anti-diuretic hormone (ADH) in the bloodstream. ADH encourages reabsorption of water into the bloodstream. This has the effect of concentrating the urine. Consequently, a reduction in ADH can result in an elevated daily production (more than 10 times the normal) of very dilute urine. Deficiency of ADH may result from a head injury, or tumour, or an infection such as encephalitis.

Clinical signs

The animal usually appears to be quite happy in itself, but has polyurea and is polydipsic. The high urine output may cause dehydration, high blood sodium and even shock.

Diagnosis

In diabetes insipidus the specific gravity of urine is usually very low (1.001–1.005). Diagnosis may be confirmed by an ADH response test – if the animal is given ADH, the concentration of its urine returns to normal. If the animal does not respond to the administration of ADH, it is indicative of kidney disease.

Treatment

The aim of treatment is to regulate fluid levels in the body. Treatment is by administration of a synthetic intranasal or intraocular ADH preparation; anti-diuretics may assist. Ensure that the animal does not become dehydrated as it will be urinating more frequently, and in greater quantities in the process. Keep water bowls/bottles topped up on a regular basis, and vegetables and fruit may be used to boost water intake. Use barrier creams to limit damage from urine scalding. Ensure that urine-soaked bedding is removed regularly to keep the cage and animal dry.

Pregnancy toxaemia/ketosis

Pregnancy toxaemia and ketosis are common conditions in pregnant or lactating guinea pigs. Ketosis occurs when the concentration of ketone bodies in blood plasma becomes elevated. Ketosis is a metabolic (fasting) disorder, whereas pregnancy toxaemia is a toxic (circulatory) disorder.

Symptoms

The animal will exhibit the following:

- reduced activity – eating, drinking, grooming
- ruffled coat
- excess salivation
- acidosis with the characteristic smell of 'pear drops' on the breath or in the urine
- hypoglycaemia
- fits and even death within 2–5 days if left untreated.

Causes

Glucose deficiency is the primary cause of ketosis. In sows it can occur during pregnancy or lactation when the demand for glucose by the foetuses as well as the sow dramatically increases. Obesity combined with fasting, and any stress may predispose the animal to metabolic ketosis.

Pregnancy toxaemia, on the other hand, is only seen in pregnant sows. They are usually obese, and there is a massive displacement of the viscera. This may cause aortic compression and impaired blood flow through the arteries which as a result can cause foetal death from uterine ischaemia.

Treatment in guinea pigs

Prevention is preferable, as treatment is rarely successful in the advanced stages. The following have been suggested:

- Betamethasone – 0.1–0.2 ml Betsolan (Schering–Plough Animal Health) by subcutaneous (SC) or intramuscular (IM) injection.
- Dexamethasone – 0.1 ml Dexafort (Intervet UK Ltd) IM.
- Solution of 4 to 5% glucose in 0.9% saline – up to 10 ml SC.
- Dextrose-containing fluids – parenteral administration.
- Calcium gluconate.
- Magnesium sulphate – promote arteriolar dilatation and uterine perfusion.
- Vitamin B_{12} – 0.25 ml vitamin B_{12} 250 μg injected intramuscularly (may act as an appetite stimulant).

Management

Excess body weight is one of the predisposing factors for the condition. Hence it is essential to ensure that the guinea pig does not become overweight.

> **Tip:** Prevent obesity in small animals by providing the correct amount and type of diet daily and encourage exercise and activity.

Eclampsia/hypocalcaemia

Eclampsia is a condition that occasionally occurs in older female guinea pigs with large litters up to 7 days after parturition. It is similar to milk fever in dairy cattle and other animals.

Clinical signs

The animal exhibits:

- sudden depression
- muscle spasms progressing to fits
- paralysis and unconsciousness.

Cause

The cause of eclampsia is an acute calcium deficiency. As the pregnancy progresses and demands of the developing piglets upon the sow increase deficiencies tend to occur. Fulfilling the calcium requirements during gestation and lactation appears to be particularly difficult. In guinea pigs absorption appears to be proportional to intake – they have no mechanism to regulate calcium absorption at gut level. In the body calcium is required for the activity of nerve impulses and contraction of muscles. So in deficiency, these are adversely affected causing the muscular spasms.

Treatment

Normal serum calcium levels may be quickly restored by intraperitoneal injection of calcium gluconate, but the effect may only be transient. Nutritional management may be effective; dietary calcium supplementation during pregnancy and lactation aids prevention. As the pregnancy progresses the level of calcium should be gradually enhanced. This level should be maintained throughout lactation until the piglets start to wean themselves.

> **Tip:** Calcium-rich food sources include dark green leafy vegetables such as cabbage, spinach, kale and watercress. These are also rich in vitamin C, which is also beneficial during pregnancy.

Metastatic calcification

Metastatic calcification is a condition that seems to be prevalent in older animals, especially guinea pigs. There is mineralisation of the soft tissues and internal organs, i.e. kidneys, heart, liver, spleen, muscles, stomach, aorta, colon and cornea.

Causes

It is not unusual for calcium salts to be deposited in tissues other than bones – any tissue affected by injury or disease, e.g. scars, may become calcified during or after healing.

In metastatic calcification though, several tissues are affected at the same time.

The primary cause is believed to be an imbalanced diet, although hormones may be involved. In this case a mineral imbalance between calcium, phosphorus and vitamin D seems to be the cause.

Excess vitamin D alone is sufficient to cause calcium to be deposited in tissues other than bone.

Low dietary levels of magnesium and potassium levels are also thought to be involved.

In some animals (cats) an excess of vitamin A can cause a similar calcification of the joints often seen in cats fed solely on tinned fish (pilchards) resulting in a 'rigid cat'.

Clinical signs

The earliest sign of a problem is:

- weight loss
- joint stiffness
- some animals suffer renal failure or die unexpectedly.

Nutritional management

As the disorder tends to be identified only at post mortem, prevention is vital.

> **Tip:** Check the diet of the guinea pig to ensure that the ratio of calcium to phosphorus is approximately 1.5:1, and that the calcium level is 0.8%, phosphorus 0.65%, vitamin D 1000iu/kg and magnesium and potassium 0.2% and 0.5% respectively.

Pododermatitis

This is a condition that refers to inflammation of the skin covering the feet and is frequently observed in all small animals.

Causes

The occurrence of pododermatitis is often coupled with bacterial infection of *Staphylococcus aureus*. It is also associated with rough and inappropriate hutch flooring, insufficient floor litter and bedding, and poor levels of hygiene.

Obesity can also predispose to this condition; animals are inactive and sedentary, often remaining in one position, leading to formation of sores and ulcers.

Clinical signs

Swelling, redness and heat on the skin become apparent covering the feet and surrounding area, leading to ulceration. Infection may ascend up the leg causing complications with swelling of the hock joints. This may progress in severe cases to osteoarthritis and degenerative changes to the liver, spleen, kidneys and adrenals.

Treatment

Treatment is often unsuccessful once the condition has reached severe swelling and ulceration. Bathe lesions with saline water. Systemic antibiotics can be used and application of antibiotics and corticosteroid ointment topically to help control the outbreak. Dress the foot to reduce pressure on the lesions and prevent further contamination and aggravation from bedding materials. Change the animal to softer bedding materials, a smooth floored cage, and strict hygiene control of the hutch. Reduce weight, alter activity patterns and encourage the animal to exercise.

> **Tip:** Advise owners on replacing wire-floored cages, keeping adequate hygiene levels in the cage and weight reduction.

Myodystrophy

Myodystrophy is a disorder of the muscle, due to impaired nourishment, which whether caused by diet, hormonal imbalance, infection, disease or even toxic compounds results in abnormal or impaired growth. Myodystrophy tend to be seen more frequently in breeding and juvenile animals (guinea pigs and rabbits), although it has been reported in adults too. The cause of myodystrophy is vitamin E deficiency.

Symptoms

These include:

- reproductive failure
- reluctance to move, stiffness, hind-leg weakness, paralysis
- wasting (degeneration) of the skeletal muscles.

Treatment

Supplementation of the diet of breeding animals during pregnancy and lactation helps to prevent deficiency and hence myodystrophy. The diet should contain around 50 mg/kg of vitamin E. Good commercial rabbit and guinea pig foods contain sufficient levels of vitamin E.

Barbarism

Causes

As with rabbits, low levels of dietary fibre in guinea pigs and chinchillas can give rise not only to gastrointestinal disturbances and dental disorders, but also to behavioural problems such as barbarism. Guinea pigs have a relatively low boredom threshold especially when enclosed in small or unstimulating housing, with little access to space to play in and investigate.

Prevention

Reduce the energy density of the diet and provide more forage; this will increase the eating period, and lessen the time available for barbering themselves or cage mates. Hiding treats around the cage, or hanging them just within reach, can enhance their mental stimulation, and make them work for them. Provide environmental enrichment activities within the cage to reduce the boredom threshold.

> **Tip:** When suggesting accessories to enrich the animal's environment ensure they have an actual function or activity or replicate normal behaviour, and don't just look good.

Poisoning

Coccidiostats

Coccidiostats are often used to reduce the outbreak of coccidiosis in intensive rearing situations, e.g. poultry, pig and rabbit diets. Although harmless to the rabbit, coccidiostats have harmful effects on the gut flora of guinea pigs and have been associated with liver and kidney damage, stunted growth and their sudden death. Coccidiostats may inadvertently get into guinea pig food through cross-contamination of production lines. If in any doubt, always check with the manufacturer before feeding.

Poisonous plants

The diet of rodents in their natural habitats consists mainly of wild plants, seeds and grasses. It is thought that the toxic chemicals present in plants provide some protection against ingestion by predators such as herbivores and insects. Many toxic plants are not palatable, and if given a choice the animal will avoid eating them. However, in some situations, the animal may eat them.

Rodents are particularly susceptible to poisoning. Unlike cats and dogs, rodents are unable to vomit. As a result plants usually inducing this symptom in animals which can vomit may go unnoticed in the even smaller animals.

Not only are they unable to reject the material from the system quickly, but the digestive system is such that there can be recycling of toxic compound – most rodents are coprophagic and hence may eat faecal material.

As well as causing a certain amount of stress to the animal, this also poses a challenge when trying to treat a rodent that has ingested some poisonous plant, as inducing vomiting is obviously not an option.

Which plants are poisonous? Many plants (cultivated flowers and shrubs, and wild plants) are believed to be poisonous to rodents. The following list is not exhaustive, but some to avoid which are often found in the home or garden include: agave, amaryllis, anemone, antirrhinum, azalea, bittersweet, bluebell, bryony, buttercup (although harmless when dried), boxwood, caladium, chrysanthemum, clematis, columbine, crocus, cyclamen, daffodil, dahlia, delphinium, dog mercury, fig, figwort, fool's parsley, foxglove, hellebore, hemlock, henbane, holly, hyacinth, iris, ivy berries, Jerusalem cherry, juniper, kingcup, laburnum, laurel, Leyland cypress, lilies, lily of the valley, lobelia, lords and ladies, love-in-a-mist, lupin, marsh marigold, meadow saffron, mistletoe, monkshood, morning glory, narcissus, nicotiana, nightshade (all types), oleander, poppy, primrose, philodendron, poison ivy, privet, ragwort, rhododendron, scarlet pimpernel, spurges, St John's wort, tulip, wisteria, wood sorrel, yew and most evergreen trees.

> **Tip:** Always carefully identify the plants before allowing a pet to have access to them, as often harmful plants are similar in appearance to those that are not harmful.

Symptoms

Fortunately, in most cases, ingestion of plants will only result in moderate digestive upset, which is not usually life threatening. Because of the varied nature and levels of the toxic compounds within these plants the symptoms can range from a slight stomach upset to potentially death. Other symptoms may include salivation, skin allergies, difficulties with breathing, heart problems, etc.

Treatment

Treatment of poisoning depends on symptoms and is typically based on supportive care. The animal needs to be kept warm and quiet, to comfort it and minimise shock. Fluids or liquid feeds may be given to assist in diluting the poison and flushing the agent through the system. Activated charcoal is useful for absorption and use protectants to limit gastrointestinal damage.

Edible plants

Edible materials tend to fall into a number of categories: grasses, wild plants and herbs, cultivated plants, and leaves, twigs, nuts and berries.

Grasses have been eaten for many years by many different animals and are valuable not only in terms of nutrition, but also for maintaining the grinding surfaces of the teeth.

> **Tip:** Grass clippings should not be fed under any circumstance – they start to ferment very quickly and can cause digestive disturbances.

Edible wild plants and herbs

Those most frequently mentioned are: agrimony, avens, borage, bramble, buckwheats (knotted persicaria, lady's thumb, pale smartweed), burnet, caraway, chamomile, chickweed, cleaver, clover, coltsfoot, comfrey, corn marigold, cornsilk, corn spurrey, cow parsley, dandelion, dead-nettles (henbit or dead-nettle, red henbit or spotted dead-nettle, white dead-nettle), dock (bitter dock, green sorrel), echinacea, garlic, goats rue, golden rod, goosegrass, ground elder (do not use once flower buds have appeared), groundsel, hogweed (knot grass or prostrate knotweed), knapweed, mallow, marsh-mallow, mayweeds (scented mayweed, scentless mayweed), meadow horsetail, milk thistle, mouse ear, nettle, orache, ox-eye daisy, parsley, plantain (common plantain, english plantain, hoary plantain), sea beet, shepherd's purse, sow thistle, sunflower, vetch, wheat, wild carrot, wild parsnip, wild rose, wild strawberry and yarrow.

Cultivated plants

Edible cultivated plants include: lucerne, wheat and barley, flowers of aster, daisy, geranium, geum, marguerite, marigold, michaelmas daisy, nasturtium, rose, sunflower and wallflower.

Leaves and twigs

Leaves from a number of different trees and plants may be fed including apple, beech, birch, blackberry, cherry, hazel, horse chestnut, oak, pear, raspberry, strawberry, vine. It is best to feed young leaves as they are believed to have a higher nutritional value.

In addition twigs from apple, birch, blackberry, hawthorn, hazel, maple, pear, raspberry cane and willow tree may be provided. These can be especially useful for inappetent animals during illness or post-operatively.

CASE HISTORY 1

Patient

A 3-year-old male guinea pig suffering from development of calcium carbonate stones in the bladder. The guinea pig has been fed on a popular brand of alfalfa-based diet, which may have led to a build up of crystals in the bladder and the resultant formation of stones. Although the aetiology is not entirely clear, predisposing factors for urolithiasis include: atypical calcium metabolism, high dietary levels of digestible calcium, other dietary factors which influence urine pH, chronic underlying cystitis, and low water intake. Obesity, limited exercise, neutering and breed are also suspected to contribute, as in other animals.

Condition

The guinea pig arrived having passed blood in the urine observed by the owner and crying in obvious discomfort during urination. Other observations over the previous week were polyuria, polydipsia, perineal irritation due to urine, and straining to urinate. In addition, the animal appeared depressed and was anorectic. The animal was dehydrated, necessitating fluid therapy.

Treatment

The guinea pig was immediately given fluids orally and subcutaneously to assist in rehydration. Pain relief was given to control the discomfort and antibiotics administered. An X-ray of the bladder revealed three to four small uroliths formed that would require surgical removal.

Two days later the animal had the stones removed from the bladder and recovered from the operation well. The following treatment was provided to assist in prevention or reformation of uroliths:

- **Cranberry juice** is reported to have exceptional benefits on urinary crystal dissolution, and prevents bacteria sticking to the bladder wall. Bacteria can cause the bladder wall to inflame and thicken, which is very painful to the animal. Initially, syringe feed cranberry juice (fresh, not cordial) then add to the drinking water daily. Syringe about 5–10 ml twice a day. Add cranberry juice to the water. Add about 10% cranberry juice initially; gradually increase each day, until you are adding 30% cranberry juice. This can be continued permanently following treatment as an inclusive part of the diet.

- **Promote diuresis;** diets should be supplemented with lots of fresh vegetables. These supply essential vitamins, minerals and water. Feed only fruit and vegetables that contain low levels (<50 mg/100 g) of calcium, such as cucumber, carrots, cauliflower, tomatoes, apple, lettuce (in moderation) and celery. These vegetables also contain high levels of water, which helps to prevent the animal getting dehydrated. They produce small volumes of concentrated urine and tend to be predisposed to developing urinary sludge. The concentrated urine tends to sit in the bladder, and sediments. The sediment forms a sludge that is an irritant to the bladder, urethra and surrounding skin. It can also cause cystitis. By encouraging a high water intake the urine is diluted, and regularly removed from the bladder, preventing sedimentation.
- **Avoid feeding dark green, leafy vegetables** such as kale, spring greens, broccoli and spinach as these are extremely high in calcium (all contain >50 mg calcium/100 g, some as high as 200 mg calcium/100 g.
- **Review the animal's current dry diet** – they should have calcium:phosphorus ratio of 2:1 to ensure an appropriate level is being provided. Try to feed diets that are within the region of 0.8 calcium to 0.4 phosphorus to prevent excess dietary levels; diets such as Burgess Supa Excel are perfect and provide the correct dietary levels.
- **Restricting the animal's access to dry food** is advisable, especially if there are any uncertainties over the calcium level or form. Many manufactured feeds are rich in alfalfa, which is extremely high in calcium, and contain limestone (calcium carbonate) and calcium di-phosphate. In addition, the vitamin and

mineral supplements may contain other calcium salts, e.g. calcium pantothenate (vitamin B_5) and calcium iodide, all of which contribute to the total calcium level.

- **Vitamin C** – it is advisable to supplement with additional vitamin C and also vitamin B (the water-soluble vitamins). Vitamin C (ascorbic acid) has the added advantage of being a urine acidifier, and is reported to aid dissolution of uroliths in guinea pigs.

CASE HISTORY 2

Patient

A 2-year-old rat that had been suffering from a skin condition for approximately 8 months. The owner was distressed at the rat's loss of condition and discomfort. He has always been fed the same diet since ownership and is also given a treat of additional mixed nuts that he adores.

Condition

The rat's coat was in very poor condition and was causing irritation to the animal. Small red pustules were observed on the surface and a scurfy appearance was obvious. There were also superficial wounds to the body that were self inflicted through scratching. The animal was losing a little weight, but was overweight for its size anyway. However, other than the coat the animal appeared healthy with no obvious cause for the problem.

Treatment

The initial assumption was that there would be a problem with mite infestation from contaminated bedding. On thorough examination and following a skin scrape all the results were negative. It was considered that the reaction might be an allergy or nutritional problem. Rats are very sensitive to food high in protein and fat, and can't tolerate these in high levels in their diet. Many diets contain high levels of seeds and nuts. These should not be an inclusive element of rats' daily dietary ratio; however, they can be fed in small quantities as treats.

The diet was immediately evaluated and found to contain high levels of these with supplementary nuts being fed too. The diet was immediately changed to a complete rat food with the exclusion of seeds and nuts. Fresh vegetables and fruit were provided daily as a treat to replace the mixed nuts, and these were given as a weekly treat in minute quantities.

Within a week there was a dramatic reduction in inflammation and irritation of the skin overall. The red pustules had disappeared completely. Over the next couple of weeks the rat's coat returned to normal and no signs of allergy were observed, and it remained clear after the owner maintained the animal on the new diet. The new diet also assisted in weight reduction, as rats are prone to obesity.

SECTION 2

Snakes, lizards and chelonia care

SECTION 2

Snakes, lizards and chelonia care

Introduction

REASONS FOR ADMISSION

In practice one should always expect the unexpected, and this usually arrives in the waiting room in the form of a writhing pillowcase or a moving cardboard box. When the contents of these carrying vessels are examined further the nurse is usually presented with a manic lizard desperate to escape from its temporary imprisonment or a writhing snake doing a vertical take off from its container.

The following chapters set out to provide the nurse with information that will help with the care and treatment of a range of reptilian species. Topics covered include: the identification of species commonly being presented for treatment at the veterinary practice, the reasons for their arrival, handling, general nursing, care, and the basic principles of housing and husbandry.

As more and more people become reptile owners there is an increasing demand on the veterinary practice to be able to provide advice, treatment and care for reptiles. It is important to remember that many of the commonly encountered problems have poor husbandry as a root cause, so when any reptile is being admitted a full and accurate case history must be obtained. Candid questioning must be carried out to establish how the reptile is housed, the environmental conditions, details of feeding, etc.

It must also be highlighted that a snake, lizard or chelonia may have been ill for some time before presenting with noticeable clinical signs, and that their demonstration of pain and discomfort is also not fully understood.

Reptilian conditions commonly seen in veterinary practice

- Anorexia
- Metabolic bone disease
- Endo- and ectoparasites
- Necrotic dermatitis (shell or scale rot)
- Stomatitis (mouth rot)
- Wounds caused by bites or burns
- Dysecdysis (difficulty shedding)
- Dystocias
- Respiratory infections
- Malnutrition.

The above list provides the nurse with an idea of the type of conditions that may be presented for treatment, and how important it is for staff to be able to demonstrate knowledge on these conditions, and procedures to be carried out when managing such problems.

COMMON SPECIES ENCOUNTERED

Lizards

The most common species of lizard that will be encountered include:

- geckos, of which the leopard gecko is probably one of the most commonly kept species
- bearded dragons
- skinks
- water dragons
- iguanas
- monitors.

Snakes

The most popular snake species to be kept as pets include the following:

- corn snake
- kingsnakes
- common boa
- Burmese python
- royal pythons.

Chelonia

Below are the species of chelonia that are most commonly kept as pets:

- Mediterranean tortoise
- red eared terrapin
- map turtles.

It should be highlighted that this list identifies a small number of the species seen and it is often the case that once people have got the 'bug' of keeping reptiles they want more challenging and unusual species. Therefore, in preparation for what may come through the surgery door, every practice must invest in a few good reptile identification books.

RECEIVING A SICK REPTILE

Many reptile illnesses can be attributed to poor husbandry, environmental conditions and inadequate diet; therefore, the principal objectives when dealing with a sick reptile are to:

- Establish the species; if possible confirm the Latin name as this will help you find out specific information on the animal's needs, such as temperature and lighting requirements, feeding preference, and if nocturnal or diurnal species. **Remember reptiles are ectothermic – cold-blooded – and rely on their surroundings to provide warmth for their bodies. Each species has a preferred optimum temperature; this is the temperature the reptile needs to reach for its metabolism to work correctly.**

- Establish the sex of the reptile if known.
- Establish the nature of the problem, signs observed and the length of time the reptile has been sick. The owner must be encouraged to give details on how the reptile is housed and notes must be taken on:
  - vivarium set up
  - heating used and how regulated
  - lighting
  - furnishings and substrates used
  - hygiene protocols
  - humidity levels.

The owner must also clearly describe diet, frequency of feeding and supplementation used.

Information supplied by the owner can be used by the nurse to identify any errors in husbandry and provide advice and help on how these can be corrected.

It should also be noted that many reptile conditions take months to develop and will equally take time to be rectified.

EXAMINATION
Prior to handling

1. Obtain a full history of the patient.
2. Ascertain the temperament of the patient and if used to being handled.
3. Get assistance if a large aggressive species and make sure all necessary handling equipment is readily available.
4. Ensure room is escape proof and all people in attendance are confident with the type of animal about to be examined.
5. Protect yourself and be prepared for the unexpected; remember, medium to large snakes can deliver a painful bite and constrict. Lizards can scratch, bite and lash out using their tail. Some species of chelonia, especially terrapins and turtles, can issue nasty bites.
6. If confronted with a really aggressive species then allow it to 'cool down' by placing it in an environment lower than its preferred option temperature range. This will make the reptile lethargic and allow examination to continue.

7. Collect or observe faecal material or urate passed for any abnormalities or further laboratory tests.

Examination whilst handling

1. Reptiles must be restrained correctly using appropriate methods and equipment.

2. The body can be checked for parasites, burns, wounds and irregularities or discoloration to the scales or the shell. Signs of dehydration (i.e. tenting and lack of elasticity of the skin) and lack of body mass (anorexic snakes appear triangular in shape, lizards suffer tissue loss near base of tail and pelvic bones are prominent).

3. Examine soft tissues – mouth: look for signs of discharge or discoloration; eyes and nose: observe retained shed, infection or signs of dehydration; cloaca: observe for swelling or discharge.

4. Check limbs for wounds, swellings and abnormalities, etc.

5. As we are lacking reliable data for the assessment of shock in reptiles the following may prove useful:
   - Heart rate (beats/per minute) 20–100, but this varies according to temperature, size and condition of the reptile.
   - Respiratory rate varies according to stress, handling, temperature and size but approximately 4 breaths per minute.
   - Temperature – as reptiles are ectothermic, species have their own individual preferred body temperature that will need to be confirmed once the species is identified.

Once the initial examination has been completed and initial treatment administered, the reptile will need to be placed in a suitable hospital vivarium with temperatures set at the higher end of its preferred optimum temperature range as this will aid:

- immune response
- response to drug therapy
- general recovery.

Lastly, all the veterinary team's efforts and dedication during the treatment of the reptile patient will be lost if the animal is discharged without the owner being provided with clear, concise information on how to continue to care for the animal. In addition, where appropriate to ensure the patient's continued good health, the nurse must emphasise necessary changes to be made to the husbandry, environment, feeding and accommodation.

Chapter 3

Lizards and snakes

Beverly Shingleton

These belong to the order *Squamata*, which is split into *Sauria* (lizards) and *Serpentes* (snakes).

Lizards usually possess four legs (exception being the slow worm *Anguis fragilis*), a tail and moving eye lids; whereas snakes are limbless and have fused eyelids.

INTRODUCTION

Nursing the reptile patient requires a different approach to that applied during the care of companion animals. So the first step in achieving effective nursing protocols is understanding some of the basic differences in the biology of lizards and snakes compared to that of the dog and cat. Table 3.1 identifies some of the main anatomical and physiological characteristics of the reptile patient. Table 3.2 lists some of the more common species kept.

HUSBANDRY AND GENERAL CARE OF THE HOSPITALISED PATIENT

To reduce stress and potential spread of pathogens a separate area or ward should be designated for the care of the reptile patient. Ideally, this area should be subdivided into two: one for the care of the sick, injured and non-contagious reptile, and one for the contagious patient.

Hospital cage (vivarium) (Fig. 3.1)

The major cause of sickness in reptiles can be attributed to poor husbandry and nutrition. Therefore, it is imperative that the accommodation provided in the hospital be suitable for the species

to be housed and the following taken into consideration:

- the natural history of the reptile patient
- the preferred body temperature (PBT) of the reptile
- environmental conditions, i.e. is the snake or lizard a desert or tropical species?
- is the species nocturnal crepuscular or diurnal?
- does the species require a terrestrial, arboreal, aquatic or semi-aquatic set up?

Providing the wrong environment can stress the patient and this, in turn, can cause immunosuppression and infections. Therefore, the following text outlines some of the important factors to be considered when setting up a vivarium for a sick reptile.

A selection of housing should be available to suit the needs of the patient; one standard cage to

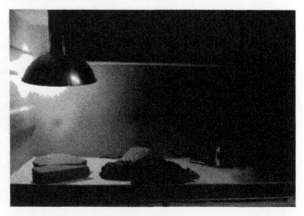

Fig. 3.1 The hospital cage (vivarium).

Table 3.1 Main characteristics of snake and lizard anatomy and physiology

Anatomical structure/system	Features
Cardiovascular	Three chambered heart, left and right atrium and one ventricle. Ventricle receives blood from both atria; muscular ridges, and timing of contractions prevents the mixing of the blood so that de-oxygenated blood is sent to the lungs and oxygenated into the systemic circulation.
	Diving causes blood to be diverted away from the pulmonary circulation and into the systemic circulation therefore bypassing the lungs. **This can cause a problem during anaesthesia; if the patient has a period of apnoea and is not ventilated, inadequate transfer of anaesthetic gases into the body will occur making stabilisation very difficult.**
	No diaphragm, which leaves the heart fairly mobile in the rib cage possibly to aid the passage of large prey items. Running through the ventral abdomen is a very large vein that needs to be avoided during surgery.
	All circulating blood cells are nucleated. Leukocytes (WBC) of snakes and lizards do not have neutrophils but heterophils; these play a similar role in defending the body against invading pathogens. These cells lack lysosomes and this is why reptilian pus is usually more solid than mammalian pus.
	Renal portal system – the external iliac veins drain blood returning from the hindquarters into a large renal portal vein which in turn flows directly into the kidney.[1] This must be considered when administering drugs into the hind legs of reptiles. Drugs given in this area could converge at high concentrations in the kidney before being distributed around the body, potentially predisposing to renal damage. A second consideration is that if the drug is excreted via the kidneys, it may be excreted before having a chance to take effect.
Respiratory	Snakes normally have one lung, the left being absent or vestigial. The right lung normally extends from near the heart to the right kidney (cranially). The lung itself is a very simple sac-like structure with ridges on the interior surface in a reticular pattern to increase the surface area for gaseous exchange. **Lungs are very fragile and care must be taken not to overinflate during positive pressure ventilation.** Lack of diaphragm means reptiles are unable to cough. They also lack the ciliated epithelium that would remove debris and pus away from the lungs (as occurs in mammals) to be swallowed; this means that if an infection of the respiratory tract occurs mucus and pus collect and pneumonia could ensue. The trachea is made up of incomplete rings of cartilage. The glottis is easy to see and is positioned on the floor of the mouth posterior to the tongue. **The visualisation of the glottis makes intubation a relatively easy task.** When snakes are feeding on large prey items the glottis moves to one side allowing breathing to continue. (Physiology of the respiratory system is discussed under Anaesthesia.)
	Lizards can inflate their lungs to make themselves look larger. Green iguanas posses a nasal salt gland that excretes excess sodium chloride and this can be seen as white powder around the nostrils or fluid when sneezed.
Digestive	This extends from the mouth to the cloaca. In the oral cavity mucous glands secrete mucus to lubricate the food; in some species of lizards and snakes these are modified to produce venom. They posses teeth that are continually being replaced (except Agamid lizards). Snakes have six rows of teeth. In most lizards teeth are attached to the mandible without sockets but in the chameleons and Agamids the teeth are arranged on the biting surface. A vomeronasal organ (Jacobson's organ) is found in the roof of the mouth and receives scent particles from the tongue for taste and 'smell'. In snakes and some lizards, i.e. monitor and tegus, the tongue is forked; chameleons have projectile tongues, and green iguanas have a red tip to their tongue. **In bearded dragons the mucous membrane lining the oral cavity appears yellow-orange and is normal (not to be confused with icterus [jaundice]).**
	Dark pigment can be seen in some species of gecko, chameleons and monitor-lizards. The digestive tract has a simple stomach and a relatively short and unconvoluted small intestine with enzymes being secreted to aid the digestion of foodstuffs. Excess fluid is absorbed in the large intestines and this is where faeces are formed. In herbivorous lizards the caecum is enlarged and used to ferment and break down the otherwise indigestible fibre to release energy. Micro-organisms that aid this process are found in the caecum and these can be affected by the use of antibiotics.
	The digestive tract terminates at the **cloaca**. The cloaca is a three-chambered structure – the digestive, urinary and reproductive tracts all emptying into here. The three chambers are as follows: **coprodeum** – receives the faecal matter, **urodeum** – receives the urethra, the ureters and genital papilla, and **proctodeum** – the mixing vat. The exit from the cloaca is the vent. **The vent is a good place to**

Table 3.1 (*continued*)

Anatomical structure/system	Features
	observe capillary refill time and mucous membrane colour and to position monitoring equipment for anaesthetics and temperature taking.
Urogenital	Kidney – no renal pelvis, pyramids, relatively few nephrons and most importantly no loop of Henle, therefore, being unable to concentrate their urine. In most terrestrial reptilian species urea is excreted in the form of uric acid (thus reduced amount of water being lost). Uric acid is insoluble and if the reptile becomes dehydrated the uric acid will crystallise and be deposited in the body tissues, especially the kidneys. If this condition is not treated promptly then the reptile will die. Snakes have paired elongated, lobulated kidneys that sit dorsally in the caudal abdomen, the right being more cranial. They are usually dark chocolate brown but this can change according to the breeding season. They have no urinary bladder but urine can be stored in the ureters. **Care should be taken when handling large constrictors especially if the cranial portion of the snake is raised above the caudal portion, as gravity acting on the weight of the stored urine can cause it to be expelled in large quantities down the handler. Try to keep the snake horizontal!** In lizards the kidneys are similar to those described for the snake but are short and have few lobules; position varies according to species. Some species do have a urinary bladder.
	Reproductive organs – male snakes have two paired invaginated hemipenes that are located in the vent and run ventrally in the tail base. These are inserted into the female's cloaca during copulation and sperm is passed into her reproductive tract. The hemipenes can be used to sex snakes.
	Lizards possess similar structures also known as hemipenes; they are sac-like and do not contain erectile tissue. They are kept in an inverted position in the tail base and can be seen externally as bulges just below the vent. During breeding only one hemipenis is used at a time. Female snakes and lizards have paired ovaries, and a left and right uterine tube. Egg binding is a problem associated with both and this is covered in more detail under common problems. Here either the shelled or non-shelled ova sit in the oviducts (shelled) or ovaries (non-shelled).
Skeletal	Snakes are limbless, but some like boas and pythons have ventral spurs (remains of claws from vestigial hindlimbs) near the vent, thought to be associated with courtship. The snake has a bony axial skeleton consisting of skull vertebrae and ribs. The ribs are flexible to allow for the passage of whole prey. The jaw of the snake lacks the mandibular symphysis, therefore allowing it to consume prey much larger than its head. Lizards have an appendicular and axial skeleton; the ribs extend off all but the tail vertebrae. One outstanding feature is some species of lizards' ability to carry out autotomy (tail loss), a process developed to escape predators (details given under common conditions). This is achieved because there is a vertical fracture plane (connective tissue or cartilage develops after ossification) through the body and neural arch of the caudal vertebrae. If the tail is handled roughly it will be shed.
Integument	**Shed in pieces (most lizards) or one whole piece including eye covering or spectacle (snakes)**. During shedding the skin appears dull; this is because a milky lymph fluid is secreted between the old and the new skin. The spectacle protects the surface of the cornea; a tear-like secretion flows between the spectacle and cornea. Infections can gain access via the lacrimal gland resulting in subspectacular abscess or if blockage and infection 'bullous spectaculopathy'. In lizards eyelids are present but modified according to species. Snakes do not have a tympanic membrane or middle ear cavity, therefore, have little airborne hearing but are able to sense vibration through the substrate. Boas and pythons have heat sensitive pits on their labial scales to help locate prey. In lizards the ear has both auditory and vestibular function. The tympanic membrane can be seen in a depression at the side of the lizard's head. Some species of lizard, e.g. green iguana and water dragon, have a parietal eye. This is found on the dorsal midline of the head; it has no visual function but has a role in thermoregulation and hormonal production. Some lizards have chromatophores in their skin; these react to light, heat and hormones giving them the ability to change colour. Dewlaps, crests and spines are all well developed in the male affording protection and acting as secondary sexual characteristics. Also femoral pores can be seen along the ventral aspect of the thigh in species such as iguanas, tegus and bearded dragons (more pronounced in sexually active males). Geckos have precloacal and femoral pores, and bilobed swelling at the base of the vent.
	Many species have developed small bones just below the surface of the skin called dermal bones or osteoderms. These serve to give extra protection to the reptile, help to retain body water and in crocodilians aid with thermoregulation.

[1] Research is still continuing into the renal portal venous circulation and how drug therapy is effected.

Table 3.2 Commonly kept species and food preferences

Species	Food
Snakes	
Boas Common boa (*Boa constrictor*) Rainbow boa (*Epicrates cechria*) Emerald tree boa (*Corallus caninus*) Rosy boa (*Lichanura trivirgata*) Sand boa (*Eryx jaculus*)	Depending on the size of the snake: rodents (mice, rats, gerbils), chicks (day old), birds
Pythons Royal python (*Python regius*) Blood python (*Python curtis brongersmai*) Children's python (*Antaresia childreni*) Reticulated python (*Python reticulatus*) Burmese python (*Python m. bivittatus*) Green tree python (*Chondrophython viridis*)	Depending on the size of the snake: mammals, rabbits, birds, chicks
Colubrids Rat snake (*Elaphe obsoleta* spp.) Corn snake (*Elaphe guttata*) Milk snake (*Lampropeltis triangulum*) Hognose (*Heterodon* spp.) Bull/gopher/pine snakes (*Pituophis melanoleucus* spp.) King snake (*Lampropeltis getulus*)	Mice, rats, gerbils, birds
Garters Common garter snake (*Thamnnophis sirtalis*)	Earthworms, fish, small rodents, pinkies
Lizards	
Geckos Leopard gecko (*Eublepharus macularis*) Day gecko (*Phelsuma cepediana*) Fat tailed gecko (*Phelsuma laticauda*)	Insects, (crickets, hoppers, locusts) neonate mammals Day gecko: also offer fruit purée, baby food
Agamas Agama (*Agama agama*) Water dragon (*Physignathus cocincinus*) Uromastyx or dab lizard (*Uromastyx acanthinurus*)	Agama: insects, (crickets, hoppers, locusts) some fruit/veg matter Water dragon: insects, crickets, locusts, small rodents, pinkies, some fruit/veg matter Uromastyx: fruit/veg matter (foliage-, leaf-based diet), occasional insect
Chameleon Jackson's chameleon (*Chamaeleo jacksoni*) Panther chameleon (*Chamaeleo pardalis*) Veiled chameleon (*Chamaeleo calyptratus*) Plated lizard (*Gerrhosaurus* spp.)	Winged insects, occasional pinky, waxworms Insects, offer some vegetable matter
Iguanas Green iguana (*Iguana iguana*) Anoles (*Anolis carolinensis*) Collard lizard (*Crotaphytus collaris*)	Green iguana: fruit/veg matter (foliage-, leaf-based diet) Anoles: insects (crickets, hoopers) Collard lizard: insects, small rodents
Monitors/tegus Tegu (*Tupinambis* spp.) Monitor (*Varanus* spp.)	Mammals, eggs, birds
Skinks Blue tonged (*Tiliqua gigas*)	Insects, snails, mammals

suit all is not adequate and as mentioned above the accommodation **MUST** suit the individual's needs.

The main points to consider in selecting suitable accommodation are as follows:

- ease of access
- durable
- secure
- easy to clean.

Allowing the client to provide the housing is not recommended as it, in itself, may be incorrect or harbour disease.

In the hospital ward the cages should be easy to clean and disinfect. Security is another feature, especially as many reptiles are 'escape artists', and you do not want the 40-kg, 14-foot Burmese python exercising itself around the ward!

The ability to observe the patient without unnecessary disturbance is important and this can be achieved by surrounding glass or glass sliding doors with non-reflective material as used on car windows.

Vivarium materials (Table 3.3)

Hygiene is a major consideration and recommended materials are either fibreglass or moulded plastic, both of which are quite expensive but if the practice is considering widening its interest in reptile medicine and care they are a long-term investment. Table 3.3 looks at the various materials available on the market.

Shape and size

As mentioned earlier, reptiles do not conform to a set size, habitat preference or activity level, therefore, ranges of different dimension cages are essential.

Terrestrial or ground dwelling species would require a horizontal vivarium, arboreal animals require a taller vivarium, and the burrowing species will require a deep base to hold much substrate.

Substrate (Table 3.3)

This is the medium that sits in the bottom of the vivarium to absorb faeces and urine, and in the

Table 3.3 Substrates and vivarium materials

Material for vivarium construction	Substrates
[1]Melamine chip board	[6]Peat
[2]Moulded plastics	[4]Wood chip
[3]Glass tanks	[6]Vermiculite
Marine Ply	[4]Bark chip
[2]Fibreglass	[4]Corn cob
Plastic tanks (fauna boxes)	[5]Repti/calci sand
Small plastic tubs (hatchling snakes)	Newspaper
	Gravel
	Alfalfa pellets
	[4,7]Wood based cat litter
	[8]Sphagnum moss

[1] Not ideal for species requiring high humidity.
[2] Excellent for cleaning; can be jet washed.
[3] Good for aquatic species and species requiring high humidity. Poor insulation, poor security, difficult to attach fittings.
[4] Substrates if eaten can cause gut impaction or get stuck in mouth so should be avoided.
[5] Only sand produced specifically for reptiles should be used as others contain silica, which will dehydrate the animal. Sand is used for desert species.
[6] Good for retaining moisture and humidity.
[7] Only litter free from pine oils should be used.

case of burrowing animals, allows them to display their natural behaviour.

When choosing a substrate one would normally select a substrate that was comparable with the animal's natural habitat, and looked aesthetically pleasing. In veterinary practice the aesthetics are not an important factor, and in these circumstances the substrates used should **display faecal and urate materials easily; be hygienic, cheap and readily available; and if ingested should not cause impaction or complicate medical problems**. Newspaper or thick white paper like that used at the 'fish and chip' shop is ideal. Table 3.3 lists the common substrates.

Cage furnishings

In the hospital vivarium these need to be kept to a minimum.

One of the main provisions should be a series of hides, as these will make the reptile feel safe, secure and reduce stress. As a guide for the size of hide, when the snake or lizard is in situ it should be able to touch three sides of the hide; this is

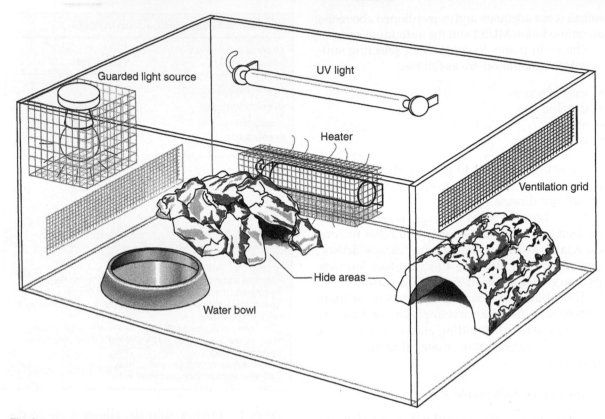

Fig. 3.2 Schematic diagram of a typical vivarium.

reported to reduce stress. Other furnishings can include secured, textured branches that can support the weight of the reptile (especially important when hospitalising an arboreal species).

> **Tip:** Plants can look nice, but are difficult to keep clean. A word of warning: lizards will ingest plants and if these are plastic or silk they can cause intestinal impaction and will not show up on X-ray.

If using stones or large heavy objects in the vivarium, make sure that they have a smooth flat base to prevent them rolling onto the snake or lizard and causing injury. A large heavy ceramic bowl will be needed to provide drinking water and bathing.

As a general rule keep all furnishings to a minimum as this will aid in maintaining the cage, make cleaning easier, and it also gives the nurse or veterinary surgeon ease of access when handling (Fig. 3.2). Trying to handle and restrain an emerald tree boa (*Corallus caninus*) can be a task in itself, but when you have to fight through a forest canopy to get to the animal it can be a stressful experience for the snake and handler.

GENERAL ENVIRONMENTAL CONDITIONS

The four main environmental considerations here are:

1. ventilation
2. heating
3. lighting
4. humidity.

Each one will be discussed separately as it relates to the reptile patient.

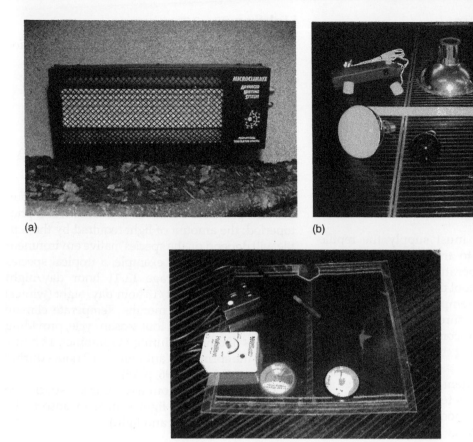

(a)

(b)

(c)

Fig. 3.3 Heating equipment. (a) Ceramic heater. (b) Reflector bulbs. (c) Heat mat and rocks.

Ventilation

Like mammals, all reptiles require air in order to survive. Ventilation is achieved by providing housing that has holes positioned at the back or sides of the cage.

To achieve good through flow of air and prevent drafts, vents should be placed opposite each other but at different levels, i.e. one at the top and one at the bottom.

Heating (Fig. 3.3a,b,c)

The provision of heat in the vivarium is essential and this is where an understanding of snake and lizard biology is important (Table 3.1). Snakes and lizards are classed as being 'ectothermic', meaning they rely on external heat sources to

warm up their internal body temperature. So for the reptile's body to function correctly a heat source has to be provided in the animal's accommodation.

Heat can be provided in many forms (see Fig. 3.3a,b,c), but the main ones are as follows:

- ceramic heaters (Fig. 3.3a)
- reflector bulbs with or without UVB content (Fig. 3.3b)
- heat mat and rocks (Fig. 3.3c).

Tip: Make sure all heat and light sources are guarded as reptiles can suffer serious burns from sitting on lamps. Snakes have few nerve endings in their ventral scales and will not realise they are cooking themselves!

Regulation of temperature

Snakes and lizards have a **preferred body temperature** (PBT) or **preferred optimum temperature zone** (POTZ); this relates to the *ideal* or optimum temperature that the species requires for its metabolism to function correctly (movement, feeding, digestion, enzyme activity, reproduction, etc.).

> **Tip:** To aid their immune system, sick or injured reptiles will seek out the high point of their POTZ.

The heat provided must supply the reptile with an opportunity to thermoregulate (move between different temperature zones to allow the reptile to warm up or cool down as required).

When providing a temperature gradient, the positioning of the heat source is important, as this will allow the reptile to control its body temperature at different times of the day (see Fig. 3.2 for vivarium set-up).

A temperature gradient can be regulated by observation of thermometers and correctly positioned thermostats. A good instrument to measure temperature is a laser heat gun (Peregrine), which can be aimed at an area within the vivarium and a reading taken and recorded.

Overheating the reptile can be just as detrimental to its health as underheating.

Diurnal cage temperatures should be in the following ranges:

Tropical species	26.5°C–37°C (80–98.5°F)
Temperate species	24°C–29.5°C (75–85°F)

Please note: this is only a rough guide and many species require hotter or cooler temperatures depending on the time of year and seasonal fluctuations. So the individual species' requirements must be researched. More detail on preferred temperature ranges for commonly kept species can be found in Mader (1996), p. 12, Table 2.1.

Another consideration is that drugs' absorption and utilisation by the snake or lizard is influenced by their POTZ, so when reptiles are receiving medication or anaesthetics the provision of heat is essential.

Lighting (Fig. 3.3b)

There are three main types of lighting used for reptiles (see Fig. 3.3b):

1. incandescent bulbs, e.g. light bulbs, coloured light bulbs
2. ultraviolet (UV) strip lights with UVB and UVA content
3. reflector bulbs (can be combined with UVA and UVB).

Lighting not only stimulates natural behaviour, but also provides the lizard or snake with a photoperiod; the amount of light required by the reptile will depend on the species' native environment and time of year. For example, a tropical species will require on average 13/11 hour day/night (summer) cycle and 11/13 hour day/night (winter) cycle, each lasting 6 months. Temperate climate species should be on a four season cycle, providing 15 hours of daylight during the summer, 12 hours during the spring and autumn, and 9 hours during the winter (Mader 1996, p. 16).

Lighting also encourages diurnal species to bask (sit under the light source to absorb the energy from the heat and light).

> **Tip:** UVA stimulates behavioural and physiological effects.
> UVB is necessary for calcium metabolism and the activation of vitamin D.
> UVC is not important in reptile husbandry.

Full-spectrum light (such as that produced by sunlight UVA, UVB, UVC) is important for all tropical, subtropical and desert, diurnal lizards and also some snakes. Although allowing our captive reptile to bask in natural sunlight would be the ideal, given our climate and the fact that it would be unsuitable to allow an iguana recovering from an operation to bask in the neighbour's 20-foot pine tree, it will have to be supplied by artificial means.

There are a number of UV lights on the market that supply an adequate amount of UVB. At present *Zoo Med Reptisun 5.0* is one of the best strip lights on the market. For use in larger enclosures (minimum of 4 foot), the Powersun (Active Mercury

Box 3.1 Calcium metabolism in reptiles

UVB rays are necessary for the production of vitamin D_3 and calcium metabolism in lizards and chelonia. The process is a complex one and the nurse should have some understanding of the relationship between UVB and calcium metabolism in reptilian species.

Process
The process starts in the skin of the reptile:

1. UVB rays from the sun or UV lamp in contact with the skin start a chemical reaction that results in **provitamin D_3** being converted into **previtamin D_3**.
2. The previtamin D_3 is then converted into vitamin D_3 (this stage is dependent on the skin reaching sufficient temperature).
3. The **vitamin D_3** (cholecalciferol) is then absorbed into the bloodstream and transported to the liver where it undergoes further change, before being sent via the bloodstream to the kidneys.
4. It is in the kidneys that the active form known as **1,25 dihydroxyvitamin D** (calciferol) is produced and this chemical will travel via the bloodstream to the small intestines where it will aid in the transportation of calcium across the wall of the small intestine and into the bloodstream.

Vapour) UV is effective, which gives off 5–8 times more UVB than strip lights.

The role of UVB and calcium metabolism is explained in Box 3.1.

It should be highlighted here that UVB lights do not have an infinite life span and, although the white light may be seen, the UVB content is generally exhausted within 6–9 months of use. For satisfactory vitamin D synthesis, the UVB light needs to be on for 10–14 hours daily and be positioned approximately 24 cm above the reptile.

Tip: Positioning of the UVB light is very important. The height should be measured from where the rays will be landing on the animal and not the base of the cage. Also, to maximise UVB utilisation, the height can be reduced for young animals.

Replace UVB lights every 6 months if young growing stock is housed.

Humidity

This is the amount of moisture in the air and the humidity requirements will depend on the species'

natural habitat; for example a rainforest species will require a higher humidity than their desert counterparts.

Most species do well at a humidity of 50–70% and humidity can be achieved by frequent spraying of the vivarium using a plant mister or placing damp sphagnum moss or tissue paper in a small ice cream tub or plastic sandwich container. Correct humidity is necessary to allow normal ecdysis (shedding of the skin). Decreasing ventilation should not be used as a means of increasing humidity as this can lead to an increase in temperature, which in turn can cause a rapid bacterial and mould growth in the cage.

CLEANING AND HYGIENE

As when dealing with companion animals this is of paramount importance. When a patient is in situ attention should be given to:

- removing and disposing of all soiled areas as soon as they are identified (the hospital cage should be checked at least twice a day for faecal and urate matter)
- using a detergent, wash and rinse food bowls and water receptacles
- using a detergent or mild disinfectant, clean areas and any furnishings that have been soiled
- rinsing and drying cleaned areas
- replacing substrate
- thoroughly disinfecting all equipment used and storing it correctly.

Tip:

Good cleaning agents
Skin contact
- Chlorhexadine (Hibiscrub)
- Povidone-Iodine (Pevidine).

Use on inanimate objects
- Trigene
- Virkon
- Hypochlorites.

Whilst cleaning the cage the occupant can be placed in a holding pen like a pen pal. The removal of the patient will help to minimise stress to the snake or lizard and also prevent potential attack.

If the cage is to be cleaned after the patient has left, then the following protocol should be observed:

• All furnishings and substrates must be removed and, if possible, disposed of.
• All organic material must be removed and correctly disposed of.
• If objects are to be used again, i.e. water bowls, rocks, these must be thoroughly cleaned and disinfected, as must any items that have been used during the reptile's stay, e.g. feeding tongs.
• The empty cage must be cleaned using copious amounts of hot water and detergent, paying particular attention to the corners, non-removable fixtures and fittings, and glass sliding doors.
• The entire cage must be rinsed before applying the disinfectant.
• Leave the disinfectant in contact with the cage for the recommended period before rinsing.
• Whilst cleaning the cage, the nurse must observe her own health and hygiene, and wear protective clothing such as latex gloves and aprons. Hands must be washed after any contact with the reptile or its vivarium (see Box 3.2).

FIRST AID

The principle of providing first aid to reptiles is very similar to that applied to companion animals. The main areas to be considered are:

• Reptiles' differing biology compared to that of companion animals (see Table 3.1).
• Reptiles' environmental needs. As all reptiles are ectothermic (cold-blooded), the provision of heat is paramount in treating the first-aid emergency (thermal regulation is discussed under general environmental conditions).
• Suitable containers must be available for placement of the casualty until further veterinary assessment and treatment can be given. Figure 3.4a,b,c shows a range of temporary accomodation and environmental set up suitable to house a small reptile patient.

Box 3.2 Reptile zoonosis

As veterinary nurses we are familiar with the mammalian zoonoses, but reptiles harbour a host of very different pathogens as set out below. To prevent human infection and potential serious illness strict hygiene protocols must be employed when dealing with any reptile.

Salmonella
This organism is excreted intermittently in the faeces of most reptiles and can be passed on to humans via ingestion of faecal matter! Good hygiene is required here; hands must be washed after handling or cleaning reptile accommodation. Symptoms of human infection include abdominal pain, diarrhoea, vomiting, nausea and high temperature.

Campylobacter
This has been isolated from pet turtles and human infection manifests itself as gastroenteritis.

Aeromona spp., *Citrobacteria* spp., *Enterobacteria* spp., *Klebsiella* spp. and *Proteus* spp.
These are a group of potentially pathogenic enteric bacteria commonly isolated from both healthy and sick reptiles. In humans they can cause inflammation of both the small and large intestine.

Arthropods
The following group of **ectoparasites** has been known to bite humans and cause skin irritations:

• Snake mite – *Ophionyssus natricis*, Trombiculid mites, e.g. *Neotrombicula autumnalis* (harvest mite), *Eutromicula alfreddogesi* (common chigger).
• Ticks – newly imported reptile species are often found harbouring ticks and if these bite humans can cause the following infections.
  —Lyme disease (*Borrelia burgdorferi*).
  —Siberian tick typhus (*Rickettsia siberica*).

This box aims to highlight some but not all of the potential reptile pathogens encountered so general care and sensible hygiene precautions should always be taken when handling reptiles.

• Clear concise history of the reptile is required. When dealing with the reptile emergency it is essential that the nurse gather as much information as possible on the problem (the importance of taking an accurate history is highlighted further in the text).

The scope of first-aid treatment is limited and can be further hindered by the lack of valuable

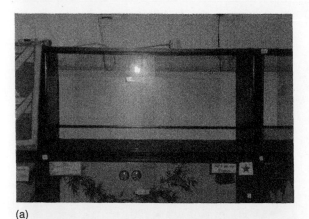

(a)

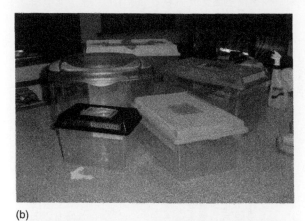

(b)

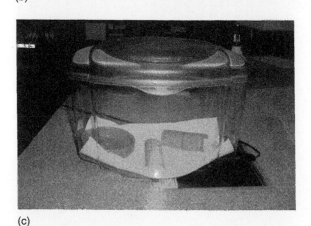

(c)

Fig. 3.4 (a, b, c) Suitable temporary accommodation.

physiological parameters on which to assess the degree of shock. Unlike our companion animals where we have reliable data on respiratory rates, rectal temperature ranges and heart rate, when

assessing the reptile patient the following information may be helpful:

- Heart rate (beats/per minute) 20–100, but this varies according to temperature, size and condition of the reptile.
- Respiratory rate varies according to stress, handling, temperature and size, but approximately four breaths per minute.
- Temperature – as reptiles are ectothermic species, they have their own individual preferred body temperature, which will need to be confirmed once the species is identified.

Assessment of shock

Using capillary refill time and colour observations can be quite difficult, especially if the jaw is clamped shut and the rest of the body covered in shell or scales. Behavioural response to shock varies according to species, ranging from aggression in a large male iguana to flaccid unresponsiveness in some chelonia or snakes.

It is not uncommon for traumatised reptiles to have a delayed response to stress, taking days or weeks to show signs.

Common first-aid emergencies

The following is a list of more common emergencies that may require some first aid (many of the conditions are detailed in Table 3.4:

- Bite wounds in lizards usually caused by fighting amongst dominant males
- Burns in snakes and lizards, caused by reptile getting too close to an unguarded heat source
- Collapse through metabolic bone disease
- Collapse due to anorexia in snakes and lizards
- Dystocia
- Tail autotomy in lizards
- Respiratory distress.

Whatever the condition requiring first aid and your limitations because of the species being presented, your priority, *apart from your own safety*, must be to ensure that:

1. the airway is free from obstruction and any discharge is removed from or around the oral cavity

Table 3.4 Common medical conditions

Common problem	Cause	Signs	Treatment	Other
Stomatitis (mouth rot)	Seen in both lizards and snakes. Normally caused by poor husbandry and injury to rostal (nasal) area due to fighting, or running against glass front of vivarium. Bacteria, viruses and fungi invade site and set up an infection.	Decrease in appetite, pinhead haemorrhages and fluid build up on the gum. If not treated the infection will rapidly spread and pus will be seen. If untreated can lead to osteomyelitis of the jawbone.	Clean mouth with povidine-iodine 2.5–5% solution applied daily to affected area. Bacteriology swab taken to determine pathogen. If severe the reptile will require an anaesthetic and area treated. Antibiotics may be given in severe cases.	Look at hygiene and husbandry. Environmental conditions. Overcrowding.
Necrotic dermatitis (scale rot)	Seen in snakes. Usually due to poor environmental conditions such as vivarium temperature too low, poor ventilation, too much moisture in the cage. Ectoparasites.	Small blisters usually appear on the ventral surface, which can become infected. If left can go necrotic.	Transfer reptile to a clean, dry vivarium and change substrate daily (newspaper ideal) with a relative humidity of 60–70%. If antibiotics needed then will have to be given via injection. **Wound will need to be cleaned at least once or twice a day using povidine-iodine or dermisol solution.** Wound must be kept as dry as possible.	If reptile very sick will require supportive therapy. Environment must be corrected before patient returns.
Burns	Unguarded heat source, hot rocks, heat pads.	Signs depend on severity of burn. Superficial – pain erythema, discoloration of scales or loss of scales, wrinkling of scales. Blisters and exudate. Deep burns would present as massive tissue damage (eschar) that may slough and require surgical debridement.	Treatment will depend on severity of the burn and general condition of the reptile. Bandaging may be necessary using dressings recommended for burns patients. Fluid therapy to replace lost body fluid and electrolytes. Antibiotics if infection or septicaemia present. Surgery to debride damaged tissue.	Healing by granulation can take a month to a year. Each time species sheds some improvement to wound should be seen. Scarring seen with loss of regular scale pattern. The area round scar may shed incompletely and may require soaking and manual removal. Ensure all heat sources are guarded and thermostatically controlled.
Fractures	Metabolic bone disease (pathological). Trauma (falling, poor handling, cruelty).	Usually closed: ● swelling ● deformity ● pain ● loss of use	Depends on type of fracture, complications and general health status of the reptile. Any metabolic disorders must be rectified immediately.	Bone healing seems to take longer in reptiles compared to mammals and birds: 6–18 months for traumatic fractures and 6–8 weeks for pathological

		• irregular movement • behavioural changes.	The same fixation techniques apply to reptiles as to mammals, and include: • immobilisation and splinting • internal fixation • external fixation and as a last resort amputation.	fractures when receiving corrective treatment to rectify hypocalcaemia.
Dystocia – snakes (egg binding)	Obstructive – fetal/maternal. Non-obstructive – poor husbandry, poor nutrition. Lack of physical activity due to captive environment.	Oviparous (egg laying) species: seen as a caudally located mass or able to palpate in thicker set species (large pythons). Viviparous (live bearing) snakes are more difficult as fetus malleable, which makes them difficult to locate. Prolonged straining or cloacal prolapse demonstrates unsuccessful parturition. Ultrasound can be useful in identifying presence of fetuses in viviparous snakes.	Intervention should be considered necessary 48 hours after the cessation of the incomplete parturition or oviposition (egg laying). Techniques include manual manipulation but this carries many risks and not generally advised. Hormonal stimulation using oxytocin or similar agents. Aspirate contents of egg, followed by an injection of oxytocin; snake can be left to pass the smaller egg naturally. Caution must be taken not to contaminate the coelomic cavity with egg yolk. Surgery: once snake anaesthetised gentle manual manipulation can be attempted. If this fails, a salpingotomy (making an incision into the oviduct) can be performed and eggs and fetus removed from the oviducts.	Oxytocin or related drugs must not be used if a snake has an obstructive dystocia.
Dystocia – lizards (egg binding)	Obstructive – fetal/maternal. Non-obstructive – poor husbandry, poor nutrition. Lack of physical activity due to captive environment. Lack of suitable nesting sites common in lizards.	Although anorexia is a common sign in the reproducing lizard, the lizard that is not eating and displaying lethargy, cachexia (loss of muscle and fat tissue from pelvic girdle, limbs and tail base) suggests further investigation.	Lizards do not tolerate prolonged periods of dystocia and it can cause death within several days. Prompt treatment following diagnosis is necessary with supportive treatment given prior to any surgical procedure. Oxytocin or similar drugs can be administered to help the passage of the eggs. Surgery to perform a salpingotomy or salpingectomy or ovario-salpingectomy.	Many lizards, including iguanas can produce a clutch of eggs without a male present. Good pre- and post-operative care is essential for the survival of lizards or snakes undergoing surgery.

(continued)

Table 3.4 *(continued)*

Common problem	Cause	Signs	Treatment	Other
Endoparasites	Mainly seen in wild caught or farmed species, but will affect any captive snake or lizard. Numerous and varied infestations although some are self limiting as will need an intermediate host to complete life cycle which captivity does not provide. But the following have been seen in snakes and lizards: • protozoans, flagellates • coccidia • flukes • cestodes • nematodes.	Some infestations go unnoticed until disease or loss of a reptile occurs. Signs: eggs or oocysts are seen in faecal smears. Reptile appears listless, failure to thrive, weight gain, dull, inappetant, weight loss. Visual signs of the parasite in adult form.	Anthelmintic drugs. Usually given orally once or twice a year. Good hygiene protocols and do not feed wild caught foods.	Suggested drugs: metronidazole for flagellates and febendazole (panacur) for nematodes.
Ectoparasites	Mainly seen in wild caught or farmed species, but will affect any captive snake and lizard. Ticks – *Ixodes* spp. Mites – *Ophionyssus* spp., *O. natricis* (mainly seen in snakes and some lizards). Both are parasitic and feed off animal's blood.	Ticks – relatively easy to spot, can blend in with scales, favour areas near recess of ear, skin folds of the vent (lizards), cavities such as the nostrils or labial pits in some snakes. Mites – smaller than the tick, hide under the scales. Colour: tan, reddish brown to black depending on engorgement. Common sites: between and under scales, especially around eyes, under chin, cloaca, axillae and inguinal regions. Other signs: snake rubbing against furnishings in cage, spending much time soaking in the water bowl. Mites may be noticed in the cage, floating in the water or crawling onto their skin. The mite causes the reptile to appear dull and lacklustre. In severe cases can become depressed, anorexic and very sick.	Ticks – manual removal. Mites – no treatment proven 100% safe for reptiles and keeper. *Isolate reptile until the vivarium is totally clean* (corners crevices, lips and furnishings). *Cover reptile in a thin layer of olive oil* (suffocates the mite). Caution: reptile becomes slippery and difficult to handle. *Bathe animal* in warm water for 30 mins, kills mites on the body but not the head. *Ivermectin* injection in small doses, topical use less effective. Spray vivarium with 1 ml propylene glycol/1 L distilled/deionised water, repeat weekly. *Frontline* (fipronil) topically on reptile and on the vivarium. Reptile weight of >500 g small bottle, six sprays per kg (concentrate on susceptible areas), <500 g dilute spray	Ticks – remove all mouthparts; any remaining parts can lead to abscess. Mites – hygiene is essential to prevent the spread (1 mite = 90–100 eggs). Dichlorvos (vapona) was off the market, but reportedly making a comeback, (changed ingredients?). Ivermectin and Frontline both alcohol based so inflammable. Frontline not licensed for reptiles. If treating eye carefully apply to scales around the eye with cotton bud. If spraying head place ophthalmic ointment on spectacle (snakes). Place reptile in a warm well-ventilated place to prevent chill from evaporation of alcohol. Consider reduced first close. Reported successful use on: Burmese, royal pythons, green iguanas and monitor lizards,

Condition	Aetiology	Clinical signs	Treatment	
			50:50 with alcohol. Apply by a cloth or dipping from an insulin syringe over animal's body (concentrate on susceptible areas). Post spraying: keep animal in well-ventilated cage for 2–3 h (fumes damaging to lungs), ensure reptile has access to a high humidity hide box in case of cutaneous water loss. Burn disposable or replaceable furnishings, spray rest and vivarium (cracks/crevices). Raise closed vivarium temperature (95–100°F, 3–4 h), desiccates nymphs, stimulates eggs to hatch. **Frequent obs (alcohol vapour = fire risk)**. Ventilate cage 3–4 h to ensure all traces of alcohol dispersed. Repeat every 3–4 weeks, 3–4 times to kill 2nd- and 3rd-generation mites.	but adverse effects have been reported, therefore, use with caution.
Thiamine (vitamin B_1) deficiency	Mainly seen in fish-eating snakes such as garter snakes, when fed thawed frozen fish. An enzyme called thiaminase present in raw fish destroys thiamine (vitamin B_1) leading to a deficiency disease.	Neurological signs such as incoordination, convulsions, loss of righting reflex.	Treatment is administration of vitamin B_1 by injection or stomach tube. Dietary correction is essential and all raw fish must be blanched/poached before feeding (ideally taking water temperature to 80°F for 5–10 minutes); this will kill the anti-vitamin thiaminase.	Fish-eating snakes should be encouraged to take other food stuffs such as pinkies, earthworms and commercially prepared diets such as 'garter grub'.
Respiratory disease	Bacterial invasion, viruses, fungi, poor husbandry, inadequate nutrition, poor ventilation, draughts. Low temperature, endoparasite. rhinitis (inflammation of the nasal cavity).	Dyspnoea, abnormal elevation of the head, open mouth breathing, wheezing, nasal discharge, problems during sloughing, debilitated. Severe cases cyanotic membranes.	Very sick animals will require hospitalisation and much supportive therapy, such as fluids and assistance with feeding. A bacteriology swab for culture and sensitivity will aid in identification of pathogen and necessary treatment. Antimicrobial therapy is recommended. Treatment for endoparasites and any other suspected cause is essential.	The patient should be maintained at the higher end of its POTZ; humidity needs to be maintained at the animal's normal range. Parenteral vitamin supplements (especially water soluble ones) have been shown to be beneficial in some cases. In severe cases prognosis is guarded and aggressive therapy recommended.

(continued)

Table 3.4 (continued)

Common problem	Cause	Signs	Treatment	Other
Tail autotomy (tail loss)	Occurs as a defence mechanism in many species of lizard, geckos, green iguana, water dragons. In many cases the tail will keep wriggling to maintain the predator's attention while 'lunch escapes'. In captive reptiles usually caused through rough handling, grasping the tail or stress.	Loss of tail and if occurs in the surgery due to poor handling a distressed owner and embarrassed staff.	The environment the reptile was living in will need to be evaluated and identified changes made. In time the tail will normally grow back, but never the same and generally less impressive. Daily bathing in povidone-iodine solution will prevent infection; continue until re-growth is established. If sutured will not re-grow.	
Dysecdysis (difficulty with sloughing) (Fig. 3.5)	Dysecdysis should be considered as a sign of a problem not the primary problem. Main causes can be attributed to poor environmental condition: • low temperature • low humidity • no water bowl or too small so prevents the snake from bathing • insufficient cage furnishings – logs, rocks for rubbing to initiate shedding • poor nutrition.	Retained flaky dry skin over body, limbs and digits, also spectacles (snakes) If not treated retained slough can cause infection or act as tourniquets around small limbs, tail tips and digits.	Skin will need to be hydrated: increase humidity in the vivarium and make sure snake has access to a large water bowl for soaking; snake can be placed in a bag (pillowcase or duvet works well) with wet towels so it can rub against the towels; the moisture should help to soften the skin allowing it to be shed. If pieces retained gentle manual removal. If the spectacle (eye caps) are retained in the snake then it is possible to leave the snake to see if they are removed during the next shed; if that fails then the spectacle needs to be softened using Hypromellose (false tears) and gentle manipulation with a cotton wool bud. Forceps or tweezers should not be used for fear of permanently damaging the delicate eye tissues. Before the patient is discharged the owners must be made aware of the need to improve environmental conditions.	This is a continual lifetime cycle. Snakes shed as one single piece, lizards shed in pieces with the exception of geckos. Frequency depends on age and health status and duration is 7–14 days (snakes). *Signs:* snakes Skin lacks lustre and shine. Eyes appear cloudy and skin dull. Snake will often refuse food. Generally quieter, hiding or sitting for long periods in the water bowl (best not to handle). Very vulnerable as vision impaired and may strike if handled. Dulling over is followed by 3–4-day period where skin and eyes appear clear. When ready to shed snake will rub its nose against rough objects to break skin and then slither out of the skin. The shed should be in one complete piece and be checked to see that spectacles and tail tip have been removed.

Information regarding treatment of mites gained from information supplied by the Reptile Trust and an extract by Ian Calvert MRCVS 'Suggested protocol for using Frontline in reptiles'.

2. haemorrhage is stemmed; bandages can be applied to hold fragments of shell in place or protect wounds from further damage
3. anorexic or dehydrated reptiles can be bathed in warm water; this may encourage them to drink and warm their bodies. Many reptiles absorb water through the cloaca.

Tip:

Dehydration in reptiles
Depending on the severity, the following signs can be seen:

- The reptile appears dull and listless
- The skin loses its elasticity and has a wrinkled appearance
- Some snakes have a single skin fold that runs the length of their body
- As dehydration progresses the eyes appear sunken and the reptile has a fixed expression
- Mucous membranes are dry and tongue appears 'sticky'
- The anorexic reptile appears thin with bones prominent and a gaunt sunken appearance.

---

4. Debilitated reptiles may put up little resistance to being stomach tubed either Hartmann's/lactated Ringer's or 0.18% sodium chloride in 4% dextrose, dose rate of 20–25 ml/kg/day, range 10–40 ml/kg/day, depending on chosen route.
5. If no other first-aid treatment can be offered the nurse must place the patient in a warm, dark cage and monitor frequently until further veterinary assistance can be sought.

The importance of keeping a sick or debilitated reptile at the higher end of its optimum temperature range can not be overemphasised as this aids:

- **immune response**
- **response to drug therapy**
- **general recovery.**

MONITORING THE REPTILE PATIENT (SNAKES AND LIZARDS)

As with any hospitalised patient routine checks should be made and information recorded on the health status of the patient and, in the reptile's case, environmental parameters. The reptile patient will not be as responsive to the nurse's TLC as will the dog or cat and it should be remembered that most reptiles find handling quite stressful. The frequency of checks will depend on the reasons why the lizard or snake has been hospitalised but morning and evening checks are recommended.

Morning

The following checks should be carried out in the morning:

- Locate patient and carry out necessary patient observations (refer to clinical history).
- Record temperature at both cool and hot end of the vivarium.
- Record humidity (if appropriate).
- Turn on lighting and basking lamp (if not regulated by a thermostat or timer).
- Check all thermostatic or heating equipment to make sure it is operating correctly, especially heat pads.
- Check cage for any abnormal discharges and remove faeces, urate and clean.
- Clean and replenish water bowl.
- Check for live food (crickets, locusts, etc.) still in cage; remove if necessary. A record should be made of food eaten compared to that offered.
- Spray the cage to provide humidity and check moss boxes and dampen if needed.
- If herbivorous lizard then supply fresh foods.
- **Before offering any live food or rodents allow reptile to reach its POTZ.**

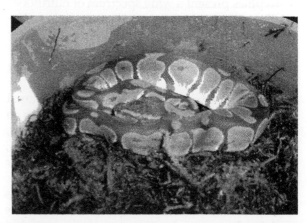

Fig. 3.5 Royal python shedding.

Late afternoon

The following checks should be done in the late afternoon:

- Carry out necessary patient observations.
- Record temperature at both cool and hot end of the vivarium.
- Record humidity (if appropriate).
- Turn off lighting and basking lamp (if not regulated by a thermostat or timer).
- Check all heating equipment to make sure it is operating correctly, especially heat pads.
- Check cage for any abnormal discharges and remove faeces, urate and clean.
- Record food eaten and remove any uneaten food, unless animal is nocturnal and prefers to take food items overnight.
- Check animal has access to water and humidity levels are correct for that species.
- Ensure cage is secured, ideally locked.

This list is only meant to provide the nurse with a guide to the checks that need to be carried out and will need to be adapted to suit the individual reptile's needs.

NUTRITION AND FEEDING

As mentioned earlier problems with poor husbandry and inadequate nutrition can be attributed to most cases that are presented for treatment at the veterinary practice.

Reptiles present a wide spectrum of nutritional challenges mainly because there is little information about their natural diet and we can only assume, rightly or wrongly, that what we offer the captive reptile goes some way to mimicking its natural diet.

The only way to understand what an animal naturally eats is either to study that species in the wild for years recording everything it eats, or to trap and euthanase a number of that species, dissect them, and then examine and record their stomach contents.

Some work has been carried out to progress this issue and information is available for some species. However, for the nurse trying to select

suitable foods for the hospitalised patient he or she will have to research the animal's natural history and select foods that are as naturalistic as possible to the reptile's preferred diet.

FEEDING SNAKES

Snakes are carnivores and should be offered a whole prey item. See Table 3.5 for food types offered to snakes and nutritional value.

Guidelines for feeding snakes

Always select a food item that is as near to the animal's wild diet as possible, i.e. offer brown mice rather than white mice to potential wild caught species. Make sure to select prey items that the snake can swallow.

If offering frozen foods defrost in the refrigerator using separate containers. When the food is **thoroughly** thawed warm it through by sealing the food item in a plastic bag and then immersing the bag into warm water (this will ensure the food is heated to the proper temperature).

Always offer the dead prey head first using feeding tongs (Figs 3.6 & 3.7) as this will keep the nurse's smell off the food and will help to prevent the feeder being bitten. It may be necessary to slightly wriggle the food item in front of the snake to stimulate the strike response (this method is especially helpfully with reluctant feeders or arboreal species).

To prevent accidental cannibalism NEVER feed snakes together. They may try to consume the same prey item. Also, to prevent regurgitation once the snake has accepted its prey item it should be left alone and not handled for 24–48 hours.

Snakes are opportunist feeders and DO NOT require feeding EVERY day and may have periods of FASTING. Frequency of feeding will depend on the age of the snake and species. As a guide feed as much as the snake will consume in one meal then wait until the meal has been digested and faeces passed.

There is no need to feed live vertebrate prey in the UK, as most captive snakes will readily eat dead prey. It is probable that anyone found

Table 3.5 Nutritional value of some commonly offered foodstuffs

Food item	Water (%)	Energy (kcal/g) As fed basis	DM	% kcal Protein	Fat	Carb	mg/kcal Calcium	Phosphorus
Representative energy and nutrient content of invertebrate food items								
House cricket	68	1.0	3.1	40	53	6	0.3	2.7
Commercial cricket	62	1.9	4.8	50	44	6	0.2	2.6
Locusts	71	1.1	3.8	58	30	12	NA	NA
Mealworm larvae	58	2.1	5.0	37	60	3	0.1	1.2
Waxworm larvae	63	5.1	2.7	27	73	0	0.1	0.9
Representative energy and nutrient content of vertebrate food items								
Adult mouse (27 g)	65	1.7	4.8	48	47	5	5.0	3.6
Mouse pup (1.5 g)	81	0.8	4.2	57	40	3	3.8	3.7
Rat pup (4 g)	71	1.7	5.9	29	69	2	2.4	2.2
Adult rat (330 g)	66	1.6	4.7	55	43	2	4.4	3.2
Day-old chick (40 g)	73	1.3	4.8	52	44	4	2.7	2.0
Adult chicken (380 g)	66	1.6	4.7	47	49	4	4.0	2.9

NA = not available.
Waxworms are very high in fat and very palatable to many insectivorous species; therefore, these should not be fed exclusively, but as a part of a varied diet. Many lizards can become addicted to these.
Day-old chicks have very little nutritional value especially to snakes.
Feed mice pups (pinkies) that have had their first feed as this will increase their nutritional value especially in terms of calcium and vitamin A content.

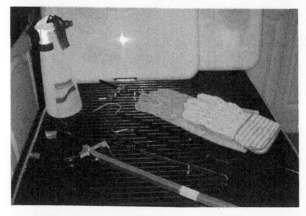

Fig. 3.6 Handling equipment.

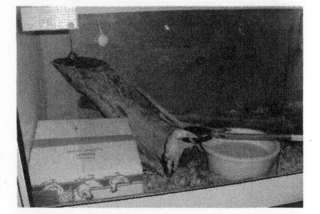

Fig. 3.7 Using feeding tongs.

feeding live vertebrates could be prosecuted under the 1911 Protection of Animals Act.

When feeding raw fish to snakes such as garter snakes the fish must be blanched in hot water for approximately 10 minutes to destroy the anti-vitamin (thiaminase). Thiaminase will destroy the B vitamin thiamine and cause convulsions and loss of righting reflex.

When NOT too feed a snake

A snake should never be fed at the following times:

1. prior to an anaesthetic
2. when it is shedding
3. when it is in brumation (hibernation) or getting ready for brumation.

FEEDING LIZARDS

Lizards present more of a challenge when trying to meet their dietary demands. Lizards' feeding habits can be classified accordingly:

- **Carnivores** – eat whole prey items such as rodents, birds, amphibians and other small lizards.
- **Insectivores** – eat a range of invertebrates such as crickets, locusts, mealworms and waxworms.
- **Herbivores** – eat a range of plant, fruit and vegetable matter.

- **Omnivores** – eat a mixture of both vegetation and animal matter.

When presented with a lizard for hospitalisation the nurse will have to establish the feeding preference of that species.

Guidelines when feeding lizards

Establish whether carnivore, omnivore, etc.

Herbivores

These include iguanas (*Iguana iguana*), chuckawallas (*Sauromalus obesus*), and uromastixs (*Uromastyx acanthinurus*).

If the lizard is a herbivore offer a variety of fresh leafy vegetables, fruits, etc. to meet the lizard's needs (see Table 3.6 for a range of plant materials and nutrition information). A green iguana up to 2 years of age needs to be offered a diet consisting of 80% green leafy matter and 20%

Table 3.6 Calcium:phosphorus ratio in some of the more commonly used vegetables and fruits

Food item	Calcium:phosphorus ratio	Food item	Calcium:phosphorus ratio
Broccoli leaves	3:9	Cucumber	1:1.1
Cauliflower florets	0:6	Lettuce, romaine	0:8
Celery stalk[1]	1:4	Lettuce, iceberg[3]	0:9
Spinach raw[1]	2:0	Tomatoes	0:3
Alfalfa sprouts	0:5	Watercress	4.3:1
Broccoli stems/florets, chopped	0:7	Apples	0.7:1
Cabbage[1,2]	2:0	Bananas	0:3
Chinese cabbage (Pak choi)	2:8	Grapes	0:7
Red cabbage	1:2	Melon (flesh)	0.6:0.9
Carrots, shredded	0:6	Strawberries	0:7
Parsley, chopped	3:3	Pears	1:0
Green peppers	0:2	Peaches	0:4

[1] Oxalates occur in spinach, cabbage, celery, rhubarb, peas, beet, greens. They bind to calcium and trace minerals preventing their absorption from the gut. Although these are high in calcium they should only be offered infrequently and in smaller amounts (once a fortnight).
[2] Cabbage, cauliflower, bok choi, kale should be fed in small amounts (once a month) as they contain goitrogens that block the production of thyroxine and utilisation of iodine, causing hypothyroidism and goitre.
[3] Lettuce is considered not an ideal food item for many reptiles, especially tortoises and iguanas, because of its poor nutritional value, but it is no worse or better than many vegetables and better than many fruits. The mixed bag lettuces as sold ready prepared in supermarkets are probably the best choice and should be part of a varied diet.

fruits and root vegetables, compared to a green iguana of over 2 years of age, which should be provided with a diet consisting of 95% green leafy matter and 5% fruits and roots.

Always ensure all foods offered are fresh, free from pesticides and thoroughly washed. If food is taken out of the fridge allow it to reach room temperature before offering it to the lizard.

Apply necessary supplements onto food; there is a range of calcium supplements on the market (Fig. 3.8). Be careful when supplementing with preparation that contains added vitamin D_3 vitamins and minerals, as it is possible to overdose and cause metabolic bone problems and calcification of soft tissues. The frequency of supplementation depends on the frequency of feeding, but as a general rule calcium carbonate powder can be added to each meal, whereas those that contain vitamin D_3 and other supplements should be offered once/twice a week.

> **Tip:** Supplementation of vitamin D_3 should not be used to overcome inadequate provision of UVB lighting. Therefore, if UVB lighting is provided, correctly positioned and replaced at appropriate times, vitamin D_3 synthesis should be adequate and oversupplementation of D_3 can harm the lizard.

All food offered should be of a size that the animal can easily ingest.

Care should be given not to offer food that can be 'addictive' and to encourage selective feeding such as banana.

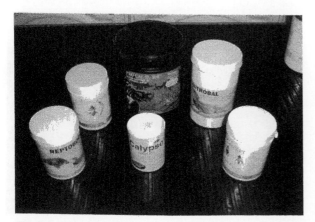

Fig. 3.8 Calcium/multivitamin supplements.

Insectivores

These include leopard geckos (*Eublepharus macularius*) and water dragons (*Physignathus cocincinus*) and they eat a range of live invertebrate foods.

When selecting foods make sure they are of appropriate size for the lizard to catch and consume.

If newly purchased live foods are to be offered, e.g. crickets and locusts, the food should be placed in a pen-pal and offered foods such as cereals, fruit, vegetables and water (to prevent insects drowning, soak cotton wool in water and place in a small dish). Leave the insects for 24–48 hours before offering them to the lizard, as this will allow them to re-hydrate and be more nutritious.

It is important to dust live food with a calcium or vitamin and mineral supplement (Fig. 3.8).

Calcium/phosphorus ratio. Many invertebrate food items offered have an inverse calcium/phosphorus ratio. Ideally, calcium should be offered in the diet at **a higher ratio of calcium to phosphorus**; if not then calcium will be removed from the animal's own stores causing metabolic bone disease, and resulting in animals producing poorly calcified eggs and dystocia. The rules for frequency of supplementation are as for herbivore nutrition.

- Method used for dusting invertebrates: live food is placed in a pot and supplement added; the pot is agitated to cover the live food in supplement powder. The live food can then be placed in the vivarium.
- It is acknowledged that one of the problems associated with dusting live prey is that much of the supplement 'falls off' the prey before it is consumed and it is difficult to monitor exactly how much of the supplement the lizard ingests. A tip is to chill the live food in a refrigerator for a few minutes, this will slow the insect down and give the reptile an opportunity to catch the prey plus supplement!
- Feed as many insects as the lizard will eat at once, do not add too many crickets, etc. to the vivarium as the live food could actually frighten the lizard and prevent it from eating.

• Large locusts have sharp barbs on the hind legs that could get lodged in the lizard's mouth or oesophagus. Some advocate removal before feeding them.

Carnivores

These include monitors (*Varanus* spp.) and tegus (*Tupinambis teguixin*).

They will eat a range of prey items ranging from rodents to other small lizards (see Table 3.5). The prey should be offered whole; as such the need to supplement is reduced, unless it is necessary because of illness. If frozen foods are to be offered, they must be prepared and offered as suggested under snake nutrition.

Caution must be taken when offering food to large lizards, especially the monitor family. To prevent injury, tongs or graspers must be used (see Figs 3.6 & 3.7).

Frequency of feeding will depend on the species of lizard, age and size. As a guide, smaller or growing lizards should be fed daily, but mature, larger species (Fig. 3.9) should only be fed two to three times a week.

Omnivores

These include bearded dragons (*Pogona vitticeps*), blue-tongued skinks (*Tiliqua gigas*) and plated lizards (*Gerrhosaurus* spp.).

This group of lizards will eat a variety of animal and plant matter so the guidelines given under the previous sections should be applied when dealing with such a species.

Water

As with our companion animals snakes and lizards require free access to water. When providing water for snakes, the water bowl must be large enough to allow the snake to submerge itself in the water. This also helps when the snake is shedding.

Tropical or arboreal snakes, such as emerald tree boas (*Corallus caninus*) or green tree pythons (*Chondrophython viridis*) require daily misting with lukewarm water. The spray should be on fine mist and directed toward the species' head; this will allow them to drink the water as it beads off or as it collects in their tight coils. Their entire body should be sprayed daily to keep them from becoming too dry as this results in dysecdysis (difficulty shedding).

Non-tropical arboreal species and terrestrial species should only be misted if they are getting ready to shed.

Some lizards such as arboreal species, for example anoles, day geckos and some chameleons, will not drink water from a bowl, but prefer to take their water in the form of droplets off a leaf. This can be achieved by misting the foliage in the vivarium using a hand-held spray, setting up an elaborate misting system, or adapting a drip system so that droplets fall on a leaf or branch. To prevent substrate from becoming saturated a

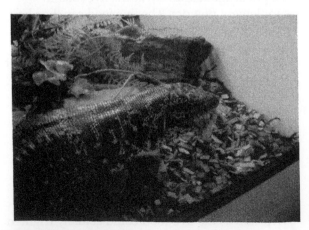

Fig. 3.9 Large lizard eating.

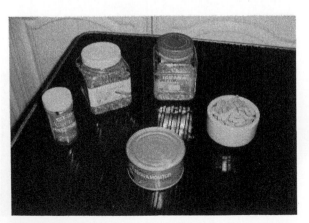

Fig. 3.10 A selection of proprietary diets.

receptacle will have to be placed under the drip tube to collect excess water.

Most chameleons need to be 'rained on' daily and some species need to feel the dripping water before they will attempt to drink. Day geckos will drink from a shallow bowl, but individuals will require misting once or twice a day.

Water containers should be cleaned and water replenished daily or sooner if contaminated with faeces and urate.

No water bowl should be so deep that the species is unable to climb out. Small pieces of slate can be angled in the bowl to allow small lizards a way in and out of the water. In the same way, if insects are being fed, small stones should be placed in the bottom of the bowl to prevent them from drowning and contaminating the water.

Box 3.3 General rules for feeding lizards and snakes

1. 'Variety is the spice' of life and everything should be done to offer the reptile a varied and balanced diet; although this is limited for the carnivore, the common boa (boa constrictor) will appreciate a gerbil now and again.
2. Always feed dead vertebrates; apart from the humane aspect, live rodents could actually attack the snake or lizard, and inflict nasty wounds as well as cause much stress to the cage occupant.
3. The quality of vertebrate and invertebrate prey will depend on its age, environment kept in, food fed and health status.
4. It is not acceptable to use wild rodents as prey items as they can carry disease and parasites. If collecting invertebrates then make sure they are non-toxic and free from pesticides.
5. There are a variety of commercially prepared diets on the market and these are fine to use as part, but should not make up the main part of the diet (Fig. 3.10).
6. Non-reptilian foods generally are not advised because they have been manufactured for animals with different nutritional needs, metabolic processes and stress levels.
7. However excellent the diet provided for the reptile is, if the environmental conditions are incorrect and optimum lighting, humidity and temperature are not available the lizard or snake will not be able to reach its POTZ and its metabolic processes will be severely compromised resulting in non-digestion of food or anorexia. Any undigested food in the gut will become a source of nutrition for gut bacteria and a massive bacterial overgrowth, with potentially fatal consequences.

NUTRITIONAL PROBLEMS IN SNAKES AND LIZARDS

The provision of a correctly balanced diet is as important as the providing the reptile with the optimum living environment. If one or both are neglected then severe problems can be seen.

One consequence of the inadequate provision of diet and environment is anorexia. Anorexia should be **seen as a sign rather than a disease** and it is, therefore, essential to correct the underlying problem as well as managing the anorexia.

Causes of anorexia (mainly seen in snakes but can apply to lizards):

1. Animal kept in an unsuitable environment
   - Temperature too high or too low.
   - Incorrect humidity.
   - Incorrect photoperiod (if a light is left on for 24 hours this will cause much stress).
   - Lack of suitable hides so reptile feels very vulnerable and stressed.
   - Cage size too large or inappropriate dimensions, e.g. arboreal snakes not given the opportunity to climb.
   - Glass vivariums can make the occupant feel exposed so cover three sides and place a towel over front when feeding.
   - Tank positioned in a very public place where reptile is exposed to much 'through traffic'.
2. Unsuitable foods being offered
   - Some snakes have very specialist feeding requirements and might refuse to eat the usually offered rodent preferring a bird or frog.
   - Prey offered is of the wrong size.
   - Prey is the wrong colour, i.e. wild caught snakes will have never seen a white mouse before and will not identify it as a food item.
   - Human scent on prey.
   - Prey offered at the wrong time of day; – a nocturnal animal will refuse to eat a rodent offered during the day.
   - Some require more stimulation before feeding, e.g. emerald tree boas (*Corallus caninus*) and green tree pythons (*Chondrophython viridis*) sometimes like to

be 'taunted' with the prey before feeding will take place (sometimes this can take 30 minutes or more).

- The position of feeding is incorrect – arboreal species will expect to catch their prey either as it flies past or climbing up the branch so placing foods on the ground will do little to stimulate the snake to strike.
- Food offered is at incorrect temperature – try offering food at room temperature.

3. The reptile
   - A wild caught species will have undergone a stressful experience, will need time to settle into its new surroundings and will not be used to eating killed prey (refer to foods offered). 'Maladaptation syndrome' has been used to describe those wild caught animals that although they appear healthy are so stressed that they fail to eat.
   - Some species are known problem feeders, such as royal pythons (*Python regius*) and some of the tree pythons and boas. Also hatchling (newly born) snakes may refuse to eat.
   - The reptile going into **brumation** or seasonal hibernation will stop eating during this period.
   - A reproducing female – during gestation a female snake may stop eating.
   - Also those pythons that incubate their own eggs, such as the Burmese, will refuse food.
   - An animal that is bullied or in a set hierarchy may be prevented from eating (seen in some lizards).

4. Diseases or mismanagement including:
   - Stomatitis
   - Respiratory disease
   - Parasites
   - Blockage in the intestines due to ingested substrate or silk plants
   - Metabolic bone disease
   - Trauma or stress
   - Overhandling.

Treatment

To be able to commence treatment it will be necessary to identify and correct the reason why the reptile is not eating. This is where a thorough case history is essential and the owners of the reptile need to describe the animal's enclosure, feeding and husbandry routine. The nurse or veterinary surgeon will have to gain an understanding of the animal's natural history such as what it would eat in the wild, and when and where it would eat.

Sometimes once modifications to how the animal is fed and kept are carried out, the lizard or snake will resume feeding. Appetite stimulants can be used such as vitamin B complex.

If anorexia is the result of a disease then this will have to be treated along with the anorexia. Diagnostic testing such as blood tests and faecal checks should be carried out.

Options

If after general manipulation of the lizard's or snake's diet the animal does not resume feeding the following can be carried out.

Non-invasive techniques (snake)

Remove water bowl from cage for 48 hours, then place rodent (food item) in water and stroke prey across snake's face – the snake should strike and consume prey.

> **Tip:** Offer freshly killed rodents; these will be offered at blood temperature as well as having enhanced smell (male mice smell more than females, and there are products on the market that are made to enhance the smell of rodents!).
> Non-rodent eating snakes can be fooled into eating rodents by smearing the mucus from a frog or gaining the scent from preferred prey item.
> The smell of blood can also stimulate the reptile to eat: in hatchlings, crushing the skulls of newborn mice (pinkies) will stimulate a young snake to eat by increasing the odour.

Invasive techniques

If the cause for the anorexia cannot be established or the patient is too weak to eat on its own then force-feeding may be attempted.

This ranges from placing the prey item in the snake's or lizard's mouth to actually placing a tube or manipulating the prey item down the animal's oesophagus. Only an experienced practitioner should attempt force-feeding.

Steps (for a snake – can be adapted for lizards). Ensure the snake is hydrated and replacement fluids and electrolytes given. Do not overfeed the anorexic patient; as a guide and as suggested by Mader (1997), the non-critical patient should receive 75–100% of their nutritional requirements over the first 24–48 hours, while critical patients should receive 40–75% of their nutritional requirements over the first 24–48 hours. This will help prevent metabolic and digestive imbalances.

Force-feeding whole prey. The whole prey can be offered but this is very stressful to the snake and it has been suggested that mild sedation should be considered.

A small prey item needs to be thawed, any sharp claws or beaks removed and lubricated (in liquid paraffin or vegetable oil); then with the snake restrained, mouth opened and holding the prey with long forceps insert nose first into the mouth of the patient and gently down the oesophagus. The food can be gently massaged down the oesophagus to the level of the stomach (one-fifth to one-third of the way down the body).

Note that some individuals may find this process so stressful that it negates any benefits. In this case, alternative methods should be considered.

There is a chance that the snake will regurgitate. Once feeding is complete the snake needs to be placed in a warm dark cage and left to rest. Subsequent feedings should not be attempted until the undigested remains of the last meal have been passed.

Tube feeding. This involves using specially formulated liquid diets (enteral) such as **Critical Care** and **Liquivite** (Fig. 3.11) or a liquidised rodent.

Select suitable tubing (urinary catheter or drip tube); these can be lubricated and passed into the distal oesophagus or stomach. When in place the fluid diet can be passed. The patient should be cared for as suggested under feeding whole prey.

It may take several attempts before the snake resumes independent feeding if at all.

METABOLIC BONE DISEASE

Prolonged malnutrition due to a lack of dietary calcium and poor environmental conditions causes metabolic bone disease (MBD).

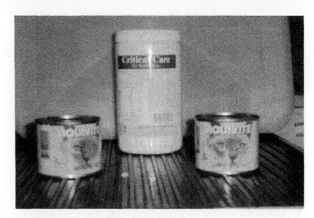

Fig. 3.11 Formulated liquid diets.

It is a condition mainly associated with lizards especially the green iguana (*Iguana iguana*).

Cause

Causes include:

- dietary deficiency of calcium or vitamin D_3
- inverse ratio of calcium to phosphorus
- no or poor exposure to UVB light
- organ dysfunction such as kidneys and liver that will inhibit synthesis and utilisation of vitamin D_3.

History

A lizard presenting with this disease will have a history of malnutrition; for example, the carnivorous lizard being offered muscle meats rather than the whole prey (muscle meat is high in phosphorus and low in calcium), the insectivorous lizard being fed insects that are mainly high in protein and low in calcium (see Table 3.5) or live food not properly supplemented, lizards not offered any alternative food items such as whole fish or pinkies, or herbivores that are offered foodstuffs generally lacking in calcium with little or no calcium supplementation (see Table 3.6).

A lizard may exhibit signs because of inadequate exposure to UVB light and consequent inability to synthesise vitamin D_3 (see Box 3.1).

General signs

The general signs include:

- Osteoporosis (loss of bone mass)
- Osteomalacia (failure of bone calcification in adult)
- Fibrous osteodystrophy (excessive bone re-absorption and secondary fibrosis)
- Rickets.

Young animals can come to the surgery presenting some or all of the following clinical signs:

- Lizard unable to raise body off the ground, severe cases unable to walk
- Pliable mandible and maxilla
- Malformed skull – giving lizard juvenile appearance (especially in green iguanas)
- Lameness or reluctance to move resulting from fractures. Fracture sites are commonly proximal to mid-shaft femur, mid-shaft humerus, distal radius and ulna
- Fibrous osteodystrophy seen in long bones or jaw.

More uncommonly seen signs include:

- Kyphosis (posterior curvature of the spine, humped back)
- Lordosis (abnormal curvature of the lumbar spine)
- Scoliosis (lateral deviation of the spine).

These can cause rear limb paresis (but this generally improves with treatment).

Less specific signs include:

- Poor growth rate in young lizards
- Loss of appetite
- Weight loss
- Lethargy
- Depression
- Animal wanting to eat but can't; this is due to demineralisation of bone tissue in the jaw.

Diagnosis by radiographs

The signs on radiograph would include:

- Bone density is decreased
- Poor contrast between bone and soft tissues

- Fibrous osteodystrophy causes uneven cortical widening
- Transverse folding fractures of long bones
- Compression fractures in the vertebrae
- Ends of long bones radiolucent.

Blood tests

Blood tests will show low calcium levels.

Treatment and management

The dietary and husbandry problems must be corrected.

It must be remembered that care needs to be taken when handling these creatures, as bones are very brittle and prone to fractures. Keeping this in mind, the cage should be sparsely furnished so the animal cannot climb or fall and fracture limbs.

If the patient is still eating, the correct diet and UVB provision should be arranged in addition to oral supplements of calcium in the form of calcium glubionate liquid (1 ml/kg) orally every 12 hours. Continue the oral calcium until the reptile is gaining weight and eating supplement on food (can take 1–3 months). Unless a carnivorous species is being treated and receiving whole prey, supplementation of calcium carbonate (powder) on food must continue.

For very debilitated patients or those with hypocalcaemia and displaying nervous signs (tremors, convulsions), injection of 10% calcium borogluconate 100 ml/kg should be given intramuscularly or ICe (see Table 3.7) every 6 hours or as needed to stop muscle tremors. Once the tremors have stopped, move onto oral liquid calcium as above (Mader 1996, Ch. 46).

Prognosis

If caught in early stages prognosis is very good, as long as the diet is maintained and owners are fully committed to caring for the lizard.

In more severe cases some permanent disfigurement will be seen, especially around the mandibles.

It should be noted that, as it took months to develop this disease it will take months to rectify the deficiency.

Table 3.7 Drug administration via parenteral routes

Route	Species	Sites	Uses
Intramuscular (IM)	Snake	Intercostal muscles of the body	Injectable anaesthetics, agents, premedications, antibiotics, anti-inflammatory drugs Ecbolics
	Lizard	Foreleg Between shoulders Pectoral muscle mass	As above
	Chelonia	Pectoral muscle mass Lateral side of the forelimb nearest the neck	As above
Intravenous (IV)	Snake	Ventral tail vein Palatine vein (in mouth) Cardiocentesis	Blood samples Anaesthetics Fluid therapy
	Lizard	Ventral tail vein Cephalic Toe nail clipping	As above
	Chelonia	Jugular vein (right hand side) Cardiocentesis, brachial vein, ventral coccygeal vein, orbital sinus and toe nail clipping	As above
Subcutaneous (SC)	Snake	Loose skin over ribs	Limited to small amounts of medicants
	Lizard	Loose skin over ribs	Lizards with tough plated scales quite difficult; also presence of osteoderms (see Table 3.1)
	Chelonia	Upper aspects of the hindlimb	Very limited, only small amounts
Intraosseous (IO) (into the bone)	Snake	Not used	
	Lizard	Shaft of femur	Fluid therapy Anaesthetics
		Humerus Tibia crest	Does not work well in active lizards Needle inserted into medullary cavity
	Chelonia	Cancellous bone bridge between the carapace and the plastron	Fluid therapy
Intracoelomic (ICe)	Snake	Lower region of the abdomen but cranial to the cloaca so avoiding the lungs	Large volumes of fluids Medications
	Lizard	Right lower region of the abdomen at a level even with the cranial surface of the rear leg	Large volumes of fluids Medications
	Chelonia	Near skin attachment to the shell just cranial to the rear leg	Large volumes of warmed fluids Medications

From Mader (1996), Chs 24, 28.

PRE-, INTRA- AND POST-OPERATIVE CARE

The reptile patient can pose a significant challenge to veterinary staff when requiring sedation or a general anaesthetic. Prior to selecting a suitable anaesthetic or premedication drug the varying biology and adaptations of many lizards and snakes have to be taken into consideration. There are various reasons why a chemical anaesthetic or premedication may be administered to a snake or lizard:

- For restraint especially when having to examine very large or aggressive species.
- To perform surgical procedures
- To carry out diagnostic sampling procedures.

When assisting or caring for the lizard or snake that is to receive a premedication or anaesthetic, some consideration should be made in respect of the reptile's biology and how this may alter the effects of the drug and dose given.

There are a number of anatomical points to remember (see also Table 3.1), for example, that the lungs of reptiles are much simpler in structure to those seen in mammals. They have a larger tidal volume, but smaller surface area. In many species of snake the left lung is absent or vestigial, the exception being boas and pythons, which have a fully developed right lung and smaller left lung. The lungs in reptiles are very fragile and care must be taken NOT to overinflate and rupture the lungs during positive pressure ventilation.

The larynx is generally located rostrally in the mouth at the base of the tongue making it easy to identify and intubate.

Reptiles do not have a diaphragm; this means that pressure changes and movement of air in and out of the lungs is produced by:

1. using intercostal muscles to generate a negative internal pressure.
2. contraction of smooth muscle in the wall of the lungs which alters the volume of the lung and causes air movement.

The above points are very important when monitoring anaesthetic and as skeletal muscle function is lost when surgical plane of anaesthesia is reached this will necessitate the need to carry out assisted ventilation. Also if the patient is positioned in dorsal recumbencey pressure from the internal organs on the lungs will reduce tidal volume and assisted ventilation may be necessary.

PRE-ANAESTHETIC PREPARATION AND PROCEDURES

1. It is recommended that the reptile patient be fasted for 24–72 hours prior to surgery. This is not through concerns of aspiration (the glottis remaining closed), but to reduce pressure from the gastrointestinal tract, which may affect the tidal volume and necessitate assisted ventilation.
2. A thorough physical examination including weight of patient and biochemistry will determine if the snake or lizard is a suitable candidate for the elected procedure.
3. To ensure the patient is hydrated prior to, during and after surgery fluid therapy should be considered (see p. 59, common first-aid emergencies, point 4) at a preferred rate of 10–40 ml/kg/day or for severely shocked patients or undergoing surgery 5 ml/kg/hour for 1–2 hours (Mader 1996). Routes can be intravenously (IV), intracoelomically (ICe) or subcutaneously (SC) (see Table 3.7). The use of infusion pumps, electrical or spring action, are very good for delivering small volumes of fluid at an accurate rate.
4. To prevent hypothermia and to ensure body systems continue to function correctly supplementary heat must be provided.
The operating theatre should be maintained at an ambient temperature of 21°C, humidity 51% and op-site prepared using a solution of either chlorhexidine or povidone-iodine diluted in warm water. Surgical spirit should be avoided as this evaporates and causes heat loss. A toothbrush can be used to pre-prep scales. Plastic disposable drapes provide good visibility of the patient and prevent bacterial 'strike through' during surgery.
5. The patient's POTZ must be maintained thoughout the procedure as a full and rapid recovery may depend on this.

Premedication

A variety of drugs are available to provide chemical restraint or sedation, but many have limited use in reptiles and benefits are not widely acknowledged.

INDUCTION
Injectable agents

The main concern when using injectable anaesthetics is their unpredictable effect on a metabolism that is very slow, resulting in some patients taking hours or days to fully recover from the anaesthetic. If injectables are used then one of the preferred routes is the IV or intraosseous (see Table 3.7).

One of the most widely used and supported injectable anaesthetics is **propofal** (Rapinovet™

Schering-Plough); this can be administered at a rate of 10/14 mg/kg IV or intraosseously.

Inhalation agents

These have several advantages over injectable forms of anaesthesia especially when the patient is intubated and connected to a calibrated vaporiser and anaesthetic circuit.

For induction of anaesthesia an Ayres T-piece and facemask can be used or the patient can be placed in an anaesthetic chamber. Problems can arise if the species holds its breath or struggles when the face mask is applied making induction very difficult and prolonged.

Isoflurane (Isoflo: Schering-Plough) seems to be the inhalation agent of choice as it provides quick and smooth induction, good depth of anaesthesia and rapid recovery especially when compared to injectables and other inhalation agents available. It is also licensed for use in reptiles.

Once the patient is anaesthetised it should be intubated and an endotrachael tube secured and maintained on oxygen and inhalant agent (2–4% isoflurane being used as a suggested rate).

The benefits of maintaining the lizard or snake on an inhalant agent are as follows:

- The depth of anaesthesia can be controlled.
- Supplementary oxygen is being supplied and if necessary allowing for positive pressure ventilation.
- Recovery once anaesthetic gas flow is terminated is more rapid compared to injectable agents.

Monitoring the anaesthetised patient

Like any mammal the reptilian patient must be closely monitored and findings recorded throughout the surgical procedure and period of anaesthesia.

Suggested routine checks include:

- The temperature of the lizard or snake must be maintained; a low wattage heat mat or waterbed to maintain a core preferred body temperature is recommended.

- Taking the cloacal temperature of a patient using a fine tipped rectal thermometer.
- Observation of certain parameters can be used to check the depth and plane of anaesthesia and condition of the patient.

Surgical plane of anaesthesia has been achieved when:

1. Ribs fail to elevate as a finger is moved down the patient's back.
2. In snakes, the tail fails to move when the cloaca is stimulated.
3. Lizards lack the pedal reflex when the foot is squeezed.
4. In lizards, the corneal reflex should be present, if not the patient is excessively deep.
5. In snakes, the tongue withdrawal reflex should be present, if not then the patient is too deep.
6. At a surgical plane many patients will lose the ability to ventilate spontaneously so positive pressure ventilation has to be undertaken.

Useful equipment in monitoring the anaesthetised patient

Electrocardiograph (ECG) can be used to monitor the heart's electroconductivity but the QRS pattern is somewhat different to that seen in mammals. The heart rate should remain steady throughout the procedure.

Pulse oximeter (cloacal or oesophageal), which measures the pulse and arterial oxygen saturation, is also proving useful in veterinary practice and can be adapted for reptiles.

The mucous membrane colour can be observed by looking at the cloacal tissue at the vent.

> **Tip:** As an average, lizards and snakes have a heart rate of 40 beats per minute and a respiratory rate of four breaths per minute or less. Therefore, intermittent positive pressure ventilation is essential in such patients and should be carried out at a rate of two to four breaths per minute. This will ensure the patient is well oxygenated and remains anaesthetised.

GENERAL SURGICAL NURSING AND POST-OPERATIVE CARE AND NURSING

The general techniques applied when nursing surgical feline and canine patients can be used for reptiles:

• Warmed pre-operative fluids are important, especially for very sick or dehydrated patients.
• Any intra-operative fluids must be warmed to prevent hypothermia.
• Preparation and surgical time must be kept to a minimum to reduce period of anaesthesia.
• All surgical procedures much be performed using an aseptic technique.
• Sterile waterproof plastic drapes are a good alternative to cloth as they can be cut to size, fenestrated and, if moulded round the patient, allow observations of respiration, etc. to be carried out. They also prevent the patient from getting wet.
• Blood loss should be kept to a minimum using diathermy, radiosurgery or hemoclips.
• Pre- and post-operative analgesia can be administered; opiates seem to have little beneficial effect on the reptile patient compared to non-steroidal anti-inflammatory drugs that seem to provide the most appropriate level of analgesia.
• Antibiotics can be given pre- and post-operatively; choice will depend on the individual and condition treated.
• Recovery should be in a quiet environment with temperature and humidity set at the higher end of the snake's or lizard's POTZ. Care must be taken NOT to overheat the patient as this will raise its metabolic rate and increase its demand for oxygen.
• Observations and records should continue especially if fluid therapy, drains or feeding tubes have been employed.

Summary

To ensure proper metabolic function the patient should be maintained within its optimum temperature range. During anaesthesia the patient should be intubated and assisted ventilation performed. The patient's depth of anaesthesia and vital signs must be carefully monitored and recorded throughout the surgical procedure.

HANDLING AND RESTRAINT OF THE REPTILE PATIENT (SNAKES AND LIZARDS)

The methods are shown in detail in Box 3.4.

SPECIFIC DISEASES OF SNAKES AND LIZARDS

Table 3.4 sets out some of the more commonly encountered problems, their cause, clinical signs and suggested treatments. Many of the conditions described have poor husbandry as a root cause so when any reptile is being admitted a full and accurate case history must be obtained. Candid questioning must be carried out to establish how the vivarium is set up, environmental conditions, monitored equipment used and provision of UVB in diurnal lizards.

It must also be highlighted that a snake or a lizard may have been ill for some time before presenting noticeable clinical signs, and that how reptiles demonstrate pain and discomfort is not fully understood.

CASE HISTORY 1

Patient

Female green iguana (*Iguana iguana*) named Brontie, approximately 4 years of age (rescue animal so exact age not known).

Presenting signs

Decline in appetite over past 4 weeks and now anorexic, restless, weight loss over pelvis with some abdominal distension.

Examination

Gentle palpation revealed rounded masses in the dorsal abdomen.

Radiograph identified the presence of unshelled ova (eggs) within the ovaries, confirming **pre-ovulatory ova stasis** (more details see common problems Table 3.4).

Box 3.4 Basic restraint and handling methods

Equipment (see Fig. 3.6)
Gauntlets
Gardening gloves
Thick towel
Snake hook, various sizes
Snake stick
Cat grasper/dog catcher
Pillowcases
Duvet covers
Perspex tube

Transportation

Snake and lizards are best transported in a tied pillowcase or duvet cover depending on size of reptile. This method makes the snake or lizard feel secure and safe.

Another transportation method is a ventilated polystyrene box. The reptile can be placed in the box within the pillowcase providing extra insulation. Heat is an important factor and body warmer packs available from chemists are a safe way of providing supplementary heat, as are microwave heat pads, but take care that these do not get too hot. Hot water bottles can be punctured by large, sharp claws and should be avoided.

Snakes

Method will depend on the temperament of the snake and its size. Large snakes of 6 feet plus should be handled utilising two people and SHOULD NEVER BE PLACED AROUND THE NECK.

Friendly non-venomous snake

1. If you can guarantee the snake is friendly it is best handled using minimal restraint supporting the weight of the body in both hands.
2. Snakes do not like their heads and tails being grasped so keep hands to the middle.
3. Snakes tend to imagine your hands are 'branches'.
4. If the snake is in a pillowcase **do not** put your hands in the bag; this is a sure way of being bitten. If friendly, then allow the pillowcase to fall open and handle the snake as already mentioned. Have a snake hook ready to move the snake and be prepared for the snake to emerge rapidly!

More aggressive or larger snakes (reticulated pythons, anacondas, tree pythons/boas)

1. If in a cage/box locate the snake.
2. Use the snake hook to move the snake into a position where it can be grasped.
3. Place a thick towel over the snake and grasp at the back of the head through the towel, then pass the head into the other hand so the rest of the body can be restrained. The same method can be applied if the snake is in a pillowcase; you just need to locate the head and grasp it through the pillowcase.
4. If the snake is particularly fractious then it can be guided into a clear plastic tube with a diameter large enough for the snake to fit in but not to turn around.
5. Snake hooks and sticks should be used to manipulate the snake rather than for restraint, as damage can be done if too much pressure is exerted on the snake's body, particularly behind the head; snakes have a single occiput and the neck can be dislocated. Bruising is another factor of poor handling and this can lead to weakness. The bruised muscles leak myoglobin (haemoglobin), which can impair kidney function.
6. When restraining a snake for examination or injection, the head has to be restrained to prevent biting/striking. The thumb and the first finger can be placed either side of the occiput and the forefinger on top of the head.
7. After any stressful procedure the snake should be placed in a warm dark vivarium and allowed to recover from the ordeal.
8. Beware, snakes love to hide in dark places, and sleeves and pockets are ideal, so when handling concentrate on where the head is going!
9. If bitten by a snake as the teeth angle back toward the head do not pull off, rather hold the head in place and get an alcohol-based substance and spray in the mouth (isopropyl alcohol); snakes hate the taste and will release. Also recommended is plunging the handler and the snake into cold water! The wound should be flushed and cleaned using chlorhexidine (Hibiscrub) and any shed teeth removed. Antibiotics and medical treatment may be required.

Lizards

Even the smallest lizard can inflict a nasty bite, especially some of the lizards that belong to the gecko family, such as tokays (*Gekko gecko*) and day geckos (*Phelsuma* spp.).

Rough handling or grasping of the tail can lead to autotomy (tail loss).

Method for handling small lizards

1. As these can be fairly delicate creatures, a gentle but secure hold is necessary.
2. Grasp the thorax between the thumb and the first two fingers; the remaining fingers and hand can support the abdomen.
3. A net can be used to catch agile species such as day geckos (*Phelsuma* spp.) and anoles (*Anolis carolinensis*). The net can be placed gently over the lizard and the lizard can be handled through the net using the method described.
4. If handling tokay geckos (*Gekko gecko*) always wear protective gloves as they are known for their ugly demeanour.

Medium-sized friendly lizards, e.g. blue-tongued skinks (Tiliqua scincoides), *plated lizards* (Gerrosaurus), *bearded dragons* (Pogona vitticeps)

1. The same method as for small lizards can be applied but using the free hand to support the rest of the body and tail.

Medium to larger lizards

For those more aggressive individuals or those with sharp nails and long lashing tails, e.g. green iguana (*Iguana iguana*), smaller tegus (*Tuppinambis teguixin*), water dragons (*Physignathus cocincinus*), or monitors (*Varanus* spp.).

1. Restrain the front legs against the animal's thorax and hind limbs against the pelvis and tail. To help control the tail, position it under your arm and use your elbow to keep in against your body.
2. Tails are like whips and will slice through flesh. When handling any species with sharp nails and a long whipping tail have arms well protected and wear gauntlets.
3. They can also be wrapped in thick towels and limbs restrained in this manner. Always keep them away from your face. Large iguanas, although vegetarians, will quite happily take a chunk out of the handler's ear lobe!
4. Many of these lizards have the ability to crocodile roll and once this has started they are very difficult to control and the injuries to the handler can be great.

Very large aggressive lizards, monitors and iguanas

1. A quick release dog catcher can be placed around the neck and one of the forelegs, positioning the tail against the pole to prevent thrashing and rolling.
2. From this position the lizard can be moved.
3. If the lizard is being aggressive and difficult to restrain a chemical intervention should be sought.

Chameleons (Chamaeleo spp.)

1. Most chameleons are friendly and actually prefer to climb onto the handler's hand, using it as a twig.
2. They will panic if they are unable to feel the ground underneath them and, therefore, when examining make sure at least three feet are tightly holding onto a finger or twig.
3. If examining the mouth be aware that they have a very long tongue (it is quite amazing to see it 'packed' into the mouth) and ensure that it is not entwined or dislodged making it difficult to return to its normal position.

In general, always handle over a table and keep both snakes and lizards away from the face. It is also worth remembering that arboreal species will try and move upward, especially certain species of boas and chameleons. A chameleon is probably happiest sitting on the handler's head!

After discussions with the owner it was decided to surgically remove the ovaries and oviducts by performing an **ovariosalpingectomy**.

Patient care and preparation

The patient was weighed and placed in a pre-heated vivarium with basking area UV light.

The temperature was monitored and maintained to the higher end of the iguana's POTZ (30°C).

Once settled a heparinised blood sample was taken from the ventral tail vein and the following haematological tests were carried out:

- PCV
- Albumin
- Globulin
- Calcium
- Phosphorus
- Uric acid.

Aid in identifying dehydration

This revealed that the animal was slightly dehydrated.

Fluid therapy was administered using lactated ringers intracoelomonically.

Intra- and post-operatively, fluid was administered intravenously at a rate of 5 ml/kg/hour.

Pre-operative antibiotics were given: ceftazidine (Fortum) 20 mg/kg intramuscularly.

Surgical procedure

1. A pre-anaesthetic propofol (Rapinovet) was administered intravenously into the tail vein at a dose rate of 10 mg/kg.
2. The iguana was then placed in dorsal recumbence on a heat mat (which was covered by a surgical drape).
3. The animal was intubated and maintained on isoflurane (2–4%). A Doppler was taped over the thorax to monitor heart rate.
4. The patient was prepared for aseptic procedure, using dilution of povidone-iodine diluted in warm water.
5. Plastic fenestrated drapes were used to gain good vision throughout the surgery.
6. A paramedian incision was made into the coelomic cavity extending from the xiphoid process to the cranial pelvis.

NOTE: a large incision is recommended to allow clear visualisation of the reproductive organs and avoid damage to other tissues such as the bladder.

7. The ovaries are easily identified and resemble clusters of yellow-orange grapes (colour represents presence of yolk).
8. One of the ovaries was gently manipulated to identify vascular supply (the blood vessels arise from branches off the aorta and renal veins).
9. The vessels were double ligated using 3/0 vicryl, incised between the ligatures and replaced into the coelomic cavity. Observations were made for signs of haemorrhage. This procedure was carried out for both ovaries.

The right ovary is positioned very near the vena cava and the left is near to the left adrenal gland. It is possible to leave the oviduct in place but because of the possibility of infection it should be removed.

10. The oviducts were double ligated using 3/0 vicryl close to the insertion of the cloaca, and small blood vessels sealed off using radiosurgery.
11. The musculature of the coelomic wall was closed with a continuous monofilament of absorbable suture material (vicryl 3/0).
12. The skin was closed using 4/0 nylon and an everting horizontal mattress suture. This prevents the natural inverting of reptile skin and prevents dysecdysis in the future.

Post-operatively the iguana was placed in the vivarium set at a temperature of 30°C. Fluid therapy continued for a further 24 hours. Anti-inflammatory drugs were given to counteract the lizard's obvious discomfort, being seen hunched in its vivarium following recovery. The patient was discharged 2 days post-operatively, with sutures to be removed in 4–5 weeks. The owners were advised not to allow the iguana to bathe for 2–3 weeks whilst the wound was healing. Spraying frequently each day was recommended, as this aids overall hydration. The iguana returned for a check after 1 week and was reportedly doing well, with its appetite having returned to normal.

CASE HISTORY 2

Patient

Female common boa named India (see Fig. 3.12 at end of chapter), approximately 6 years of age, 2 metres in length and weighing 8.2 kg.

Presenting signs

The owners observed a clear discharge 'bubbling up' from the nares, and had seen discharge on the glass vivarium doors. India was lethargic and had not eaten for 4 weeks (normally she would eat a large rat once every 2 weeks). She had been observed resting with head raised and mouth open; sometimes she appeared to be yawning.

The owners had recently moved India into a larger vivarium and had initially considered that her disinterest in food and change in temperament were due to her getting used to her new larger surroundings. Questions regarding India's environment and hygiene were asked, especially regarding the frequency of cleaning, substrate used and heating supplied.

Examination

Due to the size of the snake, three members of staff were 'on hand' to help restrain India.

The mucous membranes in the oral cavity appeared pale pink, but there were no signs of cyanosis.

She was suffering from mild dehydration (5–8%), and the skin had a slightly wrinkled appearance.

Ausculation of the lungs presented rales due to accumulation of mucus in the lungs and bronchi.

Initial diagnosis was upper and lower respiratory tract disease.

Respiratory tract infections are particularly difficult to treat in snakes. This is primarily due to the anatomy of their respiratory tract, and the main factors that contribute to the progression of the disease are that there is no ciliated, epithelial lining present and no diaphragm. Unlike mammals, reptiles are unable to cough and remove the accumulating mucus from the bronchi and lungs. It can take weeks for the mucus to be removed from the lungs, and if environmental temperatures are below the preferred optimum temperature zone (POTZ), then the condition will persist.

India was admitted for further tests and hospitalisation. To confirm diagnosis and subsequent treatment, two radiographs were taken to evaluate the severity of the pneumonia: 1) a dorsoventral, and 2) a lateral using a horizontal beam. The two views were taken to give the veterinary surgeon a clear view of the pulmonary anatomy and how much of the pulmonary tissue was affected.

An oral swab was taken for culture and sensitivity and a mucus sample was taken for further examination for endoparasites.

Tip: Tracheal wash (this process can be performed to gain samples for further investigation)

Equipment
- An 8–10 fg sterile plastic dog catheter
- Warmed sterile saline solution (rate of 1–5 ml/kg)
- 10–50 ml sterile syringe
- Sterile containers to collect sample.

Patient preparation and procedure
The procedure can be carried out with the patient conscious or using chemical restraint. The patient is placed in a horizontal position with the head toward the end of the examination table. The jaw is held open (a small gag can be used if necessary) and the light positioned for good visibility of the glottis.

The sterile tube is inserted into the glottis and lung.

Warm sterile saline is infused into the lung and immediately aspirated back into the syringe.

To facilitate this procedure the position is changed so that the head is tilting downward over the table and the rest of body is slightly raised.

The syringe and catheter are slowly withdrawn maintaining slight negative pressure on the syringe.

The aspirate collected is placed in sterile collecting pots for further analysis.

Tests carried out

A sample of the mucus was taken for direct examination under a light microscope. This was to rule out endoparasites as a contributory factor in the cause of the respiratory disease.

A sample was sent to a laboratory for microbiology and sensitivity testing.

Patient care and drug therapy

Due to the time scale involved in waiting for the results of the bacteriology and sensitivity tests India was given an intramuscular injection of Amikin; dose 2.5 mg/kg every 72 hours for a minimum of seven doses (amikacin belongs to the aminoglycoside group of antibiotics and is a broad-spectrum antibiotic effective against most Gram-negative bacteria, making it a very useful drug when treating respiratory infections in reptiles. Fluid therapy is important when using this group of drugs due to reported nephrotoxicity.) The injection site was in the first third of the snake's body (caudal to the head) and half way between the dorsal midline and lateral aspect of the body (epaxial musculature).

Pathogens associated with respiratory disease are commonly the aerobic Gram-negative bacteria such as:

- *Escherichia coli*
- *Klebsiella* spp.
- *Pseudomonas* spp.
- *Aeromonas* spp.
- *Salmonella.*

Fluid therapy

To correct India's dehydration warmed sterile fluids were administered; a combination of 0.18% sodium chloride in 4% dextrose at 20 mg/kg. The route was intracoelomic (this route was selected as, although invasive, it was less stressful for India).

The following day, using the same fluid and dose rate as above, oral fluids (PO) were administered via a stomach tube.

India was then placed in a warm, dark vivarium set to the top end of her preferred optimum temperature zone (POTZ), 25–30°C, where she was able to recover from the procedure. (*It is important for any sick reptile to be maintained at the higher end of its POTZ, in this case 28–30°C, as this will stimulate the immune response and also allow drug therapy to be more effective.*)

She was checked every 15 min and the following observed and recorded:

- Breathing (pattern, rate)
- Environmental temperature
- Body posture (signs of respiratory distress, contortions, convulsions).

Nutritional support

India was presenting signs of anorexia but it was felt that, due to the stress she had already undergone, fluid therapy would be maintained and tube feeding with enterals would only be considered if she continued to refuse food once discharged and in her own environment.

India was hospitalised for 4 days where she received oral fluids every 24 hours and a further dose of Amikin (intramuscularly).

Discharge and advice

Before India was allowed home the owners were instructed to improve India's accommodation. The main change was to increase the temperature. The hot spot temperature needed to be increased by either suspending a guarded ceramic heater from the top of the vivarium or fixing a microclimate heater to the side. A larger heat mat had to be placed at the hot end to maintain the thermal gradient. Unfortunately, when the owners moved India to her new larger accommodation they forgot to increase the heating, and with the cold and stress of moving vivariums this had contributed greatly to her condition.

As India's state of dehydration and general behaviour improved she was discharged, returning 48 hours later for another antibiotic injection, oral fluids and results of the bacteriology and sensitivity tests.

The owners were instructed to offer food to India after her next antibiotic injection and if she failed to eat then tube feeding would be considered.

It took several weeks before India fed again and she was readmitted within that time for tube feeding.

Prognosis

This particular case responded well to treatment, but respiratory infections can take months to treat and require quite aggressive treatment. In many cases a guarded prognosis has to be given. The reasons for this are many; some of the main points include:

- The anatomy and physiology of snakes' respiratory system (as discussed earlier).
- The ability of snakes to conceal many of the clinical signs until the disease is well advanced.
- The multifactorial nature of the disease can provide a challenge in diagnosing and providing treatment, i.e. bacteria, viruses, fungi, endoparasites or aspiration or foreign bodies are contributory causes of respiratory disease.
- The compliance of the owners to improve environmental conditions, especially hygiene and temperature regulation.

Acknowledgements

Information was supplied by the Reptile Trust Burnopfield Newcastle, the Herplife web site (www.herplife.co.uk) and by David Feldmar MRCVS.

REFERENCES

Mader DR 1996 Reptile medicine and surgery. W.B. Saunders, Philadelphia
Mader DR 1997 Approach to the anorexic reptile. In: 21 Annual Waltham/Ohio State University Symposium (For the Treatment of Animal Diseases) lecture notes. Ohio State University and Waltham USA Inc, California

FURTHER READING

Beynton P, Lawton MPC, Cooper J 1992 Manual reptiles. British Small Animal Veterinary Association, Cheltenham
Divers SJ 1997 Medical and surgical treatment of reptile dystocias. In: 21 Annual Waltham/Ohio State University Symposium (For the Treatment of Animal Diseases) lecture notes. Ohio State University and Waltham USA Inc, California
Donoghue S 1997 Nutrition of companion birds and reptiles. In: 21 Annual Waltham/Ohio State University Symposium (For the Treatment of Animal Diseases) lecture notes. Ohio State University and Waltham USA Inc, California
Mader DR 1997 Reptile urogenital system and renal disease. In: 21 Annual Waltham/Ohio State University Symposium (For the Treatment of Animal Diseases) lecture notes. Ohio State University and Waltham USA Inc, California
Mattison C 1982 The care of reptiles and amphibians in captivity. Blandford Press, Poole

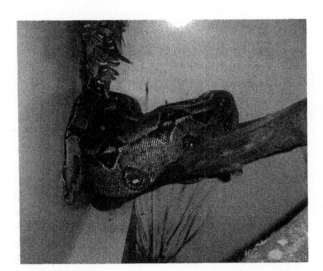

Fig. 3.12 India.

Chapter 4

Chelonia

Beverly Shingleton

INTRODUCTION

Chelonia is a term used to describe the group of shelled reptiles, which comprises the tortoises, turtles and terrapins.

In the UK, those chelonia that spend their time on land (terrestrial) are known as tortoises, those that spend their time in fresh water are known as terrapins and marine chelonia are referred to as turtles. These classifications can alter; for example in North America the term turtle could refer to either aquatic or terrestrial chelonia, and a terrapin could be a fresh-water or marine-dwelling species. Table 4.1 lists some of the commonly kept chelonia species in the UK.

The Mediterranean tortoise is one of the more commonly seen reptiles in veterinary practice and for this reason this chapter will concentrate mainly on the nursing care of the Mediterranean tortoise with references made, where applicable, to other species.

One of the first steps in managing and caring for hospitalised chelonia is to have an appreciation of its anatomy and physiology. Table 4.2 highlights some of the more outstanding anatomical and physiological characteristics of chelonia.

HUSBANDRY AND GENERAL CARE OF THE HOSPITALISED PATIENT

The chelonia patient should be nursed and cared for in a separate ward as described for lizards and snakes.

Hospital cage

Chelonia are often admitted for nursing care due to problems associated with poor husbandry and nutrition. A common reason for the Mediterranean tortoise to be hospitalised is that it is suffering from **anorexia**; this could be due to a disease such as mouth rot or respiratory infection. More likely it is because the tortoise had been ill prepared for hibernation and, as a result, is suffering from a severe metabolic disturbance.

The hospital cage should mirror the specialist requirements of the species to be housed. It is essential that the nurse is aware of the natural history of the animal and how its needs must be provided within the hospital cage.

The following must be considered:

- Natural history of the patient.
- Preferred body temperature (PBT) of the patient.
- If the species requires a terrestrial, aquatic or semi-aquatic set up.

Providing the wrong environment can cause much stress to the patient and this, in turn, can cause immunosuppression and infections. Therefore, the text below outlines some of the important factors to be considered when setting up a vivarium for sick chelonia.

A selection of housing should be available to accommodate all types of chelonia from the land-dwelling tortoise to the aquatic turtle.

Table 4.1 Common chelonia species kept in the UK

Common name	Scientific name
Mediterranean tortoises	
*Spur thigh tortoise (Greek)	*Testudo graeca*
*Hermann's tortoise	*Testudo hermanni*
*Marginated tortoise	*Testudo marginata*
Horsfield's tortoise	*Testudo horsfieldi*
East and West African terrestrial chelonia	
Bell's hinge-back tortoises	*Kinixys belliana* spp
Leopard tortoise	*Geochelone pardalis* spp
Pancake tortoise	*Malacochersus tornieri*
North American species	
American box turtle (tortoise)	*Terrapene carolina* spp
South American tortoises	
Red footed tortoise	*Geochelone carbonaria*
Yellow footed tortoise	*Geochelone denticulata*
Indian star tortoise	*Geochelone elegans*
Turtles and terrapins	
American	
Red eared terrapin	*Chrysemys scripta*
Map turtle	*Graptemys geographica*
Common mud turtle	*Kinosternon subrubrum*
Alligator snapping turtle	*Macrochelys temmincki*
Diamond back terrapin	*Malaclemys terrapin*
Florida soft shell turtle	*Trionyx ferox*
Mediterranean	
Caspian turtle	*Mauremys caspica*

Please note it is important that the veterinary practice have a library, which includes books that will give details on the individual species, husbandry requirements and nutritional needs.
*With the exception of Horsfield's *(Testudo horsfieldi)*, which is not truly a Mediterranean tortoise, all are protected under CITES legislation and are classified as Annex A. This means they require DEFRA certificates in order to be bought, sold or traded.

The main points to consider in selecting suitable accommodation are as follows:

- Ease of access
- Durability
- Security
- Ease of cleaning.

Allowing the client to provide the housing is not recommended as it in itself may be incorrect or harbour disease.

In the hospital ward, the cages should be easy to clean, disinfect and secure. Specially designed vivarium locks can be fitted to glass sliding doors.

Vivarium materials

Hygiene is a major consideration and recommended materials are either fibreglass or moulded plastic (see Fig. 3.1, Lizards and snakes); these can be quite expensive, but are a good investment if the practice is considering widening its interest in reptile medicine and care (for further information on materials see Table 3.1, Lizards and snakes).

If aquatic or semi-aquatic species are to be hospitalised, then a selection of robust glass tanks will be required with securely fitted lids. Semi-aquatic species must have access to an area of land for basking, and a way of getting in and out of the water.

Substrate

This is the medium that sits in the bottom of the vivarium to absorb faeces and urine (for further information on substrates see Table 3.1, Lizards and snakes).

Substrates should display faecal and urate materials easily, be hygienic, cheap, readily available and should not cause impaction or further complicate medical problems if ingested. Newspaper or thick white paper like that used at the 'fish and chip' shop is ideal.

If aquatic or semi-aquatic species are hospitalised then a filtration system will have to be provided to prevent the water becoming stagnant (if not the water will require changing every day).

Cage furnishings

In the hospital vivarium these need to be kept to a minimum, as this will aid hygiene and access to the patient.

Most chelonia will require a hide; aquatic and semi-aquatic species will need an area to get out of the water to bask. The basking area should take up approximately one-third of the tank leaving the rest as water.

Table 4.2 Common anatomical and physiological characteristics of chelonia

Anatomical structure/system	Features
Musculoskeletal	Shell is divided into the upper carapace and the lower plastron. This protective shell has derived from the ribs, vertebrae and limb girdles fused with dermal bones. Keratin shields called scutes cover the bony shell. The scutes are named according to their adjacent body portion and provide useful demarcation sites for surgical procedures, treatments and identification (see Fig. 4.1). Adaptation can be seen in the case of soft-shelled terrapins, where the scutes have been replaced by tough leathery skin. In some species the anterior or posterior plastron is hinged sealing the fore- or hindlimbs, e.g. Bell's hinge back tortoise (*Kinixys belliana*). As shell is living tissue, when calculating drug dosages the total body weight of the chelonia must be considered.
Respiration	Those chelonia that are able to retract their head and neck into the shell have short trachea that quickly bifurcates (divides into two) cranially into the dorsal surface of the lung. This allows breathing to continue when head is retracted into shell. Lungs attach dorsally to the ventral surface of the carapace. No diaphragm is present and lungs are large, divided into sack-like structures. The lung surface is reticular and contains smooth muscle and connective tissue. Large lung volume is an advantage for aquatic species aiding buoyancy. As chelonia lack a diaphragm they are unable to cough and have no ciliated lining so the removal of secretions and debris from the lungs is very difficult. Species of turtles and terrapins such as the snapping and side-necked during hibernation are able to gain oxygen via the cloaca. **When administering anaesthesia it must be remembered that many species of turtles and terrapins are excellent at breath holding for long periods!**
Gastrointestinal	Unlike lizards and snakes the tongue does not extend beyond the oral cavity. They have no teeth and do not chew their food. They use their beaks (rhamphotheca) to bite off pieces of food, which are swallowed whole. **Aquatic species will only eat in the water.** The stomach sits along the ventral left side of the chelonia. It has been known for some species of chelonia to swallow stones to aid in the breakdown of foods. Compared to mammals, small intestines are short. In herbivores the colon is the site for microbial activity. The time it takes for food to pass along the digestive tract can vary and factors that can interfere with transit times include temperature, foods fed, fibre content, feeding frequency and water content of food.
Urogenital tract	Paired kidneys attached dorsally to the inside of the carapace in the region just over the rear legs. No renal pelvis, pyramids, relatively few nephrons and no Loop of Henle; therefore, most chelonia are unable to concentrate their urine. In terrestrial chelonia nitrogenous waste (urea) is excreted in the form of uric acid (this reduced amount of water being lost during waste removal). Uric acid is insoluble and if the chelonia becomes dehydrated the uric acid will crystallise and be deposited in the body tissues, especially the kidneys (see Post-hibernation anorexia). If this condition is not treated promptly then the chelonia will die. In aquatic and semi-aquatic species nitrogenous waste is excreted directly into the water. Chelonia have a urinary bladder; in terrestrial chelonia it is especially large, thin walled and used for water storage. A chelonia may go long periods without passing water and uses the bladder as a reservoir allowing water to be resorbed back into the circulation. **This is why it is important that a tortoise has a full bladder prior to hibernation and if the bladder is emptied during hibernation the tortoise must be woken up.** Males have a large penis that sits in the floor of the cloaca. When aroused the penis swells and extends beyond the cloaca. This is seen often in oversexed juveniles and must not be mistaken for a prolapse. Sexing tortoises – males have longer, tapering tails and a longer slit like vent opening; females have shorter, stubby tails with a circular vent opening. In sexually mature males the plastron is more concave than that of females. Sexing turtles and terrapins – in many cases tail length can be applied. Some males have very long nails on their forefeet (red eared terrapin).
Cardiovascular	Chelonia have a very similar system to that described in chapter 3, Lizards and snakes. They are thought to have a renal portal system and, therefore, **drugs should be administered in the front half of the animal.**

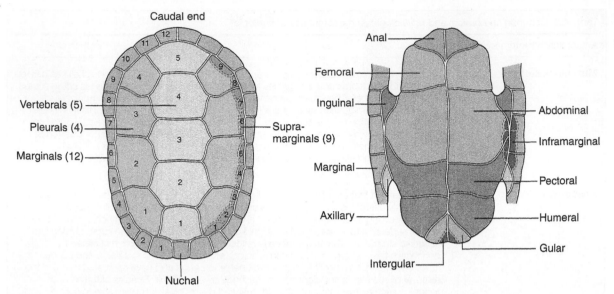

Fig. 4.1 Nomenclature of the carapace and plastron.

GENERAL ENVIRONMENTAL CONDITIONS

The four main considerations here are:

1. ventilation
2. heating
3. lighting
4. humidity.

Each one will be discussed separately as it relates to the patient.

Ventilation

Chelonia require air to survive; ventilation is achieved by providing housing that has holes positioned at the back or sides of the cage. To provide an adequate airflow the holes should be placed on opposite sides at the top and bottom of the vivarium. Vents should not be placed at the same height opposite each other as this can cause a draft.

Heating

The provision of heat in the vivarium is essential as chelonia are 'ectothermic' and rely on external heat sources to warm up their internal body temperature (for more detail on heat regulation see section under Lizards and snakes). So for the chelonia's body to function correctly, a heat source has to be provided in the animal's accommodation.

Heat can be provided in many forms (see Fig. 3.3a,b,c, Lizards and snakes); the main ones are as follows:

- Ceramic and tube heaters
- Reflector bulbs with or without UVB light
- Heat mat
- Aquarium heaters plus a guard (as used in fish husbandry).

Regulation of temperature

Chelonia have a **preferred body temperature** (PBT) or **preferred optimum temperature zone** (POTZ). This relates to the ideal or optimum temperature that the species requires for its metabolism to function correctly (movement, feeding, digestion, enzyme activity, reproduction, etc.). The heat provided must supply the chelonia with an opportunity to thermoregulate (move between different temperature zones) so the positioning of the heat source is vital and a basking area at one end of the tank or vivarium will provide a thermal gradient (see Fig. 4.2 for set up of the vivarium). Another key factor is the regulation

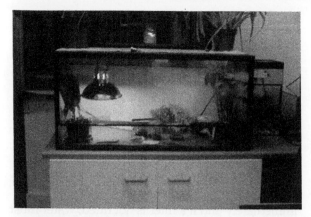

Fig. 4.2 Set up of vivarium.

of heat supplied and a correctly positioned thermostat; observations of thermometers can achieve this. A good instrument to measure temperature is a laser heat gun (Peregrine), which can be aimed at an area within the vivarium and a reading taken and recorded. Overheating the reptile can be just as detrimental to its health as underheating. For individual species' POTZ, the nurse will have to refer to specialist books providing details on that species.

Drug absorption and utilisation is influenced by their POTZ, so when chelonia are receiving medication or anaesthetics the provision of heat is essential if the drug is to be metabolised correctly.

When providing heat for aquatic and semi-aquatic chelonia, a tank heater will have to be provided. As aquatic species are very clumsy and frequently break their tank, a heater guard should be fitted.

Most good tank heaters will be fitted with a thermostat, which will allow you to adjust the temperature settings. A liquid crystal thermometer can be placed on the outside of the tank.

For those species that require a basking area, such as the red eared terrapin (*Pseudemys scripta elegans*), an incandescent light or spot light fitted with a reflector needs to be positioned over an area of land. This needs to be about 22 cm above the basking spot and reach temperatures of at least 30–35°C (85–95°F). The provision of such an area allows the chelonia to bask and aids against respiratory disease and shell disorders.

Lighting

There are three main types of lighting used (see Fig. 3.5b, Lizards and snakes):

1. Incandescent bulbs, e.g. light bulbs.
2. Ultraviolet (UV) strip lights with UVB and UVA content.
3. Reflector bulbs (can be combined with UVA and UVB).

Tip:

Sunlight
UVA stimulates behavioural and physiological effects. UVB is necessary for calcium metabolism and the activation of vitamin D. UVC is not important in reptile husbandry.

Lighting provides the chelonia with a photoperiod and stimulates natural behaviour; the amount of light required will depend on the species' native environment and the time of year. UVB lighting aids with the formation of vitamin D_3 and calcium metabolism (see Box 3.1, Lizards and snakes).

The Mediterranean tortoise would enjoy in excess of 14 hours of sunshine during the summer months, reducing to 12 in the spring and autumn.

Full-spectrum light (such as that produced by sunlight UVA, UVB, UVC) is important for most of the chelonia kept in this country. Natural sunlight is the ideal for most of the terrestrial chelonia kept in the UK. In the case of the hospitalised patient this is not feasible and a full-spectrum UVB light must be fitted in the enclosure.

Red eared terrapins are great sun worshippers and require a full-spectrum UV light 22–24 cm above the basking area. This is important for calcium metabolism.

There are a number of UV lights on the market that supply an adequate amount of light.

At present, Zoo Med Reptisun 5.0. is one of the best strip lights available on the market and for use in larger enclosures (minimum of 4 feet). The Powersun (Active) UV, which gives off 5–8 times more UVB than strip lights is recommended (the role of UVB and calcium metabolism is explained in Box 3.1, Lizards and snakes).

Tip: Inadequate provision of heat is one of the main factors contributing to poor health in the Mediterranean tortoise. In their native land the summer air temperatures are generally much warmer than in the UK and, more importantly, the average sunshine per year is between 2500 and 3500 hours compared to our average of 1500 hours. Therefore, tortoises in the UK are having their 'sun-bathing' hours reduced to about a third of what they would have gained in their natural environment, and this can have dramatic effects on their metabolism and longevity as well as depleting their energy reserves and causing a slow urate build up in the kidneys.

All owners of tortoises must be aware of the need to provide a basking area, which can reach temperatures of 35°C (95°F) enabling the tortoise to bask and reach their preferred optimum temperature zone of approximately 30°C (86°F); this will vary between species. The basking area is especially important for those all too frequent periods when the sun refrains from shining; a spot and UVB lamp over an elected area will provide the necessary daylight and basking requirements.

It should be highlighted here that UVB lights do not have an infinite life span and, although the white light may be seen, the UVB content is generally exhausted within 6–9 months of use. For satisfactory vitamin D synthesis, the UVB light needs to be on for 10–14 hours daily, and be positioned approximately 12 inches above the chelonia.

Tip: Positioning of UVB light is very important. The height should be measured from where the rays will be landing on the animal and not the base of the cage. Also to maximise UVB utilisation, the height can be reduced for young animals. Replace UVB lights every 6 months where young growing stock are housed.

CLEANING AND HYGIENE

To maintain the health and well-being of the hospitalised chelonia it is important the following steps are taken:

1. Remove and dispose of all soiled areas as soon as they are identified (the hospital cage should be checked at least twice a day for faecal and urate matter). Also, any uneaten food must be disposed of.
2. Using a detergent wash, rinse food bowls and water receptacles.

3. Using a detergent or mild disinfectant clean areas and any furnishings that have been soiled.
4. Rinse and dry cleaned areas.
5. Replace substrate.
6. All equipment used should be thoroughly disinfected and stored correctly.
7. Whilst cleaning the cage the occupant can be placed in a holding pen like a pen pal. The removal of the patient will help to minimise stress.
8. Aquatic chelonia are usually messy creatures and produce much waste that quickly pollutes the water. Therefore, solid waste must be removed immediately and if a filter is not fitted, water must be changed daily. Most filters designed for fish keeping do not cope very well with the amount of debris produced by terrapins or turtles and these must be checked daily and cleaned on a frequent basis. The best type of filtration system for aquatic chelonia is an external filter. When replacing water, make sure it is at the same temperature as that of the water removed. For some species a sudden drop in temperature could prove fatal. There is no need to de-chlorinate the water unless otherwise advised, as chlorine seems to be tolerated by most terrapins and turtles. It has been suggested that the presence of chlorine in the water can help keep bacterial levels down. If brackish water is needed, then aquarium salt can be added to the water.

It is important to stress that when cleaning out the accommodation of any aquatic species all electrical equipment must be turned off, especially heaters, as these will crack if exposed and cause electrocution.

Tip: If using a bacterial filtration system, the water does need to be de-chlorinated, as the chlorine will kill the bacteria.

When cleaning the cage after the patient has left, the following protocol should be observed:

1. All furnishings, and substrates must be removed and, if possible, disposed of.
2. Heating and filtration equipment must be removed, cleaned, dried and stored carefully (to prevent the spread of disease, filter material must be replaced).

3. All organic material must be removed and correctly disposed of.

4. If objects are to be used again, e.g. water bowls, rocks, these must be thoroughly cleaned and disinfected, as must any items that have been used during the patient's stay, e.g. feeding tongs.

5. The empty cage must be cleaned using copious amounts of hot water and detergent, paying particular attention to the corners, non-removable fixtures and fittings and glass sliding doors.

6. The entire cage must be rinsed before applying the disinfectant.

7. Leave the disinfectant in contact with the cage for the recommended period before rinsing.

8. Whilst cleaning the cage, the nurse must observe her own health and hygiene and wear protective clothing such as latex gloves and aprons. Hands must be washed after any contact with the chelonia or its vivarium, especially aquatic species, because of the risks from *Salmonella* (see Box 3.2, Lizards and snakes).

FIRST AID

See Lizards and snakes; first-aid methods are identical.

MONITORING THE CHELONIA PATIENT

It is important to routinely monitor the health of the hospitalised patient (Fig. 4.3).

The information gained must be clearly recorded and references made to the patient's environment especially temperature. Morning and late afternoon checks are suggested.

Morning

The following checks should be carried out:

- Locate patient and carry out necessary patient observations (refer to clinical history but it is advisable to weigh the chelonia daily).

Patient details					Owner details				
Name					Name				
Species and details Sex/age					Address				
Preferred temperature zone and humidity									
Diet preference					Tel no.				

Date	Temp am/pm B basking C cool end AM PM				Humidity % Indicate if sprayed	Food offered amount (F) Water offered (W)	Food eaten amount	Urate/faeces passed ✓ or ✕ **Comment**	Signs of shedding ✓ or ✕ **Comment**	Hygiene Spot clean Total clean	Comment Medications given and signature
	B	C	B	C	✓ ✕	F W ✓					

Fig. 4.3 Hospital record sheet.

- Record temperature at both cool and hot ends of the vivarium.
- Record humidity (if appropriate).
- Turn on lighting and basking lamp (if not regulated by a thermostat or timer).
- Check all thermostatic or heating equipment to make sure it is operating correctly especially heat pads.
- For aquatic and semi-aquatic patients check the heater is not damaged; if in doubt turn off the electricity supply at the mains and then check. This will prevent 'electrocution'.
- If a filter is used check it is not blocked and that water is being drawn in and out of the filter.
- Check cage or tank for any abnormal discharges and remove faeces, urate and clean.
- Clean and replenish water bowl; many terrestrial chelonia especially the Mediterranean tortoise and tropical tortoises, such as the red foot *Geochelone carbonaria*, need to be placed in a shallow bath of warm water – this will allow them to bath and, more importantly, to drink. (see under Nutrition).
- Check for uneaten foods and remove if necessary. A record should be made of food eaten compared to that offered.
- If applicable spray the cage to provide humidity.
- If herbivorous supply fresh foods.
- **Before offering any live food or rodents allow reptile to reach its POTZ.**

Late afternoon

The following checks should be carried out:

- Carry out necessary patient observations.
- Record temperature at both cool and hot ends of the vivarium.
- Record humidity (if appropriate).
- Turn off lighting and basking lamp (if not regulated by a thermostat or timer).
- Check all heating equipment to make sure it is operating correctly, especially heat pads and tank heaters.
- Check cages for any abnormal discharges and remove faeces, urate and clean.

- Record food eaten and remove any uneaten food, unless animal is nocturnal and prefers to take food items overnight.
- Check animal has access to water and humidity levels are correct for that species.
- Ensure cage is secure, ideally locked.

Obviously daily checks will differ according to the species kept and reason for hospitalisation.

HANDLING AND TRANSPORT

A healthy tortoise is very strong and can use its legs to claw and push away unwanted hands, so to prevent damage to you and the tortoise when handling it should be grasped firmly using both hands round the middle or last third of the shell. Thumbs should be placed on the carapace, the remaining fingers taking the weight of the plastron.

Terrapins or turtles require a different approach as they can inflict nasty bites and also many have long front claws that will be used to claw the handler. Many species have surprisingly long necks that seem to snake out of the shell and chase the handler's fingers. Species such as the soft shelled terrapins and snapping turtles warrant particular care when handling.

Terrapins and turtles should be rapidly scooped up from the rear, placing both hands on the shell thumbs on the carapace and fingers on the plastron. The need to keep fingers well away from the jaws cannot be overemphasised.

Transporting chelonia

Chelonia can be transported in a strong cardboard box or wooden box with air holes. Shredded or crumpled newspaper can be used to protect them. When moving aquatic and semi-aquatic species the same method can be used.

FEEDING AND NUTRITION

Many of the hospitalised chelonia are admitted because of diet-related problems and as with other reptiles, snakes and lizards included, there is much naivety about the correct foods to feed.

This section will be divided into:

1.   Tortoise nutrition, based primarily on the needs of the Mediterranean tortoise and some of the more commonly kept tropical and sub-tropical species.
2.   Terrapins and turtles, looking at the needs of some of the more commonly kept species such as the red eared terrapin (*Chrysemys scripta*).

Feeding the Mediterranean tortoise

The Mediterranean tortoise's natural terrain would be sparsely vegetated, infertile areas. The foods they would feed on comprise a variety of plant materials, leaves, flowers and fruits. In the wild the tortoise is an opportunist feeder preferring to eat the flowers of a plant and tender leaves.

In captivity the basic diet should consist of low-protein, high-fibre foods with high mineral and vitamin content, together with a large quantity of calcium carbonate.

Wild plants

Dandelions, sow thistle and clover are all favourites of the tortoise and grow widely in the UK. Ideally, the diet should consist mainly of these food types.

Grass is not digested by the tortoise and, therefore, has no nutritional value except to add bulk and fibre to the diet.

Green vegetables

Those that are commonly available, such as cabbage, water cress, cress, spinach and broccoli are all acceptable additions to wild plants, but it must be highlighted that many cultivated vegetables are high in protein and low in fibre. Most tortoises readily take salad foods such as tomatoes, cucumber and lettuce, but their nutritional value is limited and, therefore, they should be used to enhance the palatability of the food rather than make up the sole diet. Pre-packed mixed salad leaves give the tortoise a range of different leaves and can help the overall nutritional value (see Table 3.6, Lizards and snakes for nutritional value of fruits and vegetables).

Proprietary foods

Proprietary foods such as 'Pretty Pet' are available on the market – if fed to tortoises they must be soaked in water and only offered as part of the diet (Fig. 3.10, Lizards and snakes).

Meat products

These are not recommended and should not be included in the Mediterranean tortoise's diet. Protein levels in meat are far too high and can lead to severe metabolic and organ problems. As a guide, protein levels should be limited to 1–4% of the total diet fed.

Dairy products

These are not a natural food product for tortoises and should not be included in the diet. If they are offered then the liver can become diseased.

Vitamins and minerals

The quantities of these would be higher in the wild diet compared to that provided in captivity, therefore supplementation will be necessary.

The most important mineral to be considered here is **calcium**. In their natural range the soil is rich in calcium and, therefore, vegetation also contains high levels of this mineral. In comparison, soils in the UK lack the quantities seen in their natural range and this makes it necessary to supplement the diet on a daily basis.

> **Tip:** Calcium is one of the most important supplements and should be liberally sprinkled over the diet. It is far better to slightly oversupplement than undersupplement calcium. Some sources recommend supplementing calcium to approximately 10% of the total weight of the food offered, but this can be increased or decreased according to the growth of the shell.

Vitamin A is also required in the diet and a deficiency can lead to swollen eyes and loss of appetite as the animal cannot see its food.

A vitamin D_3 deficiency in the diet affects calcium metabolism, preventing calcium absorption

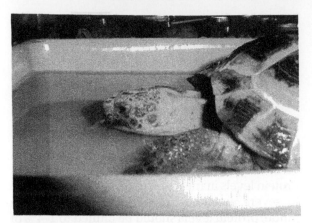

Fig. 4.4 Horsfield's tortoise having a drink/bath.

from the intestines. If present in the diet in too great a quantity it can cause excessive calcium uptake and calcification of soft tissues.

Water

As with all animals water is an essential part of the diet and the best way to provide water to the tortoise is by giving it a daily bath in 3–4 cm of warm water for 5–10 minutes (Fig. 4.4). This will allow the tortoise to take in water via either the cloaca or mouth. Alternatively, a shallow bowl of water can be offered, but this is usually trampled over and spilled.

> **Tip:** Tortoises do not have a hard palate so are unable to lap; therefore, they will drop their mouth below the water line and 'siphon up' the water until they have taken a sufficient amount.

Feeding routine for the hospitalised Mediterranean tortoise

Before feeding it is important to ensure the environment will allow the patient to reach its POTZ. If this is not provided then the tortoise will not eat or will be unable to digest its food correctly.

Sub-adult/adult tortoise

Offer a range of salad, green leaf vegetables, fruits and wild plants (see Table 3.6, Lizards and snakes for a selection of suitable food items and nutritional content). Ideally, the wild plant material should provide at least 75% of the diet, with leafy vegetables and salad making up the remaining 25% (fruits should be used as a treat – too large a quantity can cause excessive dilution of dietary protein). All foods offered should be fit for human consumption, washed and stored in a refrigerator or in the case of wild plants freshly picked. Foods should be offered on a flat dish or lid, and be of a size the tortoise can manage, especially as they prefer to bite off small pieces of food and too large pieces of fruit or vegetables can be difficult for the tortoise to eat. If using proprietary foods, make sure they are soaked and soft before offering. All food that is offered on a daily basis should be coated in calcium carbonate powder (vitamin and mineral supplement once or twice a week depending on medical history).

Be prepared to see the tortoise trample through the food scattering it about the cage; this is normal behaviour and one that has been seen in the wild. In the wild the tortoise would defecate and urinate over the plant material, not to destroy its food but to provide water and fertiliser to a sparsely vegetated land.

Once the tortoise has had sufficient it will walk away to rest and digest its food.

A note should be made of the amount of food offered and the amount eaten.

Water should also be available and, as mentioned earlier, a bath is probably the best way of achieving this.

Hatchling

The correct feeding of a hatchling tortoise is of paramount importance as poor diet can lead to various conditions such as lumpy shell, bone and shell deformities and obesity.

Many texts will concentrate on the feeding of the adult tortoise with little mention of diet for the hatchling. It is advised that the nurse becomes familiar with the dietary requirements of the hatchling, especially as more and more people are purchasing these small 50-p-sized creatures (Fig. 4.5). Various feeding regimes have been recommended, but the main aim is to balance

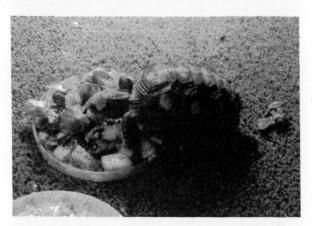

Fig. 4.5 Hatchling.

energy, protein and calcium intake, and ensure that the hatchling has access to the factors involved in calcium metabolism (heat, UVB and vitamin D).

Suggested feeding regimes

1. Feed the tortoise for 3–4 days and withhold food on the next day. This will allow for more thorough digestion of the previously eaten meals. The amount to feed will depend on how much the individual consumes at each feed.
2. Limit the amount of food offered to the tortoise at each sitting to just below the normal amount consumed. To follow this regime, observations have to be made on the quantity eaten over a period of time.

Foods to be fed

A range of foods need to be offered such as soaked tortoise pellets (Pretty Pet), mixed salad leaves, dark leaf produce such as water cress, cress, dandelion leaves, sow thistle and clover.

These foods can be fed on alternate days starting with:

- day one: soaked pellets
- day two: salads and mixed leaves
- day three: green leafed produce

and so on to match the selected feeding regime of (1) or (2).

Supplementation is very important and must be added at every meal. If using the routines suggested, calcium, multivitamin and mineral powders can be offered on a rotation basis. For example, calcium can be added to the diet on days one and two, with a vitamin and mineral powder being added on day three.

Water is extremely important and to keep the hatchling hydrated it should be observed drinking whilst being bathed in a shallow dish of warm water at least once or twice a day for 5–10 minutes.

> **Tip:** Although regarded as low in nutrititional value (except vitamin A), iceberg lettuce is a good food stuff for providing a dietary source of water for hatchling tortoises.

Remember 'variety is the spice of life' and offering the hospitalised chelonia a variety of foods will ensure it obtains the best possible nutrition.

FEEDING TURTLES AND TERRAPINS

Terrapins and turtles range from being totally carnivorous to accepting some plant material in their diet. A range of foods should be offered to the hospitalised patient including:

- proprietary terrapin and turtle pellets
- pinkies and small mice
- invertebrates such as locusts and crickets, snails, prawns in their shells
- cleansed earthworms (place worms in a tub for 12–24 hours to allow soil to pass through)
- fish, white bait, sprats
- plant material such as broad leaf watercress and romaine lettuce, oxygenating water weed
- calcium, multivitamin and mineral supplements need to be given especially to young growing terrapins and turtles
- very small quantities of the following foods: raw muscle meats, crab sticks, cockles, kidney and liver – these are very low in calcium and high in phosphorus and will require supplementation.

> **Tip:** When feeding terrapins and turtles, it is best to feed in a separate container as this will reduce pollution.

Suggested feeding regime

Quantity and frequency of feeding will depend on the size and age of the terrapin.

Young terrapins and turtles will require feeding daily, whereas adults feed every other day with a variety of foods from the list above.

GENERAL NUTRITIONAL PROBLEMS

Some of the main nutritional problems seen in chelonia are attributed to the provision of a diet that is based on too few food types. Poor provision of UV lighting, heating and little in the way of calcium supplementation.

A much-loved Mediterranean tortoise may enjoy a Sunday roast with the family, but this is not what it would eat in the wild. Owners need to be convinced that the feeding practice adopted over the past 30 years may not benefit the tortoise in the long term (a healthy, correctly fed tortoise should live for up to approximately 100 years, so many of the tortoises seen in the UK are merely surviving in the hands of well-meaning owners and probably only last one-third of their life expectancy). The role of the veterinary nurse is to find out the chelonia's present feeding regime and then help the owner to understand the need to modify the diet and the long-term benefits to the animal (very much like convincing an owner they have an obese dog that needs to go on a diet!).

Some of the more commonly seen diet-related problems are as follows.

Metabolic bone disease

This is a problem that manifests itself in many forms. The severity and signs depend on whether it is seen in the young hatchling or adult chelonia.

Signs of metabolic bone disease can include:

- Hypocalcaemia
- Soft shell

- Shell deformities (Fig. 4.6)
- Overgrown nails and rhamphotheca (chelonia beak) (Fig. 4.7)
- Abnormal gait and movement.

Anorexia

This can be associated with poor diet and lack of supplementation to the diet.

Dystocias

Some of these can be attributed to lack of calcium in the diet.

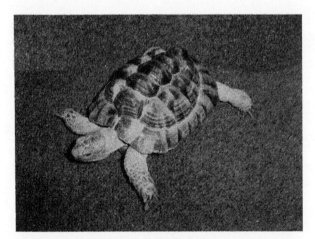

Fig. 4.6 Spur thigh tortoise with deformed shell.

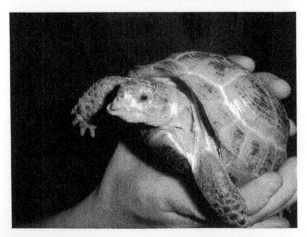

Fig. 4.7 Horsfield's tortoise with an overgrown beak.

Hypovitaminosis A

This is caused by a lack of vitamin A in the diet.

The conditions identified above will be discussed in more detail later on in the text.

PRE-, INTRA- AND POST-OPERATIVE CARE

As discussed in chapter 3, Lizards and snakes, there are many reasons for administering chemical anaesthetic or premedication to chelonia. The following reasons may apply:

* For restraint, especially when having to examine very large or aggressive species like the snapping turtle (*Chelydra s. serpentina*)
* To perform surgical procedures
* To carry out diagnostic sampling procedures
* To assist in retracting the head from the shell.

When assisting or caring for the chelonia patient that is to receive a premedication or anaesthetic, some consideration should be given to its biology and how this may affect the anaesthetic and monitoring.

It should be remembered that the lungs of chelonia are much simpler in structure to that seen in mammals. They have a larger tidal volume, but smaller surface area. The lungs in reptiles are very fragile and care must be taken NOT to overinflate and rupture the lungs during positive pressure ventilation.

Chelonia have complete tracheal rings and the trachea bifurcates shortly after entering the coelomic cavity.

When intubating, it should be noted that the tongue is thick and fleshy, so it is not as easy to visualise the larynx as in snakes and lizards.

Although reptiles do not have a diaphragm, chelonia have a membranous separation between the abdominal and thoracic cavities. Chelonia do not have intercostal muscles and, therefore, air movement in and out of the lungs is created by pressure changes brought about by altering the positioning of the abdominal organs, limbs and pelvic girdle. Chelonia do not rely on negative thoracic pressure for respiration, and if they sustain injuries to their shell and lung tissue is exposed, no obvious respiratory distress is seen. These considerations are very important when a monitoring anaesthetic and because skeletal muscle function is lost when a surgical plane of anaesthesia is reached, it may be necessary to carry out assisted ventilation. If the patient is positioned in dorsal recumbence pressure from the internal organs on the lungs will reduce tidal volume and assisted ventilation may be necessary.

Pre-anaesthetic preparation and procedures

It is recommended that the patient be fasted for 18 hours prior to surgery. This is to reduce pressure from the gastrointestinal tract, which may affect the tidal volume and necessitate assisted ventilation.

A thorough physical examination including assessing the weight of the patient and the biochemistry will determine if the patient is a suitable candidate for the elected procedure.

To ensure the patient is hydrated prior to, during and after the procedure, fluid therapy should be considered (see ch. 3, p. 61, common first-aid emergencies, point 4) at a preferred rate of 10–40 ml/kg/day, or 5 ml/kg/hour for 1–2 hours for severely shocked patients or those undergoing surgery (Mader 1996). The route used can be intravenously (IV) or intracoelomically (ICe) (see Table 3.7, Lizards and snakes, for injection sites). The use of infusion pumps, electrical or spring action, is very good for delivering small volumes of fluid at an accurate rate.

To prevent hypothermia and to ensure body systems continue to function correctly, supplementary heat must be provided. The operating theatre should be maintained at an ambient temperature and op-site prepared using a solution of either chlorhexidine or povidone-iodine diluted in warm water. Surgical spirit should be avoided as this evaporates and causes heat loss. A toothbrush can be used to pre-prep shell. Plastic disposable drapes provide good visibility of the patient and prevent bacterial 'strike through' during surgery. Drapes that adhere to the patient are also valuable as towel clips will be of little use.

Chelonia in dorsal recumbence have a tendency to roll so a towel placed in a ring around the animal will help limit movement.

The patient's POTZ must be maintained throughout the procedure as a full and rapid recovery may depend on this.

Pre-medication

A variety of drugs are available on the market to provide chemical restraint or sedation, but many have limited use in reptiles and benefits are not widely acknowledged.

Induction and maintenance

It can take up to 40 minutes to reach a surgical plane of anaesthesia in some chelonia.

Injectable agents

The main concern when using injectable anaesthetics is their unpredictable effect on a metabolism that is very slow, resulting in some patients taking hours to days to recover fully from the anaesthetic. If injectables are used then one of the preferred routes is IV.

One of the most widely used and supported injectable anaesthetics is **Propofal** (Rapinovet™ Schering-Plough) which can be administered at a rate of 10–14 mg/kg IV.

Inhalation agents

These have several advantages over injectable forms of anaesthesia especially when the patient is intubated and connected to a calibrated vaporiser and anaesthetic circuit.

Isoflurane (Isoflo) seems to be the inhalation agent of choice as it provides quick and smooth induction, good depth of anaesthesia and rapid recovery especially when compared to injectables and other inhalation agents available. It is also licensed for use in reptiles.

Once the patient is anaesthetised it should be intubated and an endotrachael tube secured, and maintained on oxygen and inhalant agent (2–4% isoflurane being used as a suggested rate).

The benefits of maintaining chelonia on an inhalant agent are as follows:

- The depth of anaesthesia can be controlled.
- Supplementary oxygen is being supplied and if necessary allowing for positive pressure ventilation.
- Recovery once anaesthetic gas flow is terminated is more rapid compared to injectable agents.

Monitoring the anaesthetised patient

As for any mammal, the reptilian patient must be closely monitored and findings recorded throughout the surgical procedure and period of anaesthesia.

Suggested routine checks include:

- The temperature of the patient must be maintained and the use of a low-wattage heat mat or waterbed to maintain a core preferred body temperature is recommended.
- Observation of certain parameters that can be used to check the depth and plane of anaesthesia and condition of patient are listed below.

Surgical plane of anaesthesia

This has been achieved when:

- there is no response when the foot is squeezed (pedal withdrawal)
- the neck can be extended without the patient pulling it back into the shell
- the corneal reflex is still present; if not the patient is excessively deep.

At a surgical plane many patients will lose the ability to ventilate spontaneously, so positive pressure ventilation has to be undertaken.

Useful equipment in monitoring the anaesthetised patient

Monitoring equipment is particularly valuable when observing the anaesthetised patient, especially in chelonia, as the shell makes it very difficult to visualise heart beat, respiratory rate, etc.

A small tipped **digital thermometer** or **rectal probe** can be used to monitor cloacal temperature.

A **Doppler flow meter** is useful for gauging blood flow, because the three chambers of the heart make little sound, making auscultation difficult. The Doppler needs to be positioned over the thoracic inlet region (base of neck in line with shoulder) and directed toward the heart at the mid-line and taped in place.

An **electrocardiograph** (ECG) can be used to monitor the heart's electroconductivity, but the QRS pattern is somewhat different to that seen in mammals. The heart rate should remain steady throughout the procedure.

A **pulse oximeter** (cloacal or oesophageal) which measures the pulse and arterial oxygen saturation is also proving useful in veterinary practice and can be adapted for reptiles.

The mucous membrane colour can be observed by looking at the cloacal tissue at the vent.

GENERAL SURGICAL NURSING AND POST-OPERATIVE CARE AND NURSING

The general techniques applied when nursing surgical feline and canine patients can be used for reptiles:

• Warmed pre-operative fluids are important, especially for very sick or dehydrated patients.
• Any intra-operative fluids must be warmed to prevent hypothermia.
• Preparation and surgical time must be kept to a minimum to reduce the period of anaesthesia.
• All surgical procedures must be performed using an aseptic technique.
• Sterile waterproof plastic drapes are a good alternative to cloth as they can be cut to size, fenestrated and if moulded round the patient allow observations to be carried out. They also prevent the patient from getting wet.
• Blood loss should be kept to a minimum using diathermy, radiosurgery or hemoclips.

• Pre- and post-operative analgesia can be administered; opiates seem to have little beneficial effect on the reptile patient compared to non-steroidal anti-inflammatory drugs, providing the most appropriate level of analgesia.
• Antibiotics can be given pre- and post-operatively; the choice will depend on the individual and condition treated.
• Recovery should be in a quiet environment with the temperature set at the higher end of the patient's POTZ.
• Regular checks of the environmental temperature are necessary to prevent overheating the patient, especially if it is recumbent and unable to move about the cage. If this occurs the patient's metabolic rate will increase as will its demand for oxygen.

Tip: During recovery, the patient may be stimulated to take a breath by pinching the tail or toes.

• Observations of the patient and frequent notes should be made about the patient's recovery, environmental parameters and checks made on indwelling catheters for fluid therapy, drains or pharyngostomy tubes if inserted.
• Suture removal can be carried out in 4–6 weeks; ideally, skin edges should be everted.
• To allow a scab to form, swimming should be avoided for at least 7–14 days with the patient being allowed access to water for feeding and hydration.
• To allow full recovery hibernation should be avoided for at least 6 months after surgery.

Summary

To ensure proper metabolic function the patient should be maintained within its optimum temperature range. During anaesthesia the patient should be intubated and assisted ventilation performed. The patient's depth of anaesthesia and vital signs must be carefully monitored and recorded throughout the surgical procedure, and post-operative checks must be made.

COMMONLY ENCOUNTERED PROBLEMS AND DISEASES OF CHELONIA

Table 4.3 sets out some of the more commonly encountered problems, their cause, clinical signs and suggested treatments. Many of the conditions described can be attributed to poor husbandry and nutritional provision. As suggested for snakes and lizards, a comprehensive case history needs to be obtained, especially regarding how the chelonia is housed and diet offered.

CASE HISTORY 1

Post-hibernation anorexia

This is one of the most common problems encountered by the veterinary nurse and in covering this particular case it is important to impress upon the nurse the need to understand why it occurs and how it can be prevented.

Patient

Male Mediterranean tortoise (*Testudo graeca*) named Trundle, in excess of 30 years of age.

History

The tortoise came out of hibernation mid-February, had not eaten for 2 weeks and was very lethargic and weak.

Trundle had been hibernating in the attic in a wooden box (that the owner had made) with air holes on two sides and with newspaper and hay as bedding materials.

There had been no pre-hibernation preparation and the owner had simply waited for the tortoise to 'dig itself' in the garden before placing it in the hibernation box (mid-October). No checks had been made on the tortoise during the hibernation period. Before bringing the tortoise out of hibernation, the owner waited until he could hear rustling coming from the box.

Post-hibernation care

The tortoise was given a bath in warm water, his eyes were bathed and the owner waited for him to evacuate the white creamy paste which was the stored urate.

The tortoise was released into the garden and offered salad foods such as lettuce, cucumber and tomato, but no other supplementation.

The owner had a specially dedicated garden for the tortoise, in which grew little gem lettuces, radishes, cucumbers, courgettes, tomatoes, nasturtiums, strawberries and weeds, including grass, dandelions, sow thistle and clover. No other supplements were given. The tortoise had free range of the garden and a wooden hide was provided but never used. The tortoise preferred 'digging in' under the apple tree.

Identifying the problem

Why post-hibernation anorexia occurs

The main reason is that the UK climate is not suitable for the Mediterranean tortoise, and the traditional methods of keeping these creatures are flawed (see references made under heating, lighting and nutrition). The majority of the wild caught tortoises that are still alive in the UK are barely surviving, and those that are, are normally the ones with darker pigmented shells, which are able to absorb heat more efficiently, therefore maintaining their body temperature to the lower end of their preferred range.

During hibernation the temperature should be kept at a constant 4–5°C; higher temperatures will cause the tortoise to stir and start to burn off valuable energy reserves. The by-product of this process is urea which is stored in the kidneys in the form of uric acid (urates). If this continues then by the time the tortoise awakes from hibernation its energy stores are depleted. It fails to get the normal glucose boost that enables the tortoise to move, bask and find food. The increase in stored urate levels will depress the appetite resulting in an anorexic tortoise.

Tip: A healthy adult can be expected to lose about 1% of its body weight during each month of hibernation. A hatchling will lose much more and, if greater than 10%, must be brought out of hibernation.

Table 4.3 Common problems and diseases

Common problem	Cause	Signs	Treatment	Other information
Metabolic bone disease (MBD) (this can take on many forms according to life stage of the chelonia and each will be discussed separately)	Poor environmental conditions including inadequate heating and poor UVB provision. Diet high in protein or high in phosphorus and lacking in calcium or vitamin D₃	Hypocalcaemia. Soft shell. Shell deformities. Overgrown rhamphotheca (Fig. 4.6) (chelonia beak) and nails. Shell deformities. Abnormal gait and movement	Correct the nutritional imbalances and environmental factors such as heat and access to good UVB	For more detail on specific signs and problems associated with MBD see separate sections
Hypocalcaemia. Common cause of death in most UK bred tortoises	Main cause is diet lacking in calcium but also associated with lack of vitamin D, high phosphorus diet and lack of good quality UVB	*Hatchlings* **Acute problem**, soft spongy shell, edges of the mouth fail to harden, inappetance. Untreated shell haemorrhages, lung collapse and death. Diet too rich in protein pyramidal growth of scutes on the carapace (lumpy shell see Fig. 4.7) *Juvenile tortoise* **Chronic problem**, shell deformities not softness, flattened shell appearance, dip in rear of carapace, scutes raised, shell feels soft/spongy, carapace can appear too small for the chelonia, edge of carapace may curl dorsally, reduced weight gain and growth, deformed beak and overgrown nails, problems walking due to plastron deformities around the hindlimbs. X-ray poor mineralisation of bone *Adult imported tortoise* **Chronic problem**, poor shell growth, shape and hardness, claws are curved or bent rather than straight, beak overgrown, shell damage prolonged poor healing or may not heal, poor	Depends on the signs and progression of the disease *Hatchlings* **Mild cases**, especially if being offered a high protein diet – increase calcium uptake and slow growth (see feeding section main text) **Moderate case**, shell is only partially soft or in severe cases that are still bright and able to move – then aggressive dietary management has to be employed with calcium, vitamin D₃ and UVB access being increased. There is a calcium-based product on the market (ESU Pro CAL D3 500) (Fig. 3.8 in Lizards and snakes) which includes vitamin D₃ and in my own experiences tortoises readily eat this powder. Be warned this condition can take months to rectify. **For severe cases** that are debilitated they will require injections of calcium borogluconate and vitamin D₃ as well as being kept in the correct environmental conditions. As jaw will be soft they need tube feeding but if the condition is so	*Juvenile tortoise* If excess protein intake a cause of the problem then consideration should be given to effect on kidney and liver. Flattening of the shell can cause respiratory problems, as expansion of the lungs is hindered. Unfortunately once the deformities are established little can be done to alter this.

(continued)

Table 4.3 (continued)

Common problem	Cause	Signs	Treatment	Other information
		locomotion animal tends to rub plastron against the ground or more severe cases unable to propel itself forward. Predispose to other disease because depressed immune system (discussed in the text)	severe and some of the more terminal signs are presented euthanasia should be considered. *Juvenile tortoise* Dietary correction and environmental factors *Adult tortoise* Dietary and environmental management as before If overgrown beak this will need to be clipped and shaped. Unfortunately once the deformities are established little can be done to alter this	
Hypovitaminosis A	Lack of dietary vitamin A Possible problems with vitamin A metabolism and utilisation from ingested sources Problem seen in tortoises and terrapins	Main function of vitamin A is to maintain the integrity of the skin and epithelium, especially that lining the respiratory tract and eye tissues Deficiency results in: flaky skin, poor wound healing and secondary infections, anorexia, lethargy, weight loss, swollen eyelids, irritation around the eyes, solid purulent matter underneath the eye lids if not treated, respiratory problems, renal and liver problems. Chronic condition can cause thickening of the skin	In acute cases injection of vitamin A weekly for 2–6 weeks depending on severity Changes to dietary regime include food stuffs rich in vitamin A such as dark leafy greens, yellow or orange coloured fruits and vegetables, for carnivorous species whole mice, fish as the prey's liver will act as a good source of vitamin A Add multivitamin supplement to the diet every other day for 2 weeks, then reduce to twice weekly for a month In mild cases the addition of multivitamin supplement in the diet every 2–3 days may suffice along with appropriate dietary management If the chelonia is anorexic and very debilitated then tube feeding and fluid support will be required Eye infections will need to be treated with the appropriate antibiotics as will respiratory infections	If an eye infection does not clear up with treatment then hypovitaminosis A should be considered Care must be taken not to overdose vitamin A as this can cause another set of problems

Condition		Clinical signs	Treatment	Notes
Runny nose syndrome Common problem in UK tortoises	Common problem in tortoises with multifactorial aetiology and untreated can be fatal Commonly identified pathogens associated: Gram-negative bacteria, *Pseudomonas*, *Citrobacteria*, *Klebsiella*, fungal agents and herpes virus Tortoises can be latent carriers so mixing tortoises from different geographical regions must be discouraged Consider general health of tortoise; poor diet and husbandry leads to susceptible immune system A secondary bacterial infection can intensify clinical signs	Clear watery discharge from the nostrils, occasionally sneezing If disease progresses to the lungs breathing becomes audible and very noisy, open mouth breathing, laboured breathing, lethargy, depression, anorexia	Severe cases will require supportive therapy such as fluids, supplementary heat and lots of nursing care Assisted feeding Parenteral antibiotics Nasal drops Vitamin A injections It may take up to 3–4 days before any significant improvement is seen	A healthy tortoise should NOT have a wet nose Hypovitaminosis must also be considered here This is a highly contagious disease and the patient should be isolated. Remember chelonia do not posess a diaphragm and are unable to cough and swallow excess mucus produced in the lungs. This can cause these types of infections to progress and cause pneumonia **Tip:** when administering nasal drops to chelonia use a small syringe and catheter or extend head, squirt drops in the mouth and simultaneously let go of the head. As the head retracts back into the carapace it will force the fluid from the mouth down the nostrils! Terrapins seen with this disease may float on one side if one lung is more affected that the other
Infectious stomatitis (mouth rot)	Common condition seen in the Mediterranean tortoise especially if in poor condition post hibernation Associated with bacterial infection (Gram-negative, commonly *Pseudomonas*) or virus such as herpes virus	Early signs are often overlooked Reddening inside the mouth, blistering which commonly occurs inside lower jaw under the tongue As problem progresses tongue becomes swollen, mouth fills with mucus and a discharge resembling cottage cheese seen Osteomyelitis if infection attacks jaw bone, inappetance and death if not treated	Mild cases – topical applications of Betadine gargle and mouthwash can be applied once a day to the affected area More severe cases will require antibiotic treatment; swabs can be taken to identify pathogen and treatment Check for fungal invasion, e.g. *Candida* Severe cases – aggressive antibiotic treatment and supportive therapy to prevent dehydration	Even if treatment successful, in severe cases where osteomyelitis seen the problem can reoccur
Shell rot	Can be seen in all chelonia Can be due to fungal or bacterial infection normally anaerobic Gram-negative	Discoloration especially around areas of shell damage. Aquatic and semi-aquatic shell appears paler.	Remove all affected shell until healthy tissue seen. The area will need to be scrubbed daily using a tooth	One of the common causes of shell trauma is oversexed males butting each other or males continually ramming

(continued)

Table 4.3 (continued)

Common problem	Cause	Signs	Treatment	Other information
	Fungus or bacteria gain entry due to shell trauma. Other contributing factors include poor hygiene in both terrestrial and aquatic chelonia, high humidity, low temperature, lack of UV light, inadequate diet, overcrowding, and lack of basking sites in terrapins and turtles	Dry flaking of shell or soft tissue. Bacterial infections: affected areas appear wet and obnoxious odour with blood and purulent discharges. Fungal infections appear dryer and less smelly than the bacterial infections. The infection can spread under scutes and lead to a deep infection with much tissue damage	or nailbrush for at least 5 minutes with antibacterial scrub such as Hibiscrub, povidone-iodine; continue for at least 4–6 weeks. Swabs may need to be taken for culture and sensitivity and antibiotic treatment administered. If abscesses form these will need to be flushed out and antibiotics given. Note: healing might take weeks or in extreme cases years. The shell can be considered free from disease when it is smooth, dry and free from odour and discharge. The animal may be permanently scarred. The very sick chelonia will need supportive therapy including assisted feeding and fluid therapy	into the rear end of the female, so it is advisable to keep chelonia separate. Environmental condition and diet must also be corrected before the chelonia can be discharged. During hospitalisation the provision of heat,[1] and hygiene and nursing support is essential for recovery. If untreated septicaemia will ensue and subsequent death. Suggested antimicrobial treatment Fungal: oral dosing of ketaconazole (20 mg/kg/day). Bacterial: amikacin (Amikin paediatric) 10 mg/kg/every other day for 3 days
Endoparasites	Large grey ascarids *Angusticaecum* spp. Small thread-like oxyurid-type nematodes	Healthy tortoise – few physical signs apart from seeing them passed in faeces. Faecal smear will show presence of eggs. Death in hatchlings with large infestations	Oral dosage of anthelmintics Panacur (fenbendazole 50 mg/kg) or Systamex (oxfendazole 65 mg/kg). Two doses will need to be administered via stomach tube with an interval of 14 days between each dose. If problems stomach tubing place Panacur granules or paste in food	Worming should be carried out on a regular basis, especially if tortoises kept in groups or small areas. Mediterranean tortoises should be wormed prior to hibernation. Advisable to keep hatchlings away from pasture grazed on by adults as this is a source of infection
Ear abscess	Seen in tortoises, terrapins and box turtles. Bacterial infections of the middle ear. Gain entry via mouth and travel along Eustachian tube. Poor husbandry, sub-optimal	Large painful swellings over ear drum (normal slightly concave). Head tilting and circling	Surgery to incise the abscess, remove pus and flush cavity. Antimicrobial therapy given by injection	Husbandry and diet will need to be re-evaluated. In some cases 'seeding out' of the blood due to septicaemia manifests itself as abscesses and these will need to be treated using systemic antibiotics

	Cause	Clinical signs	Treatment	Notes
	temperatures and hygiene, especially poor water filtration In aquatic species vitamin A deficiency Depressed immune system			Note: healthy tortoises do **NOT** get abscesses
Trauma	Trauma to the shell is often caused by: chelonia being dropped or manhandled by young children, chewed by a dog (especially if young or suffering from hypocalcaemia), tortoise coming in contact with the lawn mower or strimmer	Damage to shell, shock makes the tortoise lethargic and lowers blood pressure, haemorrhage (external haemorrhage easy to identify, internal more problematic so need to observe behaviour and other parameters such as mucous membrane colour), internal organ damage difficult to assess, lung damage quite common Secondary infection should be considered	Stem haemorrhage Fluid therapy X-rays may need to be taken to establish extent of damage When patient stabilised flush wounds using antibacterial scrub, remove debris Dose antibiotics and anti-inflammatory drugs prevent infection and aid shock Repair lung damage and consider other internal injuries. Tissue fluid will seep from wounds. This may last for a few days; once stopped shell repair will be able to commence Shell repair carried out using resin patches, which can be left in place for anything between 6–12 months depending on health status of the tortoise prior to injury Very severe damage can be repaired using orthopaedic techniques	A damaged shell can take 1–2 years to heal Chelonia that are recovering from a fractured shell should not be allowed to hibernate. Extensive trauma to the shell may never fill completely. In an adult chelonia patches can be left in place indefinitely. In young animals to allow for growth patches must be removed after 6 months
Penile prolapse	Mainly seen in juvenile tortoises that have become sexually active and spend most of the day with the penis extruded	Here the penis protrudes from the cloaca for a prolonged period	Penis can be manually replaced but usually only temporary and will prolapse again. Aim to prevent penis drying out and becoming infected by keeping penis clean and lubricated (KY jelly and povidone-iodine). Condition settles down in time If penis suffers injury or becomes infected it must be treated and kept clean and lubricated as before Addition of systemic antibiotics and manually replace once inflammation has subsided	Important not to replace a dirty or infected penis If penis continues to prolapse, may necessitate a purse string suture around the cloaca, which can be removed in a few days

(continued)

Table 4.3 *(continued)*

Common problem	Cause	Signs	Treatment	Other information
			Severe infections – some or all of the organ may have to be removed	
Dystocia	Poor environmental conditions Lack of laying sites Temperature too low for tortoise to lay eggs Overcrowding and tortoise feels stressed Poor diet, especially lack of calcium Oversized eggs	Virtually impossible to detect without use of a radiograph but signs that suggest problem include: gestation period exceeded, depression, anorexia, straining, cloacal swelling	Injection of oxytocin (5 iu/kg) should see results in approximately 1 hour, during which tortoise must be kept at its POTZ. If initial injection fails, recommended that tortoise be fed calcium supplementation for 2 days before further dose at a higher rate of (10 iu/kg) After receiving oxytocin tortoise should be placed in a bath of warm water, this has proven beneficial in helping tortoise expel eggs Surgical intervention to be considered if above therapy failed, eggs stuck or cracked in the pelvis, and only after a period of calcium supplementation and increased environmental temperatures If surgery is to be undertaken, a plastronotomy and celiotomy followed by a salpingotomy will have to be performed	Compared to snakes and lizards chelonia respond well to oxytocin injections Problems more commonly seen in tortoises due to lay in autumn Tortoise should not be allowed to hibernate with eggs inside as the eggs become larger and more calcified, making removal more problematic

[1] Sick chelonia will need to be hospitalised and kept at temperatures at the higher range of their POTZ. This will encourage metabolism of drug therapy and stimulate their own metabolism. Many of the problems identified in the Mediterranean tortoise are due to the fact that it is not well adapted to the UK climate; they are kept in sub-optimal temperatures and as a result are suffering from immunosuppression.

Normally, the activity of basking, eating and drinking post hibernation will rectify the energy imbalance and allow stored urates to be passed in the form of a creamy white paste being voided shortly after hibernation, usually after a bath and a long drink of water.

Post-hibernation anorexia can also be the result of a more gradual build up of urates in the kidneys brought about by the tortoise suffering a series of 'not so good' summers and hibernation where energy levels are slowly being reduced and urate levels increased.

The severity of the anorexia will depend on the amount of urate stored in the kidneys and loss of body tissue.

Assessing the patient

History and weight of the tortoise are probably the best indications of the severity of the problem. The Jackson ratio has been the main tool for evaluating the body condition of the Mediterranean tortoise, but a method used by many veterinary surgeons and herpetologists is shown below.

Box 4.1 outlines a method of calculating a Mediterranean tortoise's weight to length ratio and, therefore, its overall health status.

Box 4.1 Weight to length ratio calculation

- Take the measurements in centimetres of the carapace length in a straight line from the nuchal to the supracaudal scute (see Anatomy and physiology)
- Calculate the weight in grams
- Divide the weight by the length in centimetres cubed, as shown below:

$$\frac{\text{Weight in grams}}{\text{Length in centimetre cubed}}$$

- In a healthy tortoise, if the carapace length is less than 15 cm, the ratio is between 0.21 and 0.23
- In a healthy tortoise, if the carapace length is greater than 15 cm, the ratio is between 0.22 and 0.25
- Anorexia will reduce the ratio:
  - below 0.20 requires attention
  - below 0.18 requires urgent attention
  - at 0.15 death occurs.

(Pursall 1995)

Treatment

On admission Trundle was weighed and his length measured. Carapace length was 19 cm and weight was 1221 g. His ratio worked out as 0.1780 (between 0.18 and 0.17).

1. After being weighed and checked for other associated problems, i.e. stomatitis, shell rot and respiratory problems, Trundle was placed in a hospital vivarium with an ambient temperature of 27–30°C (80–86°F) and a basking area with UVB strip light temperature approximately 35°C (95°F).
2. Once the tortoise had 'warmed up' so that the shell felt warm, it was given a multivitamin injection and then placed in a bath of warm water (cat litter trays are best for this).
3. The tortoise was left in here for approximately 10 minutes and observed for drinking (see notes on fluid intake under Nutrition). *Drinking is important not only for rehydration but also to flush out the stored urate.*
4. The tortoise was weighed again and weight recorded (check for fluid intake).
5. As the tortoise had not drunk, it was stomach tubed using 10 ml of **Critical Care formula** (see Fig. 3.10, Lizards and snakes) and then placed back in the vivarium under the heat lamp. Details of stomach tubing are given in Figure 4.8a,b,c.
6. The process was repeated 6 hours later, again using 10 ml of **Critical Care formula**.
7. The lighting system was placed on a timer providing a 13-hour photoperiod and basking area. Night-time temperatures were monitored and were kept between 20 and 25°C (68–77°F) (a heat mat or red light bulb can provide this).
8. The above regime continued for 2 weeks until the tortoise started eating voluntarily and normal urate was seen.
9. In general, the anorexic tortoise needs to be kept in a quiet environment with minimal handling to reduce stress.
10. Trundle was discharged after spending 3 weeks in the surgery. His owner was sent home with a new husbandry and feeding regime, and the tortoise continued coming in for weekly weight assessments until his ideal ratio was achieved.

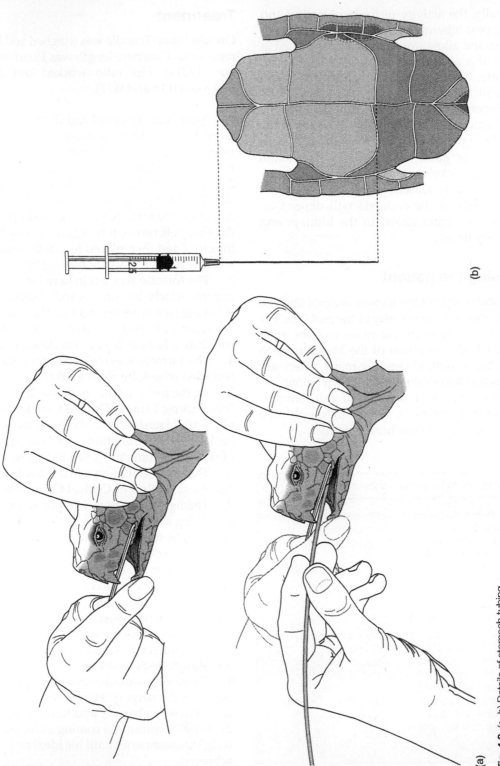

Fig. 4.8 (a, b) Details of stomach tubing.

Stomach tubing

A useful guide to help calculate the amount to feed is as follows:

$$\frac{\text{Carapace length in cm cubed}}{333}$$

Total amount should be divided and given at two separate feedings 4–8 hours apart (Pursall 1995, p. 55):

1. As the stomach is positioned midway down the plastron measure for the feeding tube (urinary catheters are ideal for this) from the caudal end of the abdominal shield to just beyond the gular notch and mark.
2. Hold the chelonia at 45° angle as shown in (a) extend the neck and hold behind the mandible.
3. The neck must be fully extended to ensure the oesophagus is straightened.
4. The mouth will need to be opened and a gag inserted. The back of a teaspoon works well and as blunt does not cause any damage; it is also a useful tool when trying to get a stubborn mouth open.
5. Insert the pre-filled lubricated tube.
6. When inserting run the tube in line with the roof of the mouth and into the oesophagus. The glottis should be easy to see and therefore avoided!
7. When the demarcation line is reached slowly depress the plunger and the food will empty into the stomach.
8. Slowly withdraw tube.
9. Care must be taken not to overfill the stomach. If this happens then food will 'well up' into the mouth.
10. Once the procedure has been completed the tortoise needs to be placed in the hospital vivarium under the lamp and left quietly to recover.
11. The process can be repeated again in approximately 4–8 hours.

Other suitable foods can be vegetable baby food, liquidised salad and green leaf vegetables that will go through a catheter.

If the tortoise is very debilitated a pharygostomy tube can be inserted and food given directly into the stomach. These are generally well tolerated by most chelonia and can be removed once the tortoise is eating on its own.

Fig. 4.8 (c) Details of stomach tubing.

Box 4.2 gives details on pre- and post-hibernation procedures for the Mediterranean tortoise.

CASE HISTORY 2

Paraphimosis in a Mediterranean tortoise

Patient

Male spur thigh tortoise (Greek) (*Testudo graeca*) named Frank, approximately 4 years of age, 125 mm in length and weighing 527 g.

Presenting signs

Frank was admitted to the surgery with a prolapsed penis; the owners initially thought it to be a rectal prolapse. Frank is housed with another Greek tortoise and the owners had seen him repeatedly mounting and knocking his friend (for more details on this condition see Table 4.3).

Examination

Male chelonia have a large fleshy penis, which appears dark purple to black. Normally the penis

Box 4.2 Pre- and post-hibernation care

All owners of Mediterranean tortoises need to be aware of good pre- and post-hibernation routines.

Pre-hibernation preparations (October)

● The tortoise should be wormed and checked to confirm good health.
● Weight should be recorded (see Box 4.1). Regarding weight ratios, if weight falls in one of the danger areas then do not hibernate.
● Food should be withheld for a minimum of 3 weeks prior to hibernation; this will ensure no undigested food is in the digestive tract (causes bacterial overgrowth)
● The tortoise should be bathed daily for 2 weeks in 1.5 inches of warm water; this will ensure hydration (see Table 4.2 for anatomy and physiology of the urogenital system)
● The tortoise should be weighed once more before placing into hibernation.

During hibernation

● The temperature has to be maintained at 4–5°C; anything above 10°C will cause the tortoise to stir and use up valuable energy stores, lower will cause the tortoise to freeze
● A maximum/minimum digital thermometer placed on the outside of the box will allow for constant checks to be made of the environment temperature
● It is also recommended that the tortoise is weighed regularly (some experts suggest every week) and if the ratio falls within the critical levels, the tortoise must be taken out of hibernation
● The position should be where the tortoise will not be exposed to extremes of temperature, exhaust fumes or rodents, and can easily be accessed and checked
● Ventilated polystyrene boxes lined with shredded paper are ideal for hibernating tortoises and for extra protection can be placed in a ventilated outer wooden box, again surrounded by shredded paper or polystyrene chips
● Attach a digital max/min thermometer to the outside
● Length of time spent in hibernation should be no more than 20 weeks, ideally 6–10 weeks.

Post hibernation

The aim is to get the tortoise feeding, so as soon as it emerges it needs to be placed in a bright, hot enclosure and bathed daily in warm water.

Hibernating hatchlings

Hatchling tortoises can be placed outside during the summer months as long as they have been acclimatised. This is achieved by slowly reducing the temperature in their vivariums before placing them outdoors. It is recommended that young tortoises do not spend the night outside, especially during early spring and autumn, and that they are placed back in their vivariums during cooler spells.

Before hibernating the tortoise, the above must be achieved and the tortoise needs to weigh at least 50 g or use the ratio calculations in Box 4.1. A short hibernating period is recommended (1 month) and checks made throughout the period, and any significant weight loss must result in the tortoise being taken out of hibernation.

Hibernation is a natural part of a Mediterranean tortoise's yearly cycle and has been reported to aid their immune system. A main consideration is that in the wild, the period of hibernation would normally be 6–8 weeks, not 4–5 months.

sits in the base of the tail, but when they become excited the penis is everted, and prolonged periods of stimulus can cause the penis to remain engorged and exposed. The chelonia penis only serves as a copulatory organ with no urethra or urinary function.

Frank's penis was swollen, dry and covered in debris; due to the excessive swelling Frank was unable to retract his penis so he was admitted for treatment.

Treatment

The penis was cleaned using a 2.5% solution of povidone-iodine. No signs of trauma were visible. To keep the penis lubricated and to prevent further drying out, the penis was covered with obstetric gel. Frank was then placed in a hospital vivarium fitted with UV light and heat source, providing a thermal gradient and basking area. Food and water were also offered. The vivarium was lined with paper so the prolapsed penis would not get soiled.

Frank was hospitalised for 5 days and started on a course of the systemic antibiotic ceftazidime (Fortum) 25 mg/kg intramuscularly every third day.

The penis was washed with povidone-iodine twice a day and lubricated frequently throughout the day.

By the third day of Frank's hospitalisation the swelling had considerably reduced and the penis was manually manipulated back into the cloaca (Fig. 4.9).

He remained in hospital for a further 2 days for observation.

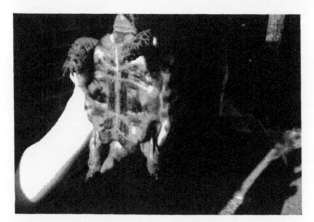

Fig. 4.9 Prolapsed tortoise penis after treatment.

The penis remained inverted and he was discharged from the hospital.

Discharge and advice

To decrease Frank's stimulus to mate, his owners were recommended to keep Frank away from the other male tortoise.

It was highlighted that this is a problem seen in juvenile tortoises and that it may reoccur.

The owners were given advice on how to treat a further prolapse:

1. To keep the penis clean using a dilute povidone.

2. To keep the penis lubricated with obstetric gel or KY jelly (Johnson and Johnson).
3. To prevent trauma, especially as other tortoises are attracted to the exteriorised organ and can bite it.
4. To return to the surgery where the prolapse will be reduced and a cloacal pursestring suture used to hold the penis in place.
5. The owners were warned that if the penis was damaged and infected then amputation of the organ might have to be considered.

Frank was discharged, but unfortunately he continued to prolapse, which the owners found very difficult to cope with, so Frank was rehomed.

REFERENCES

Mader DR 1996 Reptile medicine and surgery. W.B. Saunders, Philadelphia
Pursall B 1995. The guide to owning a Mediterranean tortoise. TFH, Havant

FURTHER READING

Fenwick H Taking care of tortoises, their eggs and hatchlings. Published by H. Fenwick, Cambridgeshire Herplife web site: www.herplife.co.uk
Mara WP Map turtles and diamond back terrapins. TFH, Havant

SECTION 3

Bird care

Bird care

Introduction

Veterinary nurse training covers many different areas and the pressure to complete the training in the required time means that some subjects are covered in more depth that others. Knowledge of birds (both wild and domestic) and their care is an area that receives less coverage than some others. For many practices, this may be reflective of the amount of avian patients treated. However, if even only a handful of birds are seen in a year, when faced with the actuality of a bird in a hospital cage, it is a comfort to have as much information as possible.

It is difficult to discuss wild and domestic birds as one category (the introduction to wildlife rehabilitation deals with wild birds more effectively); however, there are a couple of points to be made that apply equally to both.

Species identification

Whilst it is not incumbent upon the veterinary nurse to be able to recognise every species of bird that may be put before her/him, there is a need to be able to identify the more commonly encountered species for two main reasons:

1. The diet required by a quail, for example, is significantly different from that of a mynah bird. Most falcons, e.g. a kestrel, require a stump of wood for a perch, whereas most hawks, e.g. a sparrow hawk, prefer a branch.
2. It is difficult to regain kudos with a rescue centre when you have handed them what you thought was a thrush only to be told it is a young blackbird. Far better to impress Mrs Jones with your knowledge that she owns a peach faced love bird and not a large budgie.

To treat or not to treat

There is no question that over the last few years there have been huge improvements in our ability to treat avian patients and along with this comes an increased expectation by the clients as to the level of veterinary care. However, consideration must be given to quality of life. This is particularly important when applied to birds. A bird that is unable to fly is severely disabled. Some domestic species are able to tolerate this better than others, e.g. chickens; however, serious thought must be given to the question:

Just because we can treat it, should we?

This becomes even more poignant when applied to wild birds, as not only is their natural method of locomotion severely undermined, but they are condemned to a life of captivity to which they are not accustomed.

These chapters aim to give the veterinary nurse a basic knowledge of how to provide for an avian patient entrusted to her/his care as it is usually the nurses that have the responsibility of ensuring that the care, i.e. the accommodation, feeding, administration of drugs, etc., is carried out.

It cannot be overemphasised that if the nurse has the knowledge of the special requirements of these species, it will significantly improve their chances of recovery.

Chapter 5

Cage birds

Emma Brooks

INTRODUCTION

The success of treating a critical avian patient relies heavily on the environment in which the bird must recover (Loudis & Sutherland-Smith 1994). In an ideal world there should be a separate avian ward away from any noisy dogs and cats.

When housing the sick bird the environmental temperature should be between 26 and 32°C (80–90°F). Patients should be viewed easily from across a room or through a window, so as to minimise the stress of excessive disturbance. The cage size needs to be adequate for the size of the bird; a budgerigar is fine in a 'budgie' cage, but would you put a cockatoo in the same sized cage?

There must be minimal opportunity for disease transmission. Providing good ventilation and isolated air space for each bird is essential. Equipment must be separate and easily cleaned for each bird. There needs to be a good disinfection regime in place; daily changing of bedding, food, water, etc; at least daily disinfection and cleaning of the patient's cage and equipment. All infectious cases must be isolated and zoonotic diseases should be considered.

ANATOMY OF THE BIRD

Mammals and birds are endothermic, meaning warm blooded. These animals are able to maintain their own body temperatures regardless of their surroundings, within certain limits.

There are 28 different orders of bird; however the ones most likely to be presented at a veterinary practice fall into one of the following categories:

- Psittaciformes – budgerigars and parrots
- Passeriformes – perching birds, canaries and finches
- Falconiformes – hawks and falcons
- Strigiformes – owls
- Galliformes – domestic fowl and quail
- Anseriformes – ducks, geese and swans.

To nurse the avian patient, you must first understand their anatomy (Figs 5.1 & 5.2). Although they follow the vertebrate pattern, there are several differences from other vertebrates.

Skeleton and muscles

The bones have thin cortices and some are pneumatised. This means that the bones contain an air sac as an extension of the respiratory system.

The number of joints is greatly reduced to facilitate flying. However, they do have very flexible necks so that their beaks can reach all parts of their bodies.

The sternum (keel bone) is enlarged to cater for the bulky flight muscles. In addition, the weight of the skull is lightened by reducing the maxillary region and by the fact that birds have no teeth.

The pelvis is also modified to allow the passing of an egg and birds have an open pubis rather than a symphysis.

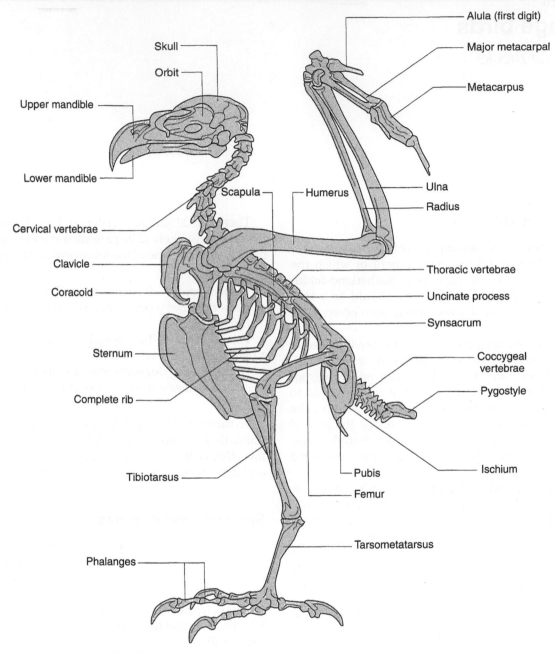

Fig. 5.1 Skeletal system of a bird.

There is a quadrate bone between each dentary and two joints between the upper and lower jaw. This allows backward and forward movement, and it is well developed in parrots. There is also a joint between the skull and upper part of the beak, which is called the craniofacial hinge.

Finally, the number of digits in the forelimb (wing) is reduced to two.

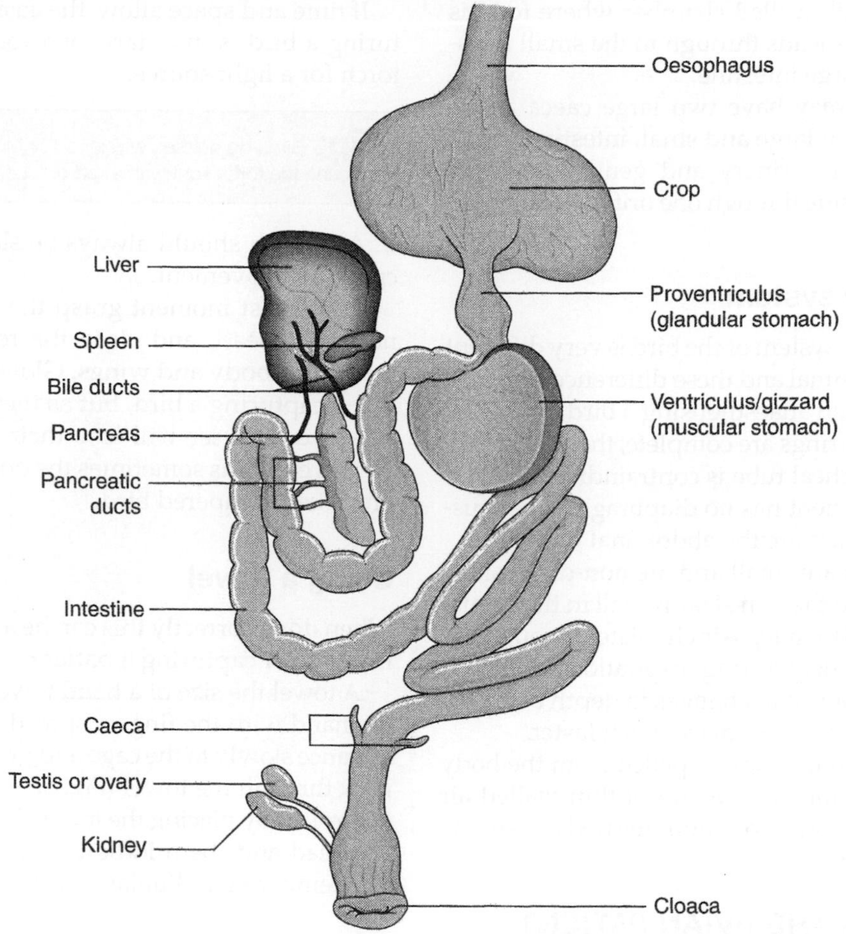

Fig. 5.2 Alimentary canal of a bird.

Feathers

Birds' plumage is composed of keratin. This provides lightweight, strong feathers, which helps insulate the bird.

The feathers are divided into several groups:

- Flight feathers – long and rigid.
- Contour feathers – make up outer layer of feathers and are shorter and more flexible.
- Down feather and filoplumes – lie beneath contour feathers and provide insulation.

To keep the feathers in good order, birds have a preen gland at the top of the tail. Some birds do not have a preen gland.

Cockatoos and cockatiels produce a fine dust from their feathers to keep their plumage in order.

It is very important to protect feathers when hospitalised so as to minimise damage to plumage.

Gastrointestinal tract

As birds have no teeth, some will hold food with their feet and tear it with their beak, whilst others swallow it whole.

In most species there is a diverticulum of the oesophagus in the ventral neck. This is called the crop and is used as a storage organ.

The stomach is divided into a proventriculus, the glandular stomach, and the ventriculus (gizzard), a thick walled chamber where food is ground up. This leads through to the small intestine, then the large intestine.

Some birds may have two large caeca at the junction between large and small intestines.

The digestive, urinary and genital tracts all open to the outside through one orifice – the cloaca or vent.

Respiratory system

The respiratory system of the bird is very different to that of a mammal and these differences must be considered when anaesthetising a bird.

The tracheal rings are complete; therefore, cuffing of endotracheal tube is contraindicated.

An avian patient has no diaphragm. The muscles of respiration are the abdominal muscles.

Birds' lungs are small and are non-distensible. They lie close to the dorsal body wall in the cranial part of the body cavity. Air circulates through the lungs continuously during inspiration and expiration. This means that changes in depth of anaesthesia are likely to take place much faster.

Air is drawn into and expelled from the body by expansion and contraction of thin walled air sacs. These extend throughout the body even into some of the bones.

HANDLING THE AVIAN PATIENT

Gentle but firm handling will keep the patient's stress levels to a minimum.

> **Tip:** Owners should be warned beforehand that a sick bird might collapse in the process of handling for examination.

Psittacines vary dramatically in size; however, they all bite. Skill in catching and handling only comes with practice and an understanding of how a patient will react. Many parrots will screech if threatened; African greys also growl. The Amazon may roll on its back and attack with its beak and feet.

In the consulting room it is easiest to catch a bird from its cage, usually by taking the bottom off and turning the cage on its side; the catcher can then approach from the bottom of the cage.

If time and space allow, the easiest way of capturing a bird is in a darkened room with only a torch for a light source.

> **Tip:** Birds do not see well in red or blue light so covering the torch light with a red or blue filter helps.

Approach should always be slow so as not to create air movement.

At the last moment grasp the bird around its neck and head, and close the rest of the hand around its body and wings. Gloves may be worn when capturing a bird, but as they are very cumbersome the user will lose their sense of touch. However, this is sometimes the only way of handling a bad-tempered bird.

Using a towel

When done correctly this can be a relatively stress free way of capturing a patient.

A towel the size of a hand towel is draped over the hand with the fingers spread out. Once again advance slowly to the cage and grasp the head and neck through the towel (Fig. 5.3). The beak can be controlled by placing the index finger on the top of the head and the middle finger and thumb over the temperomandibular joints. The rest of the

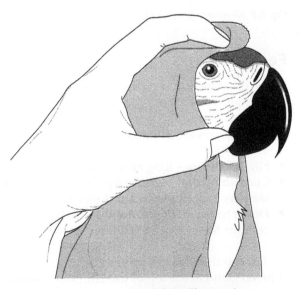

Fig. 5.3 Restraining an avian patient with a towel.

hand, or the other hand, can drape the remaining part of the towel over the bird's wings and body.

Once the patient is captured, it should be spoken to in a calm voice. Scratching or tickling of the feathers on the back or sides of the head can also help to keep the bird calm.

> **Tip:** Do not tickle the top of the head, as this will stimulate the natural allopreening of another bird.

If bitten

1. Keep calm.
2. Blow on the bird's face.
3. Try gently squeezing on the top of the bird's head.

HOSPITALISATION

The avian patient is generally presented to the veterinary practice in one of three conditions:

1. Injured – these birds can be specifically treated while supportive measures are initiated.
2. Sick – their medical needs can be addressed whilst investigating the cause or nature of the illness.
3. Apparently healthy.

When admitting a sick bird for intensive care treatment there are many advantages and a few disadvantages.

Advantages

- The bird will be under continuous observation by the veterinary staff and its condition can be monitored.
- The bird can receive regular medication as deemed necessary.
- Action can be taken if the bird's condition deteriorates.
- It can be kept under controlled conditions throughout its recovery.
- Some owners are unable to medicate their birds or give supplementary feeding.

Disadvantages

- The bird is in unfamiliar surroundings and this may cause stress.
- The bond between owner and bird may be broken, which may cause additional stress.
- There is a risk of infection to the other patients and staff members.

Equipment

Special equipment is minimal. Most veterinary practices have isoflurane anaesthesia, ophthalmic-sized surgical instruments, a 2.7 mm endoscope, microscope with oil emersion, radiosurgery unit and radiographic equipment.

Laboratory equipment is also necessary or at least a laboratory service close to the veterinary practice.

Gram scales with an accuracy of $+/-1\,\text{g}$ are necessary to monitor patients' weight changes and calculate correct dosages.

Other equipment includes small syringes and needles, catheters, small cuffed and non-cuffed endotracheal tubes, bandaging and splint materials, and protective collars.

For patient maintenance, ceramic, stainless steel or hard plastic feeding and drinking containers, and a variety of perches that can be cleaned easily. Perches must be of a non-porous material like PVC (see Table 5.1 for a summary).

Initial examination

Information should be obtained from the owner on presentation to ascertain the patient's stability. It can seem that the chronically ill bird may be closer to death than the acutely ill, but often it is the opposite way around. Birds that display signs of illness for some time often compensate for the disease, whereas those that develop serious signs acutely may be more seriously affected by the disease process. Whatever information is provided it is essential to observe the bird before handling it.

> **Tip:** It cannot be overemphasised that the bird's life may depend on the 'hands-off' assessment.

Table 5.1 Equipment needed for avian patients

Weighing scales	To +/−1 g
Syringes	1 ml, 2 ml, 5 ml
Needles	24 g, 23 g, 21 g
Catheters	24 g, 23 g
Blood tubes	Serum, heparin, EDTA
Microscope slides	–
Swabs	Plain and transport
Bandages and splints	Small sizes
Gavage tube (metal)	–
Small clean towels	–
Clinical record system	–
Metal and plastic feeding bowls	–
Perches	–
Isoflurane anaesthesia	–
Small endotracheal tubes	2.0 mm–3.5 mm
Ophthalmic sized surgical instruments	–
2.7 mm endoscope	–
Radiosurgery unit	–
Radiographic equipment	–

Observation

If possible observe the patient from a distance. Birds will often appear more alert and responsive when approached, giving an illusion of wellness.

Once visually examined, the bird may be physically examined. In the event of distress on examination, the bird should be placed in a hospital cage, and the patient's hydration and temperature should be focused on and treated before any further examination takes place.

Once fluids, heat and humidity have been supplied, a critical patient may show clinical improvement in a relatively short space of time.

After being observed from a distance the bird can be examined more closely. The vet or nurse should pay attention to the response to approach, food and water intake, the droppings and other normal or abnormal signs, e.g. blood or feather loss. All signs should be recorded on a hospitalisation form and decisions can then be made on the treatment protocol.

Laboratory monitoring

Blood samples should be taken from every sick hospitalised bird, preferably before any treatment.

0.5% of the patient's body weight may be taken and stored in a heparinised or EDTA tube (2 ml of blood from a 400 g parrot).

Blood values should then be monitored regularly after starting treatment.

Faecal examination may also be of benefit in assessing treatment response. Faecal parasite evaluation may be performed and smears may give the bacterial status of the intestines. Faecal examination can also give an indication of the caloric intake of the patient. Anorexic birds commonly have scant, slimy, dark green faeces.

The urine in the droppings of normal birds is clear and the urates white. An increase or decrease of urine or a change in colour is abnormal and should also be assessed.

Physical monitoring

The average adult bird has a temperature of 38–42.5°C. Regulation of temperature relies on many factors – feather condition, muscle condition, hydration, food intake and respiration.

Wet, destroyed, plucked feathers cause greater heat loss. Poor body condition hinders heat regulation and dehydration interferes with evaporative heat loss system. If possible overheated birds will pant to cool themselves down. It should be noted, however, that monitoring temperature is very stressful and dangerous to the avian patient.

Monitoring body weight is essential in ill birds. They should be weighed daily especially when tube feeding. Weight should be recorded at the same time each day, preferably in the morning or evening before feeding.

Medicating the avian patient

Medication may be administered orally, by injection or topically. The choice of route is usually determined by the severity of the infection, the number of birds requiring treatment and the ability of the owner.

Oral medication

This method is difficult in psittacine birds, as it is difficult to get them to open their mouths. It should not be used in critically ill patients.

Tablets and capsules. Most birds have a crop, which acts as a storage organ. If tablets are to be given then it is best to grind them down and make a suspension that is then given via a crop tube into an empty crop. Coated tablets are of no benefit to birds with a muscular gizzard as it will destroy the coating and give the pepsin and hydrochloric acid in the gizzard full access to the drug. Capsules are a good alternative but these are also best given via a crop tube into an empty crop.

Solutions and suspensions. Neither are used very often, the main disadvantage being that inhalation and/or regurgitation may result. However, if they are used they can be mixed with the food or administered as a gavage, especially when sick birds are requiring oral fluids.

Medicating feed or water. Medicating into the food is a reliable method as long as the patient is eating normally. Medication into water is a controversial area in avian medicine, but sometimes it is the only practical way. However, many birds refuse to drink water that tastes abnormal and this may then result in dehydration.

Parenteral dosage

This is the most effective way of administering drugs.

Intramuscular injection is often easier than oral administration. The main problem is the short dosing intervals required with many products. The pectoral or leg muscles are commonly used when dosing intramuscularly.

> **Tip:** The venous plexus which lies between the superficial and deep pectoral muscle must not be punctured.

Birds should be weighed and appropriate dilutions and syringes used for accurate dosing. Repeated injection into the same site or use of irritant drugs can result in muscle necrosis or atrophy.

Subcutaneous injection into the axillary area is preferable for large volumes of injection. However, because of the minimal amount of dermis and little skin elasticity, some of the injection may leak out and can cause skin necrosis and ulceration.

Intravenous (IV) sites should be saved for emergencies and single-dose administration. Haematomas are common and veins will be needed for regular blood sampling.

Topical medication

These drugs include skin preparations, eye drops and ointments. They should be used sparingly and carefully especially when using skin preparations, as they can stick on the feathers and will, therefore, be ingested when the patient preens itself.

> **Tip:** Topical steroid ointment should never be used on an avian patient as there have been several reports of death after application.

Nebulisation

This can play an important part in the management of respiratory disease. As the avian lung is very different from the mammalian lung, i.e. air capillaries are not dead end saccules, it can be a very effective treatment. Several nebulisers are available in the medical field, but it is important that they only produce very small particles if they are to have any effect. Most IV antibiotics can be mixed with saline for nebulisation. Ideally, the patient should be nebulised for 15–30 minutes twice to four times daily for any effect.

Hospital wards and cages for the sick bird

Isolation units

An avian isolation unit should be provided – separate from any small animal isolation units.

If a standard hospital cage has a floor space of at least 50 cm × 50 cm, then the average parrot cage will fit inside.

Keeping the patient in a cage inside the kennel unit has the advantage that cleaning the enclosure and transportation is possible without catching the bird.

Perches should be made of PVC and should be covered in self adherent bandage to fit the grasp of the patient's foot, to improve traction and prevent foot and leg problems.

Food and water should be provided in hard plastic or stainless steel containers and fitted at perch height.

The floor area should be covered with newspaper.

Intensive care units

An intensive care area is essential for the critically ill patient or a patient recovering from major surgery.

Aquabrooders are ideal for the sick avian patient (Fig. 5.4). They provide warmth and humidity to the critically ill, are easy to clean and disinfect, and reduce hospital contamination from discarded food and droppings. They also ensure visibility without approaching the patient.

Floor and air temperature should always be monitored to ensure that the patient is not burned or overheated.

Part of the aquabrooder can be covered with clean towels to allow privacy and prevent heat loss. If more heat is required an infrared light can be used. The advantage of infrared is that there is only heat and no light.

> **Tip:** If a standard light bulb is used, 24-hour light may interfere with the bird's hormonal pattern and cause moulting and other hormonal disturbances.

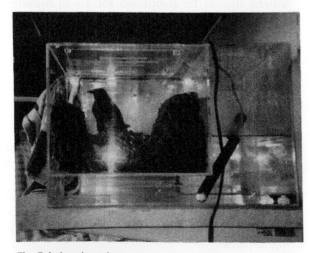

Fig. 5.4 Aquabrooder.

Commercial intensive care units are also available that have controllable heat, humidity and oxygen, but they are expensive.

It is suggested that a humidity of 50–80% should be provided in intensive care units. A simple way of providing humidity and heat is to place a bowl of hot water, covered with a plastic or rubber grill, inside the intensive care unit. The bird is then placed on the grill allowing warm steam to envelop its body.

Mental support

Avian patients undergo many changes due to stress. This can delay their recovery time. Stress can involve many factors. By following these points you can help reduce the avian patient's stress level:

- Avoid handling more than necessary.
- If possible allow recovery to continue at home.
- Cage mate may be brought in providing that there is no risk of injury to the new bird or the sick bird.
- Avoid 'high traffic' areas where the patient is exposed to unfamiliar people and pets.
- Respect the diurnal cycle of the patient and try to maintain a 12-hour light cycle.
- Consider sounds and smells as well as sight; encourage the owner to bring in familiar toy or perch.
- Barking, bird calls and predator smells can be distracting to a recovering patient.

Monitoring

It is essential to monitor and keep records of any patient that is hospitalised. It allows staff to follow progress and assess treatment. Progress may be assessed by observation and clinical signs, but for a more reliable assessment monitoring blood changes like packed cell volume (PCV), weight changes, urine and faecal output should also be monitored. Hospital forms should be produced for each hospitalised bird for daily assessment (Fig. 5.5). The following at the very least should be recorded:

- Food and water intake
- Droppings – quality and quantity

Avian Admission and Discharge Form

Bird's name		Owner		Case No		Vet
Species		Breed		Colour		
Weight on admission				Sex		Age

Clinical summary / problem list

1
2
3
4
5

Plan

At discharge Equipment left	Medication to go home with	Remove catheter / bandage

Client communication

Vet / nurse to recall / recheck

Daily assessment – Morning Afternoon Evening – to be initialled by vet

Date	Weight			Treatments					Notes / initials
	M	A	E						
Diet									
Appetite									
Crop empty									
Respiration									
Vomit									
Casting									
Faeces									
Attitude									
Special information									

Fig. 5.5 Lansdown hospital form.

- Clinical observations
- Medication – quantity and route
- Weight.

Preventing the spread of disease

Many avian pathogens are spread via aerosol and feather particles. It is imperative that an efficient ventilation system is installed within the avian unit.

All materials used on avian patients should be cleaned and disinfected between patients. However, be warned that all disinfectants are toxic to birds and must be used with care to prevent problems.

Tip: Virkon is reputed to be one of the safer disinfectants at a dilution of 10 g/1 l of water.

The order in which patients are maintained is the same for all animals – clean, feed and treat. Start with the healthiest and end with the most contagious and critically ill. When working with a contagious or zoonotic case it is advisable to wear gown, gloves and a mask, that can easily be changed. Staff should also use a disinfectant spray on their clothes and hair between patients.

Feeding the hospitalised patient

Treatment success is very much reliant on the management of the recovering patient. Anorexia often goes 'hand in hand' with many avian diseases. The route, frequency and type of food must all be decided. Nutritional management is often the most frustrating part of a case. Small amounts of highly palatable food must be given at regular intervals to encourage the appetite of a sick bird. Owners are often helpful in this part and should be encouraged to bring in the bird's favourite foods and, if necessary, help feed their bird, as the patient is usually more responsive to its owner.

Force feeding (Fig. 5.6)

Different birds require different food types. Psittacine birds do well on commercial avian dietary formulae ('Polyaid'- The Bird Care

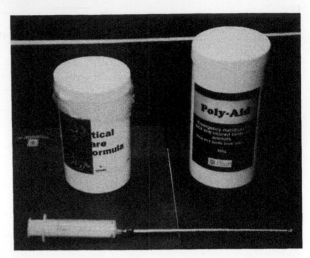

Fig. 5.6 Feeding tube.

Company or Critical Care formula - Vetark Animal Health).

Tip: If unable to obtain this, human formulae can also be used.

The main aim is to maintain or increase their weight during recovery.

If force feeding is necessary then the diet must be easy to administer, highly digestible and contain sufficient energy.

Birds that are not drinking must also have fluid supplementation.

The frequency of feeds is dependent on each case but the total daily requirement should be divided into an equal number of feeds.

Crop tube feeding

Tube feeding should not be undertaken if there is crop stasis or an impaction of the crop, ileus or gastrointestinal tract.

In psittacines, a curved, ball-tipped, metal feeding tube is a wise choice as it cannot be bitten in half.

The patient is caught and its neck extended. The tube is then inserted by the left commisure of the beak, slid over the tongue to the right side of the neck and then into the crop without causing trauma (Fig. 5.7). The crop is then palpated to

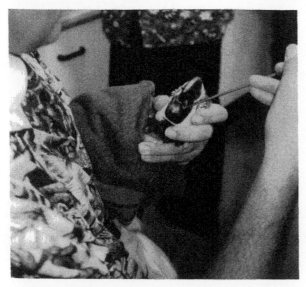

Fig. 5.7 Tube feeding.

Table 5.2 Volumes and frequency of tube feeding anorexic birds

Species	Volume (ml)	Frequency
Finch	0.1–0.3	Every 4 hours
Budgerigar	0.5–1.0	Every 6 hours
Cockatiel	1.0–2.5	Every 6 hours
Conure	2.5–5.0	Every 6 hours
Amazon parrot	5.0–8.0	Every 8 hours
African grey parrot	5.0–10.0	Every 8 hours
Cockatoo	8.0–12.0	Every 12 hours
Macaw	10.0–20.0	Every 12 hours

(Carpenter 1996).

ensure that the tube is in the correct place and that it is empty. The neck is kept in extension and the food injected.

Always feed fresh, warmed food to prevent delayed crop emptying.

If food refluxes remove the tube, let go of the bird and allow it to clear the food on its own.

Fluid therapy

Fluid therapy is extremely important in the sick avian patient. It restores blood volume, normalises cardiac output and helps with tissue oxygenation. Deciding on the route of administration very much depends on the status and co-operation of the patient. IV and intraosseously (IO) are the most effective routes in the critically ill patient.

Fluid choice

When dealing with shocked or dehydrated patients, crystalloid fluids are the appropriate choice. They are effective, inexpensive and easy to administer.

Hartmann's is favoured as it corrects metabolic acidosis, which is present in most cases.

Fluids with glucose in them are good for the anorexic patient (see Table 5.2 for feeding in anorexic birds).

Hypertonic saline (7.5%) can be used in conjunction with therapy to establish circulatory function, but it must always be followed with the administration of isotonic fluids.

Tip: Hypertonic saline should not be used in cases of dehydration or head trauma, as the risk of intracranial haemorrhage is greater.

Colloids have a similar effect to hypertonic saline, but have a longer half life.

Blood transfusions are beneficial for chronic anaemia, but only to stabilise the patient whilst the cause is being sought. Birds with a PCV of less than 20%, as a result of acute blood loss, may also benefit. One per cent of the donor's blood can be collected in citrate dextrose anticoagulant (0.15 ml/1 ml blood). The donor should be given IV saline 1–5 times the amount of blood collected.

Intravenous fluids. The basilic (wing) vein is easy to access, but very fragile. Injection into it usually results in a haematoma being formed. Some patients will tolerate a catheter being left in place, but care must always be taken due to self removal and loss of patency.

Other IV sites include the medial metatarsal vein and the jugular.

Having established your vein, IV fluids can be given as fast as the syringe, needle and catheter will allow.

Tip: Fluids must always be warmed to body temperature before administration.

Subcutaneous fluids. This route should only be used in cases of mild dehydration. Large volumes of fluid are not readily absorbed this way.

Fluid should be administered in small amounts of 5–10 ml/kg/site.

Sites would include dorsally between the wings, the axilla and the inguinal fold.

Isotonic fluids only should be used and always heat to body temperature.

Oral fluids. If the patient is bright, alert and responsive, then oral fluids are recommended as they are safe and cause little stress.

Oral fluids are given in the same manner as crop tube feeding.

Tip:

Fluid therapy summary
- Consider the following factors: hydration status, electrolyte balance, acid–base balance, blood values and caloric values
- Use a combination of routes if a large fluid volume is being given
- Fluids can be given as a slow IV or IO infusion. Give 10 ml/kg/hour to healthy patients for the first 2 hours, then reduce the amount to 5–8 ml/kg/hour to avoid fluid overload
- Fluids with dextrose added can be given for hypoglycaemia or anorexia
- Always warm fluids to body temperature before administration.

Calculation of fluids

Determine the fluid deficit (ml):

Weight (g) × % dehydration

Determine the daily maintenance amount:

50 ml/kg/24 hours (range 40–60 ml/kg/24 hours)

If possible, replace 50% of the deficit in the first 24 hours, then the remainder over the next 48 hours.

Example: a 1000 g bird is 10% dehydrated:

Fluid deficit = weight (1000 g) × dehydration 10%

Fluid deficit = 100 ml

Daily maintenance = 50 ml/kg/24 hours, therefore, daily maintenance is 50 ml

Day 1 = (maintenance + 50% of deficit)

(50 ml + 50 ml) = 100 ml

Day 2 = (maintenance + 25% of deficit)

(50 ml + 25 ml) = 75 ml

Day 3 = (maintenance + 25% of deficit)

(50 ml + 25 ml) = 75 ml

Total amount of fluid given after 3 days is 250 ml.

Anaesthesia in the avian patient

Preparing the patient

Patients should be as fit as possible prior to the anaesthetic. Dehydration should be corrected and, if possible, a blood sample should be taken to check PCV, glucose concentration and liver and kidney function. Patients with a PCV of less than 20% should not undergo a general anaesthetic, as severe anaemia is present. Patients with poor renal function should not be given ketamine as it has to be excreted by the kidney and halothane is contraindicated in patients with liver impairment.

Body weight should be taken to allow for accurate calculation of any drugs given. The average weights for some patients are illustrated in Table 5.3.

Fluids

All surgical cases must be given IV fluids warmed to body temperature. They should be given at a dose rate of 20 ml/kg as a bolus prior to surgery, then 15 ml/kg/hour during surgery.

Pre-operative starvation

Birds weighing 200 g or less should not be starved.

Table 5.3 Average avian patients' weights

Psittacine	Body weight
Scarlet macaw	1000 g
Lesser sulphur crested cockatoo	300 g
Greater sulphur crested cockatoo	700 g
African grey parrot	250–500 g
Budgerigar	30–50 g
Love bird	45–55 g
Cockatiel	80–120 g
Amazon parrot	250–700 g

Table 5.4 Analgesic dosages in avian patients

Analgesic	Dose
Butorphanol	2 mg/kg IM
Carprofen	2–4 mg/kg IM
Ketoprofen	2–4 mg/kg IM

IM: intramuscular.

Table 5.5 Commonly used injectable anaesthetic agents

Agent	Comments
Ketamine	Duration is dose dependent. Recovery is characterised by excitation, wing flapping, incoordination and head shaking. To avoid these side effects, ketamine is usually given in combination with other drugs. Poor muscle relaxation
Ketamine and diazepam	Good muscle relaxation
Ketamine and midazolam	Good muscle relaxation
Ketamine and xylazine	Good muscle relaxation. Increase in adverse cardiopulmonary effects. Xylazine can be reversed with atipamezole
Ketamine and medatomidine	Rapid reversal with atipamezole – patients are usually standing after 10 minutes
Propofol	Very short acting

In most larger birds, the time from removal of the food to recovery of anaesthesia and re-introduction of food should not be longer than 3 hours to avoid hypoglycaemia.

Analgesia

It is essential to relieve any pain that may delay return to feeding.

Analgesia is more effective if given before the onset of pain. Table 5.4 shows some of the safer and more effective analgesics.

Induction and maintenance

Injectable anaesthesia and sedation. The choice of anaesthetic agent will usually depend on the availability of the drugs and the experience of the staff. Most drugs can be given intramuscularly (IM) or IV. Although, the IV route is usually more reliable, it is more difficult and stressful. Anaesthesia can be maintained by the administration of

'top-up' bolus. Table 5.5 gives a summary of the most commonly used injectable anaesthetic agents.

Inhalation anaesthesia. When using inhalation anaesthesia it is important to remember that any surgery of the thoracoabdominal cavity or into the long bones may enter the air sacs. Anaesthetic gas is then able to escape into the atmosphere, and the plane of anaesthesia may not be steady (see Table 5.6 for a summary of the most commonly used inhalation anaesthesia).

Monitoring the anaesthesia

Depth of anaesthesia is difficult to measure in the avian patient.

The eye does not vary with the depth of anaesthesia, and palpebral and pedal reflexes are also inconsistent measures of depth.

The most reliable indicator of anaesthetic depth is the corneal reflex, which should be slow but present at a surgical plane of anaesthesia.

Breathing rate is also not consistent to the depth of anaesthesia, and, indeed, sometimes increases the greater the depth of anaesthesia becomes.

Table 5.6 Commonly used inhalation anaesthesia

Agent	Properties
Nitrous oxide	Not very potent and can be used with other anaesthetics Mix in concentrations up to 50% Should never be used if respiratory disease is present Turn off 5 minutes before the end of surgery
Halothane	Can be used as an induction and maintenance agent Induce with a mask, gradually increase concentration to desired plane of anaesthesia, so as not to overdose patient Advisable to intubate patient to maintain anaesthesia Risk of unexpected anaesthetic deaths
Isoflurane	Has now superseded halothane Considered to be the safest inhaled anaesthesia for birds Can induce anaesthesia with a mask with concentrations of 4–5% Maintenance concentrations at 2.5–3% Apnoea is still possible so intubate after induction to facilitate IPPV if necessary Recovery much faster than with halothane

IPPV: Intermittent positive pressure ventilation.

Table 5.7 Heart and respiratory rates in anaesthetised birds

Body weight	Heart rate/ minute	Respiratory rate/minute
40–100 g	600–750	55–75
100–200 g	450–600	30–40
200–400 g	300–500	15–35
500–1000 g	180–400	8–25

Generally, breathing should not drop below half of the bird's normal resting rate (see Table 5.7).

Oesophageal stethoscope. This is a cheap and effective way of monitoring cardiac output. A light plane of anaesthesia may be indicated by an increase in heart rate.

Pulse oximeters. Pulse oximeters should be used with care. The probe must be placed close to a peripheral artery to detect a problem with the peripheral circulation before problems with the central circulation. If placed incorrectly then the user will not be alerted to a problem until a fall in the central circulation, by which time the patient is likely to be in circulatory collapse and beyond help.

Various anaesthetic emergencies can occur and it is imperative that prompt action is taken to ensure the safety of the patient. Table 5.8 outlines the steps that should be taken in the event of an anaesthetic emergency.

FIRST AID FOR BIRDS

Vital signs

These are indications of existence and stability of life. They are an essential indication of the bird's well-being. They include:

- Heart rate – without a heart the rest of the body cannot work.
- Pulse rate and strength – gives an indication of how effectively the heart is pumping blood around the arteries.
- Rate and quality of breathing – even if the heart is beating, without breathing there is no exchange of oxygen and removal of carbon dioxide. Breathing is not always obvious in the bird. By opening the beak though you can observe the opening and closing of the glottis. Failure of the respiratory system is detected by a fall in the rate of breathing by 50% of normal and a fall in the depth of breathing and pale or blue mucous membranes.
- Mucous membrane colour – these membranes are the tissues lining various structures of the body. Usually their colour is pink, indicating good circulating supply of oxygen and good respiration. Changes are seen by changes in colour.
- Capillary refill time – this should be 1–2 seconds.
- Temperature – metabolism is reliant on a series of chemical changes that only occur in a limited temperature range.

Table 5.8 Anaesthetic emergencies

Apnoea	Turn off gas Increase oxygen flow Place bird in sternal recumbency IPPV once every 5 seconds	Doxapram 5–7 mg/kg IV
Cardiac arrest	Turn off gas Give rapid cardiac massage	Adrenaline 0.1–0.2 mg/kg IV
Tracheal blockage	Check oxygen flow Clear pharynx and glottis Check endotracheal tube patency Apply suction or remove endotracheal tube Place abdominal air sac tube	
Haemorrhage	Apply haemostasis	Fluids – colloids if possible IV Blood transfusion if necessary

IPPV: intermittent positive pressure ventilation; IV: intravenous.

Emergency procedures

Vital signs provide indications of a bird's well-being. If problems do arise it is important to follow the basic principles of first aid:

A – airway
B – breathing
C – circulation
D – drugs.

Airway

Check that the passage of air into the lungs is unobstructed.

- Remove any blood, foreign bodies, mucus or vomit from the mouth.
- Make sure the entrance to the trachea is clear.
- Extend the head and neck forward to maintain clear airways. If necessary a non-cuffed endotracheal tube can be passed into the trachea.
- Make sure that the tube does not become blocked.

Tip: Birds usually find breathing easier if maintained in an upright position on their keels.

Breathing

Check whether breathing. If not then artificial respiration should be given.

Artificial respiration.

- Mouth to mouth respiration – an endotracheal tube is placed and intermittent blowing into the lungs is performed. Take care not to overinflate the lungs.
- Chest compressions – intermittent pressure on the chest wall can be attempted to establish an airflow in and out of the lungs, but should not be continued for more than 2 minutes.
- Drugs – a few drops of doxapram hydrochloride (Dopram-V, Willow Francis) can be placed in the mouth to stimulate breathing. It is relatively short lived and should be repeated every 10 minutes. Injectable doxapram hydrochloride can be given IV at a dose of 1–2 mg/kg.

Circulation

- Listen to the chest with a stethoscope and feel for a pulse.
- If the heart stops, within 3 minutes the lack of oxygen to the brain will result in irreversible brain damage.
- Epinephrine can be given at a dose of 0.01 mg/kg every 3–4 minutes.

Drugs

Drugs can be useful in life-threatening situations as mentioned above. These drugs should be kept separate from other drugs in a 'crash box' so that

Table 5.9 Emergency drugs and their uses

Agent	Dosage	Use
Atropine	0.5 mg/kg IM, IV or IO	CPR
Calcium gluconate	50–100 mg/kg IV slowly	Hypocalcaemia
Dexamethasone sodium phosphate	0.1–0.5 mg/kg IM or IV	Head trauma, shock, hypothermia
Dextrose 50%	1.0 ml/kg IV slowly	Hypoglycaemia
Diazepam	0.5–1.5 mg/kg IM or IV	For sedation or to control seizures
Doxapram	20 mg/kg IM, IV or IO	CPR
Epinephrine (1:1000)	0.5–1.0 ml/kg IM, IV or IO	CPR
Fluids	Assume 7–10% dehydration + maintenance	See Fluid therapy

CPR: cardiopulmonary resuscitation; IM: intramuscular; IV: intravenous; IO: intraosseous.

they are immediately accessible in an emergency (Table 5.9).

EMERGENCY SITUATIONS

The main goal in an emergency is supportive treatment. Specific treatment can be established later. It is very important to make a plan based on the clinical observations. In the case of the sick bird perform one task at a time and wait for the effects before starting the next task.

> **Tip:** Correcting the fluid deficit and hypothermia is usually done first.

Dehydration

Dehydration can be assessed by observation of the eyes and skin on the face and keel. Are the eyes dry and dull? Is the skin discoloured and wrinkled? Any bird that is dehydrated due to illness and not injury can be presumed to be 7–10% dehydrated.

Hypothermia

Signs include:

- bird having fluffed up feathers and trembling on the perch or at the bottom of the cage
- bird having a cold beak and cold feet
- patient feeling cool to handle.

Treatment includes:

- warmed IV fluids and placing in a heated cage of about 25–30°C. This will raise core and peripheral temperature.
- warm moist air.

Hypocalcaemia syndrome

This is common in African grey parrots and is usually due to the diet being deficient in calcium, phosphorus or vitamin D_3. Diagnosis is from blood calcium levels being below 1.8 mmol.

Signs include:

- seizures
- ataxia
- weakness
- tetany.

Treatment involves slow IV calcium gluconate 10% at a dose of 0.5–2 ml/kg (50–200 mg/kg).

The diet should be changed immediately following recovery.

Cardiopulmonary arrest

There are many reasons why a bird's heart may stop. However, if it is due to a chronic illness, birds do not usually respond well to cardiopulmonary resuscitation (CPR).

Treatment includes intubation and delivery of oxygen through an open circuit. Intermittent positive pressure ventilation (IPPV) may be administered, as necessary, once every 4 seconds. Be careful not to overinflate the patient's air sacs as they can rupture.

If there is no heart beat or peripheral pulse then rapid compressions on the sternum may help.

Administer epinephrine at a dose of 0.5–1.0 mg/kg and atropine at a dose of 0.5 mg/kg IM, IV or IO.

Doxapram hydrochloride can also be useful at a dose of 20 mg/kg IM, IV or IO.

COMMON PROBLEMS AND DISEASES

Trauma

In the trauma patient, despite its condition on presentation, a complete physical examination is crucial.

Before handling the patient, attitude and posture should be noted.

Skeletal injuries are often more noticeable with the bird in its cage or standing on the examination table.

Trauma is obviously quite stressful to the avian patient, and this, in turn, results in the release of noradrenaline and dopamine. This can lead to an elevation in heart rate and peripheral vasoconstriction.

Blood glucose levels and the bird's pain threshold can also become raised.

Common traumatic injuries

Beak injury. This is usually caused by aggressive bird-to-bird interaction.

Treatment involves the control of any haemorrhage with chemical cautery or radiosurgery, and then repair of the injury under anaesthesia, as long as it is not infected.

Feather injuries. Damage to a new or developing feather can result in haemorrhage.

Treatment involves removal of the affected feather and direct pressure being applied to the bleeding. If the haemorrhage is persistent, then surgical glue can be applied.

> **Tip:** Chemical or electrical cautery should not be used as it can result in permanent damage to the follicle.

Lacerations. Treatment will depend on where and how old the injury is. To control any haemorrhage apply direct pressure, but not chemical cautery, as this can cause tissue necrosis.

Contusions. These are usually a result of window or wall crashing. This can result in skeletal, central nervous system (CNS) or visceral damage.

Treatment involves stopping bleeding if there is blood loss, and administration of IV or IO fluids, heat and corticosteroids.

Head trauma. These are also usually a result of window, wall or mirror crashing. The bird will be depressed on presentation. There may be blood loss and evidence of CNS trauma.

Treatment involves aggressive therapy in order to prevent irreversible damage. The patient should also be kept relatively cool. If there is little or no response within 48 hours the prognosis is poor.

Fractures. Fractures can result in blood loss; therefore, fluid replacement should be given to help the circulating blood volume. As there is little soft tissue on the avian skeleton, fractures are usually open fractures. It is imperative that the patient is stabilised before surgical repair takes place. Generally, analgesia is not given as the elimination of pain will encourage the patient to use the limb, and cause additional stress and subsequent injury.

Burns. This is often due to contact with hot liquids or electrical burns from chewing electric cables. If more than 50% burns, then euthanasia must be considered.

Treatment involves giving oxygen and starting aggressive shock therapy. Give IV or IO fluids and antibiotics to prevent sepsis. Analgesia is necessary for pain relief. Burns should be cleaned and debrided on a daily basis under anaesthesia.

Respiratory diseases

Treatment includes:

- administration of oxygen and establishing an airway
- ascertaining whether the disease is of the upper airway, pulmonary or air sac

- an air sac tube in patients with upper airway diseases, as this works well. The patient is placed in right lateral recumbency and a plastic tube is placed in the left abdominal or caudal air sac because of its greater size.

> **Tip:** Remember to connect the anaesthetic circuit to the air sac tube after placing it, so as to keep the patient asleep.

The oxygen flow must be lowered to 0.5–1 l/kg, so that the air sac is not overinflated.

The tube can be left in place for more than 7 days, but must be kept clean from faeces and other debris.

IV fluid should also be given to replace any respiratory fluid loss.

Psittacosis/ornithosis or chlamydiosis

Psittacosis is a very common disease that may affect all members of the psittacine family (when seen in other avian species, e.g. ducks, pigeons it is termed ornithosis). The severity of the disease will vary between species and strains of the infectious organism.

It is a disease in which birds may be infected for many years before any signs develop. A period of stress, or change in the bird's life may cause the disease to become active.

Clinical signs

Clinical signs include any respiratory signs, sneezing, coughing, eye discharges, diarrhoea, loss of appetite, sudden death or simply being 'fluffed up'. Young birds are more prone to serious disease.

Transmission

Infection is spread in feather dust, so all birds in the same air space as the one that has been diagnosed positive, will have been exposed, and are likely to be infected. Cockatiels are the most commonly affected species.

Psittacosis is also a zoonosis, i.e. it can infect and cause significant disease in humans. People over 45 years of age and pregnant women should not enter an infected area. Although it can be fatal in humans, the disease is not difficult to treat.

Symptoms include headaches, flu-like symptoms, cough, swollen glands, liver problems and pneumonia.

Salmonellosis

This is another common bacterial infection of psittacines. It is caused by large numbers of different *Salmonella* organisms. *Salmonella typhimurium* is the most common and most dangerous of the species.

It causes an enteric infection – attacking the gut and, therefore, causing enteritis.

It sometimes invades the blood, causing septicaemia and fever.

As with psittacosis, birds can remain healthy carriers of the organism and still infect others. A period of stress can cause the organisms to become active.

The organism is excreted by infected birds, therefore, readily contaminating their environment.

Everything that comes into contact with the bird must be cleaned and thoroughly disinfected. Gloves and aprons should be worn to prevent infection in humans, though there are very few reports of humans becoming infected from a psittacine.

Diarrhoea, vomiting, ruffled feathers, fever and lethargy are the main clinical signs. Infection can be acute – killing the bird within a few days – or chronic – showing a slow decline in the bird's health.

Psittacine beak and feather disease

Psittacine beak and feather disease (PBFD) is a simple virus that infects and kills the cells of the feather and beak. It also attacks the immune system, therefore leaving the bird susceptible to other bacterial infection.

PBFD usually affects young birds; however, birds of all ages can succumb to the disease.

In chronic PBFD, dystrophic feathers will replace the normal ones as they are moulted, gradually causing the bird to lose its plumage without any other signs of ill health. The powder-down feathers are usually the first to go thus creating decreased production of powder and causing the feathers to become dull and the beak glossy.

Acute PBFD can cause green or mucoid diarrhoea in the patient. These signs are often diagnosed as secondary infections, and the bird may die before showing any obvious feather lesions.

Vaccination

A killed virus vaccine has recently been developed. If given to a normal healthy bird it stimulates immunity to the psittacine circovirus. It should not be given to birds already suffering from PBFD as it can accelerate the disease.

CASE HISTORY 1

Patient

Male, 3-year-old Amazon parrot named Jerry, weighing 400 g.

Reason for hospitalisation

Idiopathic feather plucking.

Type of accommodation and bedding material used, to include: any relevant environmental factors

Metal parrot cage approximately 50 cm × 50 cm × 90 cm. The base is a detachable plastic tray for ease of cleaning. The base is lined with newspaper, and perches covered in Vet-rap bandage are placed at different heights within the cage. Half of the cage is covered with a towel to allow a convalescence area. Stainless steel food and water bowls are placed at perch height. This cage is then placed in a large kennel within the avian ward to minimise contamination from one bird to another. Room temperature is maintained at a constant 26°C with relative humidity. The ventilation system is also turned on.

Accommodation cleaning protocol, to include: type of disinfectant, dilution of, mechanical cleaning procedures, frequency of cleaning and disposal of waste

Twice daily the cage is emptied, cleaned and disinfected. The patient is placed in a temporary holding unit or taken away for medication whilst cleaning is taking place.

The cage is emptied of perches, bowls, newspaper, toys and any solid debris. Liquid debris is soaked up with paper towel. The whole cage is hosed clean with water, dried with paper towel, and then disinfected with Virkon solution (10 g to 1 l water). The cage is wiped dry.

Dirty Vet-rap is removed from the perches, and these are then washed and disinfected in the same manner as the cage. Fresh Vet-rap is placed on the perches (this it to prevent foot problems and aid traction).

Food and water bowls are emptied, washed up and then also disinfected with Virkon solution. Fresh food and water is replaced.

Feeding regime

The patient was offered fresh Harrison's complete bird food twice daily. As the patient was used to a seed mix, this was also offered and the patient gradually weaned off it.

The correct amount of food for a 400 g bird was weighed out, as the patient was being caged for longer periods than usual, and, therefore, was being given less exercise than normal.

Nursing care and monitoring of the animal: give details of grooming, wound management, cleaning, monitoring of vital signs and 'TLC'

Urine and faecal output were monitored three times daily. Any abnormalities were noted on the hospitalisation sheet. Any vomiting was also recorded.

The patient's well-being and general attitude were monitored. As behavioural problems can be factors in feather plucking patients, it was especially important to provide stimuli for the patient during his stay. Different toys were given daily and obedience training was taught as it would be in the patient's home environment.

Weight was taken and recorded at the same time each day.

The plucked areas were monitored for any soreness or further plucking.

Medication administered

One Clomicalm 5 mg tablet dissolved in 5 ml water – 0.2 ml of solution given once daily orally.

Baytril 2.5% solution – 0.5 ml given twice daily orally.

CASE HISTORY 2

Patient

Male, 12-month-old African grey parrot, weighing 500 g.

History

The patient was admitted to the hospital following a 'window crashing' accident. On presentation the patient was in shock, concussed and 10% dehydrated. The right wing was obviously fractured at the distal point of the humerus. Small cuts and abrasions were also present around the face.

Treatment and monitoring of the patient

Initially, the patient was treated for shock with IV fluids, corticosteroids and warming. Hartmann's or lactated Ringer's solution was chosen as fluid therapy. This was to correct any metabolic acidosis, restore blood volume and normalise cardiac output. The fluids were warmed to body temperature and given IV into the left basilica (wing) vein.

The patient was then placed in a pre-warmed aquabrooder. Warmth was provided at a constant 30°C. Relative humidity was also provided. Observation checks were made every 15 minutes without approaching the patient. Posture and attitude were monitored this way, i.e. was the patient standing up, fluffed up appearance, whether eating or drinking, and the quality and quantity of droppings. Respiration rate was also monitored in this way.

Every 2 hours the patient was monitored more closely, and if necessary more IV fluids were administered.

Antibiotic medication was administered every 12 hours IM (piperacillin 50 mg/500 g).

Analgesia was administered every 24 hours IM (carprofen 5 mg/500 g).

For the shock a single dose of dexamethasone sodium phosphate (0.25 mg/500 g) was administered IV.

Fluid therapy plan

Patient is 10% dehydrated:

Fluid deficit = weight (500 g) × dehydration (10%)

Fluid deficit = 50 ml

Daily maintenance = 50 ml/kg/24 hours
– maintenance = 25 ml/24 hours

Fifty per cent of the deficit should be replaced over the first 24 hours, then the remainder divided equally over the next 48 hours.

Day 1 = (maintenance + 50% of deficit)

(25 ml + 25 ml) = 50 ml

5 × 10 ml bolus evenly spaced over 24 hours

Day 2 = (maintenance + 25% of deficit)

(25 ml + 12.5 ml) = 37.5 ml

4 × 9.5 ml bolus evenly spaced over 24 hours

Day 3 = (maintenance + 25% of deficit)

(25 ml + 12.5 ml) = 37.5 ml

4 × 9.5 ml bolus evenly spaced over 24 hours

Anaesthesia

Twenty-four hours after the initial therapy the patient had improved enough to undergo anaesthesia to radiograph and, dependent on the severity of the fracture, surgical reduction of the fracture.

Pre-operative preparation of the patient

No starvation is necessary in avian patients as their metabolic rate is much higher. Therefore, food must be re-introduced within 3 hours to avoid hypoglycaemia.

IM analgesia (carprofen 5 mg/500 g) was given 1 hour prior to surgery.

Induction of anaesthesia

The patient was masked down with a mix of 2 l of oxygen and 4% isoflurane.

Intubation with a size 2.5 mm endotracheal tube followed. An oesphageal stethoscope was placed and the apnoea monitor turned on. Warmed IV fluids (10 ml) were administered.

Maintenance of anaesthesia

Anaesthesia was maintained with 1 l of oxygen mixed with 2.5% isoflurane and delivered via an Ayres T-piece. The patient was placed in sternal recumbency on a heated pad. Radiographs of the skull and right wing were taken, and showed a fracture of the distal humerus. Surgical reduction of the fracture was then performed.

Cardiac output was monitored every 5 minutes as were the respiration rate and corneal reflex.

Recovery from anaesthesia

The patient was maintained under anaesthesia for 1 hour. Isoflurane was turned off and pure oxygen delivered for approximately 2 minutes. The oesophageal stethoscope was removed, and the bird was wrapped in a warmed towel and held until fully awake.

The patient was kept hospitalised for a further 7 days to receive IM analgesia and antibiotic therapy. After this time he was discharged on strict cage rest and oral medication, to be re-assessed in 10 days.

Discussion

Depth of anaesthesia is difficult to assess in the avian patient. Monitored reflexes such as palpebral and pedal reflexes are often inconsistent. The most reliable reflex is the corneal reflex, which if touched gently with a cotton bud should be slow but present at a surgical plane of anaesthesia.

It must also be remembered that avian patients have air sacs that allow oxygen to circulate through the lungs continuously during inspiration and expiration; therefore, changes in the depth of anaesthesia happen much faster.

REFERENCES

Carpenter 1996 Exotic animal formulary. WB Saunders, London
Loudis, Sutherland-Smith 1994
Tully TN, Lawton MPC, Dorrestein M 2000 Avian medicine. Butterworth-Heinemann Medical, London

Chapter 6

Birds of prey

Sara Cowen

INTRODUCTION

Britain has a number of endemic birds of prey that may be seen in practice following injury or illness, and as a category these are defined as 'raptors'; they include falcons, hawks (falconiformes) and owls (strigiformes). However, falconry is popular in the UK and a variety of unknown species may be seen that have escaped.

The main UK strigiformes species are little owls, barn owls (Fig. 6.1) and tawny owls, all generally nocturnal. The falconiformes are mostly diurnal. The main UK species of hawk are the buzzard, the harrier, the goshawk, the golden eagle, the osprey, the sparrowhawk (Fig. 6.2) and the red kite. The main species of falcon include the kestrel (Fig. 6.3a,b), the hobby, the merlin and the peregrine.

Falcons are diurnal and spend the majority of the day in flight in search of prey, hovering and

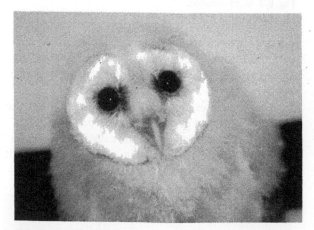

Fig. 6.1 Juvenile barn owl.

swooping. They are totally reliant on precision flying for survival and any damage to the wings, unless repaired perfectly, will result in the inability to lead a normal life and hunt.

Hawks and owls again capture prey through flight, but are less precise as they tend to sit in a branch waiting for an unsuspecting rodent to pounce on, and for this reason may tolerate an element of wing damage.

> **Tip:** When treating injured raptors you must assess whether they can return to the wild and live a normal life. Failure to do so may result in a released individual being unable to hunt, and either dying of starvation or leading a miserable life in captivity.

ANATOMY AND PHYSIOLOGY

Birds of prey feed on small mammals, catching them with their talons and tearing them apart by the use of their sharp beak.

Their eyesight is very efficient and can determine the minutest movement from their hunting position. Damaged or missing eyes will result in reduced visibility and hunting precision.

Nocturnal species are sensitive to low light conditions. Owls have ear holes present for locating prey even in darkness, which are highly sensitive. They will be observed as large holes in the skull rather than true ears with external pinnae, and in some species may be outlined with tufts of feathers.

Owls also have the ability to rotate their head by 180° as they are unable to move their eyes within the actual sockets.

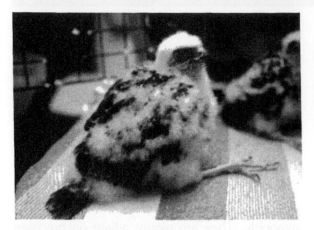

Fig. 6.2 Sparrowhawk.

All raptors have an exaggerated chest bone called the keel, which is used for attachment of large flight muscles. Always check the condition of the bird's muscle coverage; the chest should be well covered and rounded without protrusion of this keel bone.

HANDLING

On presentation of a bird of prey the less stressful method for bird and handler is to place a towel over the bird and restrain by placing hands over the shoulders containing the wings. Avoid the talons as these are likely to cause far more damage than the beak.

The bird can be gently placed on its side where it will tend to remain still. The towel can then be moved to reveal various parts of the body allowing a thorough examination to take place.

The legs can be restrained by gently holding the bird's legs together above the ankle. Alternatively they will grip onto the towel, which can be removed when the bird is placed into its cage.

It is always advisable to keep the head covered, unless examining, preventing stress to the bird and the handler being bitten. Leather gloves are the usual method of protecting the hands from the beak and talons.

ACCOMMODATION

Birds of prey are extremely sensitive to sound and movement and respond poorly to confinement. It is important to place them in a quiet, dark, warm,

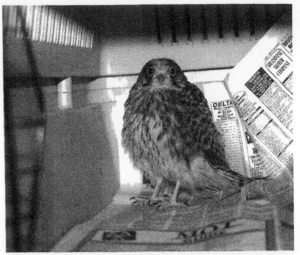

(a)

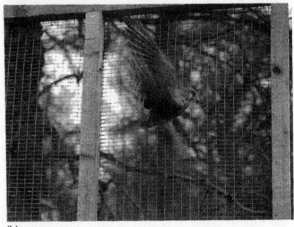

(b)

Fig. 6.3 (a, b) Kestrels.

secure container that is smooth sided. Wire cages are unsuitable as the animal will leap around and cause further damage to feathers and result in further injury.

Always cover the front of the cage to keep the animal calm and prevent threat from onlookers.

Place natural perches in the cage if able to stand allowing the animal to rest in a normal position; it would not usually stand on the floor.

Tip: *Never* place birds on hay or straw bedding material as spores present can result in the fatal condition aspergillosis. Always place in well-ventilated areas.

NUTRITION

The normal diet of a wild bird will be rodents; these are easily obtained from reptile shops. The best alternative is day-old chicks that can be fed whole or cut into smaller pieces for youngsters or weak individuals. Feeding amounts will vary, e.g. kestrel – one chick daily, tawny owl – two chicks daily.

> **Tip:** If chicks or rodents are unavailable, try strips of ox heart or beef.

If not available the birds may feed on strips of raw beef or liver. However, this would be insufficient as a staple diet in the long term, as they normally consume feathers and bones as well that are then regurgitated as a pellet, called 'casting'.

Little owls predominantly feed on insects and invertebrates such as worms and these can be provided if available.

Always check the cage for castings prior to refeeding. Check the bird's crop to see it has emptied. Failure to do so may result in a condition called 'sour crop' where the food has not left the crop and begins to decompose.

Fresh healthy road kills such as rabbits, squirrels and birds can also be a useful source of food for raptors in captivity.

Ensure that fresh water is available at all times but do not be alarmed, as a healthy individual will drink little, gaining the majority of the moisture from its diet.

> **Tip:** Consider the bird's normal pattern of activity and if nocturnal place food with bird at night.

HAND REARING

Often young birds will fall or be pushed from a nest, especially in a large clutch. These birds will require hand rearing as they are unable to catch food for themselves.

If tiny hatchlings or nestlings are found they will require a heat source such as a heat lamp to provide a temperature of approximately 30°C.

They should be placed in a small container, such as a margarine tub, lined with tissue. This will provide warmth and comfort.

Most birds will instinctively produce droppings in a sac on presentation of food. This action can be stimulated by gently wiping over the cloaca. The bird's mother would normally pick up the capsule in the beak and remove it from the nest. You can replicate this using tweezers and it will also save on the cleaning.

Hand rearing raptors is fairly easy in terms of dietary needs. Day-old chicks or small rodents such as mice can be fed. The food will need to be chopped into small pieces and can be offered using tweezers. The birds will take the meat easily, as they would normally be presented food in a similar manner by their mothers.

> **Tip:** Dipping the meat in a little water prior to feeding allows you to hydrate the patient at the same time.

If very young they will require the fur and bones to be removed for the first week and to be fed muscle only with a calcium supplement added. The fur and bones can be introduced in small amounts from week 2 onwards gradually increasing over time to fledglings (Table 6.1). The birds will take the amount they require and may return later to any that is left.

Failure to feed these birds whole animals will result in metabolic bone disease, splayed legs, hypocalcaemic fits and rickets, all of which are irreversible, and euthanasia should be considered. If caught early enough, calcium deficiencies in birds should be treated with calcium borogluconate 10% 3 ml/kg IV.

Hand-reared birds will imprint on humans and it may be necessary to find a suitable captive home. Alternatively, specialised rehabilitation can be carried out. Birds are placed long term in 'hacking houses' for a slow-release programme, so seek professional advice from rehabilitators.

> **Tip:** Never just release a hand-reared bird of prey when it has fledged, as it will have no natural instincts or knowledge of how to hunt and catch prey, resulting in starvation.

Table 6.1 Feeding guidelines		
Age (weeks)	Identification	Frequency
0–1	Bald and blind, egg sac may be present	2 hourly, meat only, no fur or bones
1–2	Soft down begins covering body, eyes open	2–3 hourly, meat only
2–3	Downy feathers cover bodies, more responsive, moving around	3–4 hourly, add small amount of bones and feathers
3–4	Fully covered in feathers, alert and standing	4 hourly, increase the amount of bones
4–5	Begin moving, around, downy feathers begin to be replaced by secondary feathers on body	Four feeds daily, chick chopped into small pieces
5–6	Begin pecking at food, appearance of primary flight feathers	Three feeds daily, larger pieces
From 6 weeks	Mainly feathers rather than down, eating on own	2–3 feeds daily, chicks halved or whole

FIRST AID

Wild birds suffer from stress easily and under certain conditions this can cause secondary problems to occur. It is important to keep initial treatment to a minimum and let the bird acclimatise before carrying out too many interventions.

Initial treatment

Initially the following should be provided:

- warmth
- darkness
- quiet
- oral fluids – Lectade
- intraosseous fluids
- corticosteroids
- sedation, if required (diazepam 1.0 mg/kg IV or IM).

ANAESTHESIA

Birds are always a risk in terms of anaesthesia as depth is difficult to ascertain through normal reflexes. They also retain the anaesthetic in air sacs dispersing it throughout the body rather than in paired lungs.

Use corneal, palpebral and pedal reflexes but these may not be consistent with response.

Pay particular attention to respiratory and heart rates throughout.

Gaseous anaesthesia can be carried out using isoflurane or halothane. Induction is by masking the patient and a concentration of 1–4% and maintain on a 0.5–1% concentration. With larger species intubation can be carried out. The advantage is induction and recovery is rapid with gaseous anaesthesia.

THERAPEUTICS

When treating birds the routes for administration are topical, orally and parenterally. Orally is often the easiest route by either tablet or crop tubing.

IM injection can be placed into the breast muscle either side of the keel or in the hind limbs. If a course of injections is required, use alternate sides daily to prevent bruising.

IV injection should be in the brachial vein or the jugular vein if possible.

COMMON ILLNESSES, INJURIES AND DISEASES

There are numerous conditions that birds suffer from and only the most common will be covered here; however, refer to Chapter 7 for additional information on diseases not specific to birds of prey.

Parasites

Capillaria infestations are often observed, with the worm being present at the back of the bird's throat. Another common nematode to be seen in raptors is the **gape worm** (*Syngamus trachea*).

Symptoms will be regurgitation of food, and thickening of the oesophageal and crop lining.

These conditions should be treated with fenbendazole 50 mg/kg orally (PO) or ivermectin 15 mg/kg IM, PO or subcutaneously (SC). This should result in killing the worms, but they may remain in the animal's throat for a few weeks possibly causing continued respiratory distress.

Antibiotics may also assist through this period following treatment.

Trichomoniasis (frounce, trick or canker)

This is observed in birds of prey and is a protozoan infection from *Trichomonas gallinae* affecting the throat and mouth, and is commonly seen in pigeons and doves. The presence of cheesy growths in the mouth and throat region will clarify.

In some cases the growths become so enlarged they obstruct the airways causing dyspnoea and possibly asphyxiation. The growth can travel down the oesophagus into the crop causing damage. Birds will usually be in poor condition and emaciated.

It is important to rehydrate the bird by orally gavaging fluids. Treatment for the protozoan is metronidazole 50 mg/kg PO twice per day for 5 days or carnidazol 10 mg/kg.

Following treatment the lesion may drop off or be carefully removed. Use a cotton bud to gently wipe away from the mouth cavity and throat area.

Contraction and spread of this condition is through direct contact so keep birds isolated from others and use a high level of hygiene with equipment.

Aspergillosis

Aspergillosis (*Aspergillus fumigatus*) is one of the most common causes of fatality in raptors, as they appear to have little immune response to this fungal pathogen. It can also be triggered whilst kept in captivity and be induced by stress, creating secondary problems that require treatment.

Aspergillosis thrives in damp conditions, and hay and straw bedding encourage this as spores may be present in dry hay.

It is believed that it may be permanently present in birds' respiratory systems without causing symptoms, but that situations such as stress, environmental change, illness, etc., may result in the bird becoming vulnerable. The fungus can then affect the respiratory system of the bird, initially without symptoms until disease has progressed.

The condition in its acute form will kill within 7 days and in a chronic form can kill in several weeks.

Symptoms may include:

- wheezing
- fluffed up appearance
- depression
- inappetance
- mouth breathing
- pneumonia
- emaciation.

Treatment is often ineffective; however, the following can be tried:

- Sporanox at 5–10 mg/kg twice per day for 2–4 weeks may assist.
- Antifungal nebuliser such as clotrimazole solution as needed.
- Oxygen, if dyspnoeic.
- Bronchodilators.

Respiratory infection

If dyspnoea is not caused by parasitic infestation it may be resultant from bacterial infection. Commonly observed forms are *Pasteurella* and *Streptococcus* spp. These can be treated with streptomycin or tylosin 20 mg/kg IM twice per day for 3 days.

Wing and feather damage

It is important to remember that if primary feathers are broken and are not able to be repaired, the bird will not grow new ones until the annual autumn moult, resulting in a long period in captivity.

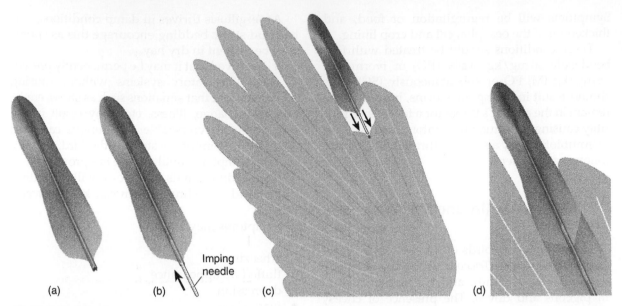

Figure 6.4a–d Imping.

Feathers can, in some cases, be repaired by attaching part of another feather; this is called 'imping', where an alternative healthy feather can be glued to the damaged one and remains until the moult. Feathers can be used from other birds that may have died and should be matched in size and length. The shafts of feathers are hollow allowing a small wooden stick, such as a cocktail stick, to be glued into the shaft of the damaged feather and the replacement feather glued to the other end (Fig. 6.4).

If the feather shaft is just damaged but intact, it can be strengthened by the application of glue onto the shaft, keeping it in place and acting as support, thus allowing it to work as a feather once more.

Fractures

Fractures of the humerus and femur are common and often concurrent with injury during flight, such as in a collision with a car.

It is vital they are repaired perfectly, as raptors are totally reliant on the wings for flight and hunting, and on their feet for capture and holding of prey.

Wings and legs can be treated in the usual way depending on the severity of the fracture. They can be splinted and cast and, if necessary,

internally fixated by pinning. (The pin should be removed before release.)

> **Tip:** If the wings and feathers are not repaired perfectly release must not be considered as it will result in starvation; in such cases, euthanasia or captivity should be considered.

Wounds

Wounds are often received during road traffic accidents or entanglement in wire resulting in laceration to the body and wings. It may often be difficult to repair the tears as the skin is very thin and withers quickly.

Treat as an open wound, placing Intrasite gel over the areas to keep muscle and underlying tissues moist and clean. Repair should be through granulation. In some areas it may be possible to apply a protective dressing; however, few birds will tolerate this and it will usually be removed.

Bumblefoot

This is a common condition seen in raptors, especially birds kept in captivity. It is normally due to penetration of the base of the foot by talons that are elongated or where perches are too thin resulting in overcurvature of the toes into the foot.

The result is swelling, inflammation and infection resulting in abscessation of the foot.

Treat with amoxycillin LA IM SID for 5 days.

If infection does not respond, surgery of the site may be required. All infected material must be removed and it may be suitable to leave the wound open to drain and heal by granulation.

The wound will require padding and dressing and may require support by splinting or casting to allow it to heal.

Poor condition and starvation

This may occur for a number of reasons including poor food availability or inability to hunt effectively, especially if a captive-bred bird escapes.

The bird will appear in poor condition, underweight and with protruding keel bone, poor muscle coverage and poor feather condition.

Treatment includes:

- rehydrating the bird with warm fluids orally
- avoiding feeding solid food immediately as the gut may be in stasis resulting in reduction of digestion of solid materials
- feeding liquid food substitutes suitable for birds for the first 24 hours, e.g. Ensure, Polyaid or liquidised minced meat and water
- providing solid food in the usual way once droppings are apparent and gut is mobile; however, avoid overfeeding, which will result in secondary problems

> **Tip:** Use mice that have been cut into very small pieces and gently holding the head in one hand open the beak and place the piece of food into the mouth with tweezers; placing near the back of the throat will assist in gaining a swallow reflex. Continue until the bird refuses food.

- providing the bird with multivitamin supplements such as Abidec and B vitamins to boost condition

- treating with broad-spectrum antibiotics as a precaution if infection is suspected, e.g. enrofloxacin orally 15 mg/kg twice per day.

CASE HISTORY 1
Patient

Adult tawny owl found on woodland path during the afternoon. On approach the bird attempted to fly and was trying to escape but was unable to get off the ground. The left wing was hanging lower than the other.

Condition

The owl was stressed and obviously suffering injury from trauma; it was frightened but alert and responsive. The bird was suffering from hypothermia and dehydration, probably due to trauma and the inability to catch and eat prey.

Capture

As the owl was unable to fly the capture was straightforward. To prevent stress a towel was placed over the bird. Placing a bird of prey into darkness is calming and enables a safe and untraumatic capture. Birds of prey often become placid and do not resist capture when covered.

Treatment

On admission the bird was fully examined, and found to be in shock and mildly dehydrated. The drooping wing was examined and crepitus in the humerus felt and it was in no obvious pain; however, this is often masked. Oral Lectade was gavaged to assist rehydration and the left wing was X-rayed to assess the degree of injury. The owl was then placed in a warm and dark enclosure to recover from shock. Dexamethasone and rimadyl were administered intramuscularly in the chest to treat shock and pain.

The following day a decision was made to pin the simple fracture with internal fixation. This would allow for the assessment of the possibility of full flight and, therefore, the ability to capture prey. The operation was straightforward and the bird recovered well. Movement was restricted for the following 2 weeks whilst the wing was strapped into position to allow the break to heal. The bird was X-rayed again 5 weeks later and an excellent mend of the break was observed; however, movement had been restricted. The strapping was removed to assess wing position; the bird had been feeding well but had lost condition and muscle coverage. The bird needed to be built up and flight status and ability assessed. After 2 weeks the bird's weight improved and it was placed into an aviary. Flight ability was poor and the muscles were weak. Flight ability was continually assessed over the following weeks and showed little improvement. The bird was unable to sustain flight and would have been unable to capture prey in the wild. At this point regardless of treatment euthanasia was the only option, as a return to the wild would have been a death sentence.

CASE HISTORY 2

Patient

An adult barn owl involved in road traffic accident, which is very common as they often fly low. The bird was collapsed and hypothermic as a result of its feathers being damp and wet from lying in the road.

Condition

The owl was unresponsive and in shock; there was obvious bruising to both wings with swelling and contusions visible on the skin. The bird was concussed with no palpebral reflex to the right eye which was half closed with swelling on the right side of the face.

Capture

As the owl was collapsed and unresponsive, it was picked up using gloves as protection against the talons and placed into a warm container to help control shock and assist in raising the body temperature.

Treatment

The bird was given Dexamethasone IM and warm oral Lectade to control both shock and dehydration. The bird was dried off as much as possible and placed in a dark container with a heat lamp.

Following a 6-hour recovery period the bird was brighter and warm. A full examination showed concussion with bruising to the right eye, although the pupil was reactive to light. The bruising of the wings was apparent but no broken bones were found. The bird was unsteady and weak and required a period of rest. The eye was treated with hypromellose drops to assist in reducing bruising and potential damage. Arnica gel can be useful in reducing bruising and can be rubbed directly onto the skin. The wings were working and all joints mobile.

The bird continued to remain in a dark and warm environment over the next few days until the signs of bruising and concussion had subsided. At this point he was placed in an aviary to assess vision, prey location and flight ability. The vision did not appear to have been affected and flight was good but not sustained due to bruising. After a few weeks the bruising subsided and the bird's condition continued to improve with increased muscle coverage. Once sustained flight was achieved the bird was released in open land near to the site of accident.

Chapter **7**

Wild birds

Sara Cowen

INTRODUCTION

Wild birds are presented to the surgery for numerous reasons including: road traffic accidents, abandonment and, more commonly, cat attacks. If a bird allows you to approach it and pick it up it is unwell. The common problems may be physical with fractures and wounds; however, they also suffer from a number of diseases that debilitate them and require treatment.

The main objective is to return the bird back to the wild in health as soon as possible.

Firstly, identify your patient so the correct diet and accommodation can be provided; the most common species seen will be pigeons, doves, blackbirds, thrushes, tits, finches, starlings and sparrows.

HANDLING

The easiest method of handling for small birds is placing a hand over the back to contain the wings. To examine closely place the bird's head between the index and middle fingers with the body gently cupped in the palm. This method will allow you to examine all parts of the bird including the wings.

Towels and blankets are used to calm larger birds.

Birds will bite; however, it is rarely painful and can be tolerated.

Swans and geese use their wings for protection and can be extremely strong. Restrain with one hand around the neck under the head and the other arm should enclose the wings and body (Fig. 7.1). Alternatively, swans, geese and other large

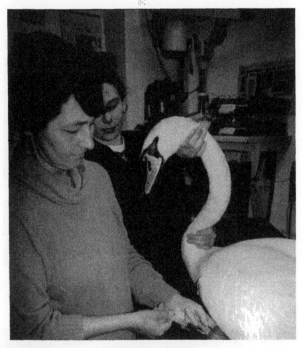

Fig. 7.1 Swan handling and investigation.

birds are restrained easily by placing them into a cloth bag with a corner removed for the head. This contains bird a the wings safely allowing transportation and treatment without damage to the handler or bird. Allow them to sit on their keel.

> **Tip:** Be very wary of water birds with long pointed beaks such as grebes and herons. They can inflict damage and will often lunge at the face. Wear protective goggles when handling.

ACCOMMODATION

Accommodation is dependent on the size of the bird (Figs 7.2 & 7.3a,b). Small garden birds can be placed in cat kennels or cat carriers as long as escape is not possible. For very small species a birdcage will be required and for larger species, such as swans, a dog kennel will be suitable.

Place newspaper in the cage and perches if a perching bird. Always ensure the cage is covered over to reduce stress; the last thing a bird will want to see is the cat opposite. If possible house in a separate, quiet room.

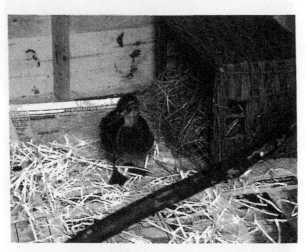

Fig. 7.2 Housing a duckling.

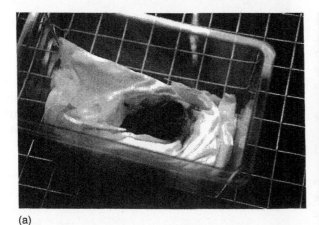

(a)

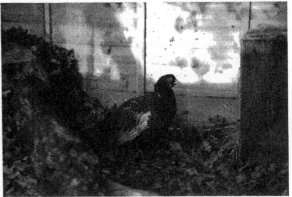

(b)

Fig. 7.3 (a) Housing a baby blue tit. (b) Housing a pheasant.

> **Tip:** *Never* place birds on hay or straw bedding material as spores present can result in the fatal condition aspergillosis. Always place in well-ventilated areas.

Woodpeckers in captivity should be provided with a log vertically in the cage for the bird to hang onto. Swifts also fare better if allowed to hang as they will not perch. Place a towel hung over the side of the accommodation for them to climb.

> **Tip:** In some cases, where birds are confined and unwilling to move, a build up of faeces around the cloaca will result in constipation or blockage. Keep the area clean and if necessary a liquid paraffin enema will assist in removing blockage.

NUTRITION

As there are so many varieties of birds it is important that you know their diet before attempting to feed, as some diets may be inappropriate.

Small birds such as finches and sparrows can be split into two categories: seedeaters and insectivores. Seedeaters can be provided with a standard mixed birdseed or wild birdseed. Insectivores are best fed on a diet of cat meat with a universal insectivorous food mixed in. Insects can be added if available, and additions such as scrambled egg and breadcrumbs will be taken.

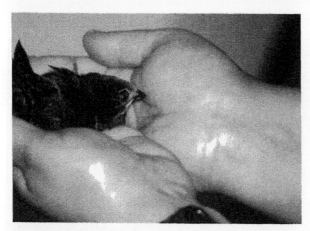

Fig. 7.4 Swift in hand.

Larger birds, such as the corvids, will feed on scraps and tinned dog meats.

Water birds will eat either fish or vegetation. Fish eaters can be offered sprats and whitebait can be placed into water. They should also receive thiamine supplementation, 1 tablet placed in the fish daily.

Birds such as swans and geese will require a mix of poultry pellets, chopped greens, corn and bread, again placed in water.

Swifts (Fig. 7.4) will need to be force-fed with mealworms regularly, as they normally feed on the wing and are unable to pick food from a bowl. Gently open the mouth and place the mealworm in.

Woodpeckers dig for their food in wood, so drill holes in a log and pack them with dog food, insects, suet, honey, etc. and place upright in the cage. The woodpecker can then feed from the log.

> **Tip:** Oral dosing of vitamin B_{12} liquid (Cytacon) weekly will help boost the bird's overall health and acts as an appetite stimulant.

See Tables 7.1 and 7.2 for the recommended diets of adult captive birds.

HAND REARING

Many birds are orphaned around spring and summer; this is only genuine where they have

Table 7.1 Captive feeding codes for common adult birds

Species	Code
Birds of prey	1
Blackbirds	2
Coots	3
Crows	2
Doves	4
Ducks	5
Falcons	1
Finches	6
Gamebirds	4
Geese	5
Hawks	1
Herons	7
Jays	2
Martins/swifts	8
Owls	1
Pigeons	4
Robins	2
Sparrows	9
Starlings	2
Swallows	8
Swans	5
Thrushes	2
Tits	9
Woodpeckers	10

fallen from the nest, if the mother has been killed or if the nest has been disturbed.

Nestlings (unfeathered) may fall from nests and it may be possible to replace them. Pick up a baby bird with a piece of kitchen roll to avoid direct contact with the hand and replace in the nest if it can be located.

Fledglings (feathered) will leave the nest before they are fully mobile and will be seen hopping around. Do not place these birds into the nest as the others may be disturbed, and the mother may well be around collecting food.

If the bird is truly abandoned and hand rearing is necessary, make up a baby bird mix (Box 7.1). Many adult seed-eating birds will eat this diet when young as it is easier to digest and richer in protein.

Feed birds using round-ended tweezers or, if extremely small, a small clean paintbrush (Fig. 7.5). The bird will open its mouth instinctively, but gently tapping on the side of the mouth will usually instigate the response. It will keep gaping until it is full (Fig. 7.6a,b). Feeding every

Table 7.2 Captive feeding chart for common adult birds

Code	Dog food	Day-old chick	Bread	Mixed corn	Mixed seed	Peanuts	Layers mash/pellets	Sunflower seeds	Whitebait/sprats	Green veg/grass	Scrambled egg	Insects/meal-worms
1		X										
2	X		X								X	X
3	X			X				X		X	X	X
4				X	X	X						
5			X	X			X			X		X
6					X	X		X				X
7									X			
8	X										X	X
9			X		X			X				
10	X				X							X

Box 7.1 Baby bird mix

- Cat/dog food
- Scrambled egg
- Universal insect diet
- Breadcrumbs
- Chopped up mealworms
- Vitamin mineral supplement
- Water

Mix up a batch in the morning that will last throughout the day.

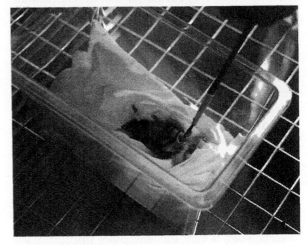

Fig. 7.5 Feeding a baby bird with a brush.

hour is required throughout the day; however, stop feeding through the night. Remove the faecal sac each time they are fed.

For very small birds unable to stand, place in a small container lined with tissue. Once birds begin standing they can be placed in cages with small perches.

They will soon begin to eat food from the bowl once fledging and will often stop feeding so much prior to this.

Tip: Once feathered and active, birds' feeding may slow down over a period of 2 days; at this point they are ready for release as they are fledged.
Always release birds in the morning and in fine weather. This allows them time to settle and rest before night time.

Some birds are born precocial (fully developed), such as ducklings, and will eat solids on their own. Place chick crumbs, egg crumbs and starter pellets into water in a shallow bowl for them to sieve through.

Tip: If they are reluctant to eat sprinkle crumbs onto their coat; the movement will attract attention and they will peck at the crumbs on the feathers.

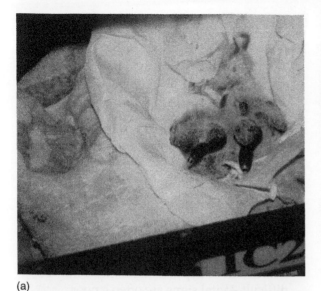

(a)

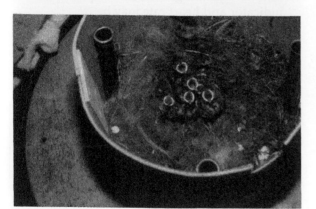

(b)

Fig. 7.6 (a) Baby pigeons. (b) Baby birds gaping for feed.

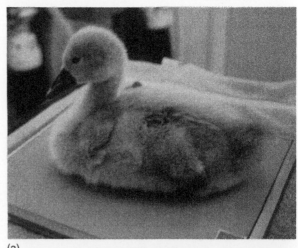

(a)

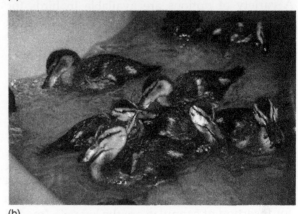

(b)

Fig. 7.7 (a) Weighing a cygnet. (b) Juvenile ducks swimming.

Ducklings, etc., although water birds, are not fully waterproofed and will be covered with downy feathers. They must not be left in water for long as they will become wet and suffer from hypothermia. Only allow them access to swimming for 10–20 minutes at a time (Fig. 7.7b) and do not leave in the cage. They will require a heat lamp to huddle under and dry off afterwards.

> **Tip:** Hang a mop head or feather duster from the top of the cage just touching the floor. This represents the mother and the birds will nestle under the mop head for comfort and warmth.

FIRST AID

Wild birds suffer from stress easily and can, under certain conditions, suffer secondary problems.

Initial treatment

It is important to keep initial treatment to a minimum and let the bird acclimatise before too much handling is done.

Birds should be provided with:

- warmth
- darkness
- quiet
- oral fluids by syringe or gavaging – Lectade or Critical Care formula

- intravenous fluids 50 ml/kg/day for maintenance
- corticosteroids – dexamethasone 0.1 mg/kg IM
- sedation if required – diazepam 1.0 mg/kg IV or IM.

> **Tip:** Gavaging is an effective method for administering liquid nutrition and fluids to birds. A tube is placed directly into the oesophagus to the crop. A useful product for liquid nutrition is Complan, a recovery diet for humans.

Fluid therapy

A variety of options are available in birds for rehydration and all fluids should be given at body temperature.

Firstly, oral fluids can be gavaged, a fairly simple but effective treatment.

They are able to take up to 25 ml/kg of fluids, and fluids should be administered warm to prevent shock. Always watch the mouth when gavaging in case of fluid appearance during the process from overadministration.

Fluids can be given intravenously; however, it is almost always impossible except in larger birds such as geese and swans. The two main sites for insertion of cannulae are the leg vein (medial tibia) or wing vein (cutaneous ulnar vein). For smaller species it is simpler to administer the fluids intraosseously in the intramedullary cavities of long bones. Only sterilised fluid must be administered.

Subcutaneous fluids are not as effective in severe cases of dehydration, but may be a useful method for maintenance fluids. A rate of approximately 5–10 ml/kg can be provided and the total quantity spread over several sites such as the hind legs, pelvis, back, etc.

PRE- AND POST-OPERATIVE CARE FOR WILD BIRDS

A physical examination of every bird should be carried out prior to any form of anaesthesia, as any health concerns may lead to complications and even death. Birds often have underlying respiratory problems and stress can promote illness following anaesthesia.

In all birds good pre-surgical preparation and intensive post-operative nursing are essential, as they are generally not good candidates for anaesthesia. A bird's respiratory system is based on numerous air sacs that are distributed throughout the body, so level of anaesthesia and overdose are concerns. It may also take longer for recovery as the anaesthesia remains residual in the air sacs for longer.

Cautions:

- If analgesia is incomplete, increasing the anaesthetic may result in overdose.
- Evaluation of depth of anaesthesia may be difficult – vital signs are often a poor indicator and heart rate may be immeasurable.
- Response is extremely variable, especially with water birds.
- Recovery can be prolonged.

> **Tip:** Birds rarely show a response to pain so do not assume because there is no sign that they are not suffering and consider analgesia for the extent of injury as for other animals.

Pre-operative checks

The following points should be addressed before any surgical intervention:

- Minimise stress by limited pre-operative handling.
- Look for oculonasal discharge – this may indicate the presence of respiratory congestion leading to further complications during anaesthesia.
- Listen to the lungs – impairment or damage may result in respiratory failure during surgery; birds commonly suffer subclinical respiratory congestion.
- If the animal is dehydrated, pre-operative fluids can be given subcutaneously or by gavaging.

Tip: Birds suffer from hypothermia and circulatory shock very easily. During anaesthesia and recovery, the body temperature should be maintained (heated mat), and the surgical area kept to a minimum, as this will be a source of heat loss.

Intensive post-operative nursing

Place the bird on a heated mat. Removal of the heat source can result in rapid heat loss. Heat lamps can be used but avoid overheating; ensure that the bird can move away from the heat if it needs to – excessive heat can cause dehydration.

Administer oxygen immediately to assist in reducing air sac anaesthetic concentration and respiratory stimulants where necessary.

Warm any fluids given to, or used upon, the bird to body temperature before use.

Ensure all excrement is cleaned up and the bird is dried to prevent hypothermia.

Encourage the bird's appetite and eating by providing the appropriate diet; see feeding guide. If appetite is poor administer subcutaneous fluids instead. Administration of an avian probiotic (Avipro) may assist in maintaining intestinal flora.

Keep the bird warm, dark and as quiet as possible to reduce stress – remember, it is wild.

Wild bird anaesthesia

See pre- and post-operative care guidelines prior to administration of anaesthetic to be fully prepared.

Induction of anaesthesia is usually through a mask and is gaseous with no premedication. Birds are fairly calm when placed into a mask and induce easily. If the bird is unsettled just cover the eyes to reduce stress.

Various sized masks are available but adaptions to equipment may be necessary to fit the bird's face and to reduce environmental contamination from the mask. Useful items are syringe cases of various sizes that can be attached to the system. Maintenance of small birds will be through the mask. However, larger birds, such as swans, geese, etc., can be intubated and placed on an Ayres T-piece; this allows monitoring of breathing from the bag. For smaller birds requiring intubation urinary or IV catheters and cannulae can be adapted. Diving birds are prone to breath holding, making assessment of patient induction level and stability difficult; this is less of a problem if the parenteral route is used.

Water birds take in water during feeding and reflux and inhalation may occur during anaesthesia. Starving for 2–4 hours prior to induction and intubation with a cuffed tube will eliminate this risk.

Tip: In birds it is not as easy to see and check movements indicating the breathing rate. If you are concerned look into the mouth and you will observe the opening and closing of the tracheal entrance, the glottis; this can be useful if the bird is covered in drapes.

Parenteral anaesthesia

Parenteral anaesthesia is possible, especially for diving birds, followed by maintenance through gaseous anaesthesia.

Weigh the bird prior to administration of a parenteral agent to prevent overdosing and a prolonged recovery period.

Ketamine in combination with xylazine or diazepam has been used successfully. Anaesthetic can be given intramuscularly.

Surgical depth of anaesthesia may last for 10–15 minutes, but can be maintained on gaseous anaesthesia for prolonged procedures.

Parenteral dose rates

Ketamine	Xylazine	Diazepam
10–30 mg/kg	0.25–0.5 mg/kg	1.0–1.5 mg/kg

Remember: bird anaesthesia is difficult and reactions of birds may vary. Dose rates are based on illness, condition, injury, body weight, etc., and each bird must be thoroughly assessed prior to induction; however, responses may vary greatly.

Gaseous anaesthesia

The preferred agent is isoflurane, with halothane as a possible alternative, as this is removed from the body quickly and has a better safety margin than halothane.

The bird's air sac system greatly increases the surface area for gaseous exchange when compared to mammals. They can also act as reservoirs for the agent following operative procedures and prolong the recovery period. Overdose is possible due to this system.

When a bird reaches the depth you require for surgery the levels may be decreased. However, the residual higher concentration still in the air sacs may actually cause further deepening than required so always monitor levels carefully and do not induce deep anaesthesia. Induction is very rapid and so is recovery if well monitored.

Induce using a concentration of 1–4% and maintain on 0.5–2%. Use palpebral, corneal, pedal and wing pinch reflexes for assessing depth during induction.

Flush the system through with oxygen during recovery to reduce air space residual concentrations.

Keep the bird warm prior to, during and after anaesthesia due to drop in core body temperature; Bubble wrap is an excellent insulate during recovery.

COMMON ILLNESSES, INJURIES OR DISEASES

There are numerous conditions that birds will suffer from and only the most common will be covered here.

Parasites

Birds suffer from the usual parasites, both internal and external. On the whole they do not suffer with heavy burdens of fleas or ticks.

Feather lice are common, living in the birds with little effect on health.

Mites can be eradicated using a topical treatment of ivermectin applying 0.1 ml placed on the bird's skin at the back of the neck.

Flat flies are often seen running over birds during handling. These lice can be removed using an insecticide powder, but pose no problem to the handler and not usually to the bird either.

Fenbendazole and thiabendazole are usual for gapeworms (syngamiasis). Infestation of this nematode worm is normal and can result in respiratory distress as they sit in the trachea. The red thread-like worm may be actually observed in the trachea or an indication of problems may be shown in mouth breathing. Mebendazole is also usual as a powder; it can be added to the food.

Alopecia

Baldness often occurs in female water birds such as ducks, especially at the back of the head, and is invariably observed during the mating season. This is usually inflicted by the drakes rather than being actual feather loss, where they pull out feathers during the onslaught of mating. The females usually require supportive treatment and peace and quiet as they can be in fairly poor condition following this.

Trichomoniasis (frounce, trick or canker)

This is observed in pigeons, doves and birds of prey and is a protozoan infection from *Trichomonas gallinae* affecting the throat and mouth. The presence of cheesy growths in the mouth and throat region will clarify.

In some cases the growths become so enlarged that they obstruct the airways causing dyspnoea and possibly asphyxiation. The growth can travel down the oesophagus into the crop causing damage. Birds will usually be in poor condition and emaciated.

Rehydrate the bird by orally gavaging fluids.

Treatment for the protozoan is metronidazole 50 mg/kg orally (PO) twice per day for 5 days or carnidazol 10 mg/kg.

Following treatment the lesion may drop off or be carefully removed. Use a cotton bud to gently wipe away from the mouth cavity and throat area.

Contraction and spread of this condition is through direct contact so keep birds isolated from others and use a high level of hygiene with equipment.

Aspergillosis

Aspergillosis (*Aspergillus fumigatus*) is one of the most common causes of fatality in birds, as they appear to have little immune response to this fungal pathogen. It can also be triggered whilst kept in captivity and be induced by stress creating secondary problems that need treatment.

Aspergillosis thrives in damp conditions, and hay and straw bedding may encourage this as spores may be present in dry hay.

It is believed that it may be permanently present in the bird's respiratory system without causing any symptoms, but situations such as stress, environmental change, and illness, etc., may trigger problems. The fungus may then affect the respiration system of the bird initially without symptoms until disease has progressed.

The condition in its acute form will kill within 7 days and in a chronic form can kill within several weeks.

Symptoms may include:

- wheezing
- fluffed up appearance
- depression
- inappetance
- mouth breathing
- pneumonia
- emaciation.

The following treatment can be offered but is often ineffective:

- Sporanox at 5–10 mg/kg twice per day for 2–4 weeks may assist.
- Antifungal nebuliser such as clotrimazole solution as needed.
- Oxygen if dyspnoeic.
- Bronchodilators.

Paramyxovirus

This is a highly contagious viral condition that is seen in feral pigeons.

Symptoms may include:

- respiratory difficulties
- ocular discharge
- watery, bloody diarrhoea
- torticollis
- head tremors
- paralysis.

However, although the symptoms appear severe, the mortality rate is low and supportive care throughout the period will usually result in recovery.

Avian pox

This is a viral condition affecting various birds.

The two forms can appear as a moist condition with lesions observed in the throat and respiratory tract, or in a dry form creating scabby lesions on the feet or beak.

It is contagious but not fatal and will often disappear without assistance, although if debilitated, antibiotics and fluids may assist in improving overall health.

Botulism

Avian botulism is caused by the bacteria *Clostridium botulinum* and is usually observed in summer when temperatures reach above 23°C and the bacteria thrive. It is usually seen in water birds such as gulls and swans, as the bacteria is picked up whilst foraging in the silt and mud.

Symptoms of botulism poisoning are:

- diarrhoea
- paralysis of the legs
- flickering of the eyes and membranes
- dyspnoea
- bradycardia
- reduced body temperature.

Treatment includes:

- IV fluids or intraosseous fluids 50 ml/kg
- corticosteroids, e.g. dexamethasone 3–4 mg/kg
- antibiotic treatment
- appetite stimulants
- activated charcoal 5–10 g
- kaolin to control diarrhoea
- force-feeding if not eating.

Wing and feather damage

A broken feather is not too much of a problem for the general bird species and only becomes a problem for specialist fliers such as swifts, which feed on the wing.

Steaming damaged or ruffled feathers over hot water will allow them to be straightened. It is important to remember that if primary feathers are broken and are not able to be repaired the bird will not grow new ones until the annual autumn moult, resulting in a long period in captivity.

Feathers can, in some cases, be repaired by attaching part of another feather. This is called 'imping', where an alternative healthy feather from the same species can be glued to the damaged one and will remain until the moult. The shafts of feathers are hollow, allowing a small wooden stick, such as a cocktail stick, to be glued into the shaft of the damaged feather and the replacement feather glued to the other end. If the feather shaft is just damaged but intact it can be strengthened by the application of glue onto the shaft, keeping it in place and acting as support, and allowing it to work as a feather once more.

Fractures

Fractures will be observed in birds as with other animals and will usually be of the wing, leg or possibly the beak. Birds show little obvious sign of pain and will often continue to attempt to fly and walk on fractured limbs (Fig. 7.8).

Wing fractures appear to be the most common (Fig. 7.9) and may often be the result of flying into windows or road traffic accidents. The obvious sign is that the wing is held drooped against the body lower than the opposite wing.

Wings can be immobilised and splinted by placing against the body of the bird and bandaging in a figure of eight across the sternum. This may well affect the bird's balance initially, but it will soon accommodate the bandage. The wings and legs can be treated in the usual manner, and splinted and bandaged to the bird's body.

Beak repairs can be undertaken using Vetseal, Vet bond or bone cement, and in some cases prosthetic beaks can be made. However, these birds must not be released and must be kept in captivity, as repair is rarely fully effective or long lasting. Birds with a missing top beak may well manage in the wild; however, they may require force-feeding.

> **Tip:** Following fracture repair, it is important to consider the species of bird. Many birds such as pigeons and ducks will cope with a damaged, repaired wing; however, birds of prey, reliant on flight and grasping to catch prey, will not. Unless full recovery is achieved it is possible that euthanasia should be considered or, alternatively, life in captivity.

Some companies now make specific splints for birds' limbs that will enable immobilisation. If both limbs are broken, birds can be suspended

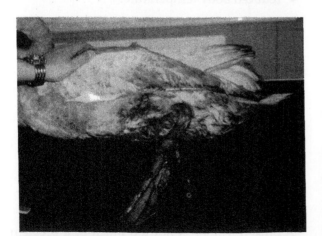

Fig. 7.8 Injured leg and wing of swan.

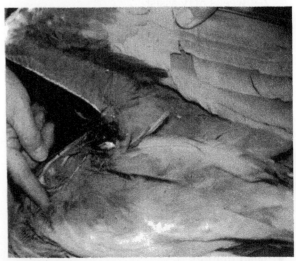

Fig. 7.9 Injured heron.

in slings to allow recovery and again some companies are now providing bird slings.

Cat attacks/wounds

Possibly the most common cause of injury to garden birds is cat attacks. Cats carry the bacteria *Pasteurella multocida* on their teeth and this can result in septicaemia and death in birds following capture. Any bird suspected or known to have been attacked should routinely be injected with antibiotics, e.g. enrofloxacin IM 5–15 mg/kg or amoxycillin LA 15–30 mg/kg IM.

The most likely wounds will be puncture wounds, lacerations, feather damage or fractures. Wounds should be cleaned and covered with Intrasite gel and allowed to heal. Larger lacerations will require debriding and suturing under anaesthetic.

> **Tip:** Birds are prey species and, as such, are not designed to exhibit signs of pain; therefore, carry out analgesia, sedation or anaesthesia for suturing, etc.

Fishing line and hook injuries

These are commonplace with water birds as the popularity of fishing increases. Many birds forage on the river floor upended looking for vegetable matter and can accidentally ingest a hook or become entangled in the process. The nature of the hook and the soft tissue in the throat lead to penetration of the oesophagus and the hook embedding into tissue (Fig. 7.10). This will not fall out as the ends are barbed. If the line is still attached this may also be ingested resulting in a blockage of the oesophagus, crop or gut. The hook may also become embedded in the feet and wings where removal is accessible.

Radiography will help locate the hook for removal. This may be easy if embedded in the mouth.

Surgery may be required if further down the tract. The end of the hook will need to be cut off before the body is pulled out.

Treat with antibiotics for secondary infection developing following removal.

Oiled birds

The main victims of oil contamination are sea birds but it can also be observed in birds inhabiting waterways and in other fresh water birds. Sources of pollution may be oil spills or contamination from riverboats.

The oil breaks down the structure of the feather barbs and barbules allowing water and cold to penetrate into the body (Fig. 7.11). The oil

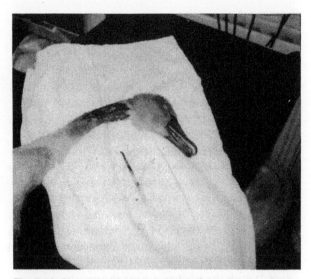

Fig. 7.10 Swan with injury to neck from fishing hook.

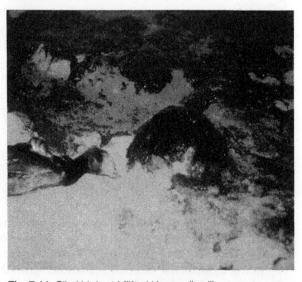

Fig. 7.11 Oiled birds at Milford Haven oil spill.

affects the bird's plumage resulting in destruction of the waterproof and insulative properties, both of which are vital to water life. The feathers no longer repel water and the bird's buoyancy becomes affected. They become hypothermic and, in the worst case scenario, drown.

The birds naturally try to preen, which is ineffective, and this results in the ingestion of the oil, leading to poisoning and damage to the intestines.

Treatment

On presentation the bird will be in shock. The bird should initially be provided with warmth and food.

Place the bird on newspaper or clean sheets with no other source of bedding such as straw or shavings and provide a heat source.

Rehydrate intravenously or orally.

For fish eaters place food such as sprats or whitebait in a shallow bowl of water for them to feed. For other birds put poultry pellets, grain, bread or vegetable matter in water for them to eat.

Try to remove oil from the eyes, mouth and nostrils using swabs and place aqueous eye drops in both eyes. Administer activated charcoal and kaolin to assist with internal damage and absorption. Weigh the bird and note the result.

Cleaning

Prior to cleaning, the bird must be bright, alert and responsive. Do not attempt to clean if still suffering from shock.

Cleaning the bird will require time and care, constant running, high-pressured warm water (approx. 42°C) and a supply of Fairy washing up liquid.

> **Tip:** Fairy or Co-op own brand seem to be the most effective at removing oil.

Start at the head region, working the washing up liquid through the feathers in the direction of the feathers, as damage to structure can be caused by going against the direction of feather growth. The head and beak can be cleaned using a small brush such as a toothbrush. Work down the back and then the chest ending at the tail. Repeat this process again and again until every residue of oil and detergent is removed.

> **Tip:** Bird feathers are water repellent due to the structure of the barbs and not to secretion from the preen gland. When fully clean the structure will allow them to be water repellent again. The water will begin beading on the feather when all residues are removed.

Once cleaned, place the bird in a clean cage with heat source and allow to dry and preen itself.

Feed the bird up and ensure all droppings are normal before considering release.

Allow the bird to swim and preen and ensure it is fully buoyant and waterproof. At the slightest sign of problems the bird should be washed again.

Lead poisoning

This often occurs when birds have ingested lead fishing weights and they have accumulated in the crop.

Symptoms include:

- lethargy
- muscle weakness
- kinked neck due to paralysis of neck muscles
- anorexia
- inability to digest food as gizzard inactive
- emaciation
- green faecal material.

Diagnosis is normally through radiography as lead weight and shot are radio-opaque.

In some cases surgical removal of the lead from the location in the digestive system may be required, normally from the gizzard; however, this is traumatic and evacuation through the alimentary canal is preferred.

Treatment involves 25% sodium calcium-edetate 0.25 mg/kg subcutaneously (SC) for 3 days. IV fluids should be given as required along with an injection of vitamin B_{12} (approximately 2–3 ml).

Recovery is often long term and advice for rehabilitation should be sought.

Metabolic bone disease

This is a condition observed when an inappropriate balance of minerals, calcium and phosphorus is received, resulting in poorly calcified bones with symptoms of bowed legs, deformity and possibly fractured bones.

In some cases calcium supplementation of the diet will assist in rectifying the problem or alleviating the immediate symptoms.

> **Tip:** If keeping birds of prey in captivity, it is imperative to feed them whole carcasses, such as day-old chicks, to provide an adequate supply of calcium, phosphorus and vitamin D.

THERAPEUTICS

Drugs can be administered to birds in a variety of ways.

Most injections are best placed IM in the chest muscles. If giving a course of injections over a few days, alternate the side for injection to limit bruising.

Medication can be given orally by liquid or tablet and is a fairly easy procedure with birds compared to mammals.

Fluids can be administered IV in larger birds and orally if necessary. The alternative route is gavaging, where the fluid is tube fed into the crop.

CASE HISTORY 1

Patient

Adult male blackbird, weighing 20 g.

Reason for hospitalisation

The bird was rescued by the client in the house having been brought in by the cat. The owner managed to catch the bird and placed it in a cardboard box. There appeared to be feathers missing, some blood spots and one of the wings appeared to be drooping.

On admittance the bird was diagnosed as having a fractured humerus of the right wing requiring splinting. There were also some superficial lacerations acquired during the attack over the body surface; also a little bleeding was observed and the bird appeared to be in shock.

Type of accommodation and bedding material used

The bird was placed in a cat carrier and placed in isolation on a heat mat to assist in combating shock. The cage was lined with newspaper and some shavings to collect droppings. Some small twigs were placed across the middle of the carrier to act as perches if required. The bird was placed in isolation to limit stress from noises of cats and dogs, a towel was placed over the front of the carrier for security and darkness during the shock and recovery period.

Accommodation cleaning protocol

The bird was fairly clean, and handling was limited to prevent injury and further shock. As birds produce solid droppings it was possible to remove them on a daily basis in the shavings and replaced with fresh shavings. No infectious disease was observed, so full cleaning and removal of all waste occurred every 3 days. The cage was thoroughly cleaned with Formula H spray and rinsed replacing newspaper, shavings and perches.

Feeding regime

As blackbirds are insectivores/omnivores the bulk of the diet comprised tinned cat food, with the addition of a dried insectivore food mixed at approximately 1 teaspoon per feed mixed in, with the addition of mealworms, with the heads removed, when available. Blackbirds are diurnal so feed was placed in the cage in the morning to follow natural feeding behaviour and the bird was allowed to feed throughout the day. Waste food was removed in the evening once dark. Fresh water was available through the day provided in shallow bowl. A sprinkling of calcium was placed daily into the feed to assist in bone repair and growth.

Nursing care and monitoring of the animals

The blackbird required daily monitoring for treatment of shock; monitoring of the puncture wounds that may result in infections, and also splinting and bandaging of the wing. Daily medication for infection and wounds was given; they were bathed and treated with Intrasite Gel for 3 days. No surgical procedures were required. The wing was splinted with an aluminium finger splint and bandaged to the bird's side in a figure of eight. The splint and bandage were changed only when soiled or if they had moved position, usually every 3 days.

Medication administered

On admission, the blackbird was given systemic antibiotics – baytril was initially given IM 0.02 ml and then one drop orally for the next 5 days during daily examination. This was to treat possible infection from the cat attack, as the bacteria found in puncture wounds often results in abscess or fatality. Wounds were cleaned with Savlon daily and treated with Intrasite Gel for 3 days.

No further treatment was required other than recuperation.

Date(s)

The thrush remained in the hospital for 4 weeks. During this period all wounds were healed within 1 week, but fracture repair took 4 weeks for adequate healing. The bird was then taken to an aviary to assess flight ability and release was 1 week later.

CASE HISTORY 2
Patient

Adult thrush found in the garden collapsed on the patio. The bird appeared very lethargic and unaware of its surroundings.

Condition

There was a swelling to the head and one eye was closed. The bird was huddled in appearance with head held close to body. Balance had been affected and the bird appeared to tilt to the left; on examination one wing was held lower than the other.

Treatment

The bird was initially examined, with swelling apparent to the head, the left eye being permanently closed and obvious signs of concussion. There was also bruising under the skin on the left wing, which appeared to have a hairline fracture in the radius.

The bird was given dexadresson to assist in controlling the shock and a drop of Rescue Remedy was placed in the mouth. The wing was splinted using a cocktail stick and strapped in a figure of eight with micropore tape against the body. The bird was placed in warmth and darkness following treatment to allow it to recover from shock. Food and water were placed in the cage.

The following day the bird looked brighter and had shown interest in the food. The bird was reassessed and the swelling and affects of concussion were reduced. The wing was left strapped up to repair, and the bird was comfortable.

The strapping was removed 2 weeks later and the bird placed in an aviary to assess flight mobility. There had been loss of strength in the muscles but the wing was in the correct position and working. The bird was left for a further week in the aviary to build up muscle coverage and was then released satisfactorily.

CASE HISTORY 3
Patient

Adult swan with fishing line hanging from mouth, being dragged behind with float attached.

Condition

The bird was active, feeding, swimming and appeared well in the water, although the line was protruding from the beak and was obviously attached in some way. There was concern that the hook may be lodged further down the throat possibly causing internal damage and infection.

Capture

Swans are extremely powerful animals and can be aggressive if threatened. The wings are more likely to cause damage to the rescuer than the beak, which may just produce a nasty nip. The bird was enticed into the bank by using bread as bait. Once at arm's length a swan hook was placed around the neck, the bird pulled to the bank and the wings quickly enclosed against the body for restraint.

Treatment

The bird was initially examined and the wire was coming directly from the mouth of the bird. By gently feeling around the beak and surrounding soft tissue a sharp point could be felt on the underside of the beak toward the throat. The fish-hook was protruding through this tissue. Inside the mouth the wire was wrapped around the tongue. The end of the hook was cut off to remove the wire. The wire was then gently unwound from around the tongue and the tongue examined for damage. The remainder of the hook, then attached to the wire, was removed from the mouth. The wire had not caused any lacerations or damage to the tongue. Betadine spray was applied to the wound, and the swan was given a shot of duphamox LA and immediately released.

SECTION 4

Wildlife care

Introduction

REASONS FOR ADMISSION

Wild animals are admitted into veterinary practice for a number of reasons and require a specialised and particular method of handling, treatment and care to survive through the critical period and to allow treatment to take place.

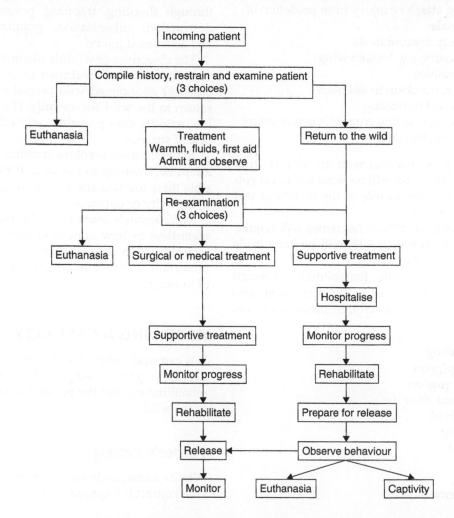

It is important to remember that whilst requiring help, they are unfamiliar with human contact and become stressed easily, exacerbating the condition and hampering the ability to treat.

The veterinary practice is often a frightening and hostile place for domestic pets and is more so for wildlife. It is important to remember that these patients require quiet, dark and secure surroundings away from the hustle and bustle of activity. It is also vital to return them back to the wild in a fit state in the fastest possible time.

Wildlife may be seen in the surgery for a number of reasons including the following:

- Orphan or abandoned young
- Road traffic accident (over 10 000 badgers a year)
- Cat or dog attack or injury from predation of wild animals
- Disease, e.g. myxomatosis
- General injury, e.g. broken wings
- Oiled casualties
- Illness, e.g. botulism in sea birds
- Pollution and poisoning
- Fishing hook and line entanglement or injury
- Cruelty from humans.

This list provides you with an idea of what type of casualties you will be faced with, and you need to be knowledgeable in the treatment and procedures for these.

Approximately 20% of casualties will require hand rearing, of which 80% will be baby birds and 20% mammals.

The British Wildlife Rehabilitation Council (BWRC) compiled a list of the top ten species likely to be treated as wildlife casualties across the UK:

1. Hedgehog
2. Feral pigeon
3. Wood pigeon
4. Collared dove
5. Blackbird
6. Starling
7. Rabbit
8. Fox
9. Swan
10. Guillemot.

However, this will be dependent on the location of your practice and the species in the local habitat.

> **Tip:** The mortality rate of wildlife casualties in captivity is approximately 60%, with the majority dying within the first 24 hours from shock.
>
> There are a number of procedures to take when admitting a patient and throughout assessment, treatment and handling, the decision should be constantly reviewed depending on the individual case.

Wildlife is an integral part of both country and urban landscape, and all forms of wildlife are essential to each other to maintain the balance of nature. Man interferes, upsetting the balance through shooting, trapping, poisoning, habitat destruction, urbanisation, population growth and accidental injury.

The objectives of wildlife treatment are to provide first aid and treatment to an injured, diseased or abandoned wild animal to enable it to return to the wild successfully. However, in reality, wildlife care probably only achieves a 20% rate of success.

Rehabilitation involves training an animal to adapt successfully to the wild. If this is not possible there are two alternatives to consider: a life in captivity or euthanasia.

Wild animals must never be treated as pets, regardless of how appealing they may be. This interferes with their natural behaviour and it is important that they maintain a healthy mistrust of humans.

RECEIVING A CASUALTY

It is extremely important to record the following details to gain a complete history assisting in rehabilitation and the possibility of release back to the wild.

Finder's details

WHO – name, address, and telephone number in case contact is required.

Casualty details

- WHAT – species, age (if known), sex (if known), marks, rings, etc.
- WHEN – when did the injury/illness happen, when was it found and captured?
- WHERE – where exactly was the animal found, landmarks, habitat?
- WHY – circumstances of finding, has the animal had any first aid, treatment, food, etc?

EXAMINATION PRIOR TO HANDLING

1. Obtain full history of patient.
2. Observe patient quietly, if possible without its knowledge.
3. Observe patient at close quarters – when handling make sure method is appropriate, positive and minimal to avoid stress to the patient.
4. Protect it and yourself, and be prepared for the unexpected. Cover the patient's head, as darkness is calming, avoid direct eye contact and beware of beaks, talons and wings.
5. Check the box it was transported in – look at droppings and any other residues that may assist diagnosis.

EXAMINATION WHILST HANDLING

1. Cover the head, allowing examination of body without inducing stress, also preventing personal damage.
2. Examine body condition – weight, level of hydration, muscle coverage.
3. Examine soft tissues – mouth, throat, eyes, nose, ears and vent.
4. Check colour, discharge, growths, foreign bodies, blockages.
5. Check limbs, wings – breaks, abnormalities, condition, etc.
6. Feet and legs – check pedal and replacement reflex, strength and condition.
7. Check coat or plumage condition.

> **Tip:** In a number of wildlife casualties pain is not exhibited; this is a natural response to avoid drawing predator attention. The patient should be treated as if in pain and analgesia should always be considered.

Chapter 8

Bats

Sara Cowen

INTRODUCTION

Bats are mammals and warm blooded, falling under the order *Chiroptera*. They are fully protected under the Wildlife and Countryside Act 1981 as the population status and habitat of these animals has declined, making the future of the species precarious.

In Britain it is illegal to disturb bats or the places where they roost.

Table 8.1 UK conservation status of British bat species (*Microchiroptera*)

Common name	Latin name
Greater horseshoe	*Rhinolophus ferrumequinum*
Lesser horseshoe	*Rhinolophus hipposideros*
Daubenton's	*Myotis daubentonii*
Brandt's	*Myotis brandtii*
Whiskered	*Myotis mystacinus*
Natterer's	*Myotis nattereri*
Bechstein's	*Myotis bechsteinii*
Greater mouse-eared	*Myotis myotis*
Pipistrelle	*Pipistrellus pipistrellus*
Pygmy pipistrelle	*Pipistrellus pygmaeus*
Nathusius's pipistrelle	*Pipistrellus nathusii*
Serotine	*Eptesicus serotinus*
Noctule	*Nyctalus noctula*
Leisler's	*Nyctalus leisleri*
Barbastelle	*Barbastella barbastellus*
Brown long-eared	*Plecotus auritus*
Grey long-eared	*Plecotus austriacus*

Tip: Being fully protected, it is normally illegal to keep healthy, flying bats, and a licence is needed to handle them. However, anyone who finds a bat that is obviously ill or injured may take care of it with the objective of rehabilitation to the wild.

Of the 16 species left in Britain, six are endangered or rare and six others are vulnerable (Table 8.1). Fifteen of these species are resident in the South of England. Only the pipistrelle (Britain's commonest bat), the common long-eared bat (Fig. 8.1) and Daubenton's extend northwards into Scotland.

Bat populations are threatened not only by loss of habitat, affecting roosting sites and feeding grounds, but also by deliberate killing and over-exploitation for food.

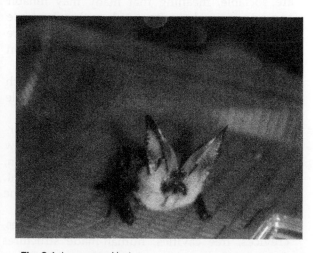

Fig. 8.1 Long-eared bat.

BEHAVIOUR

Nearly all bats are nocturnal (active at night) or crepuscular (active during dawn and dusk).

To get around in the dark, many nocturnal bats rely on a sophisticated form of sonar, known as echolocation, which helps them in navigating objects and locating prey.

Many bats, especially the crepuscular ones, have exceptionally good eyesight designed for low levels of illumination.

> **Tip:** Whilst in care keep light levels low or use a red bulb, especially when feeding, treating, etc., to prevent stress. Alternatively leave in a quiet, dark environment.

In echolocation, bats emit short pulses of high-frequency sounds from their mouths that are above the threshold of human hearing. The sound waves spread out, striking any objects in their flight path and bouncing back in the form of an echo. By interpreting the echoes, bats are able to discern the direction, distance, speed, and, in some instances, the size of the objects around them. Such information is important to avoid collision and injury such as entanglement and in catching winged insects and prey.

Bats do not build nests, preferring to hang onto cracks and footholds of buildings or caves. They prefer quiet, draught-free areas for roost sites and are sociable, meaning that many may inhabit one area as a colony. Bats such as the pipistrelle often choose modern houses as roost sites and are very commonly seen in urban areas roosting in houses.

Bats feed in flight and are insectivorous, which can cause difficulty when replicating a suitable diet in captivity.

In winter insects are scarce so bats will hibernate in cool parts of buildings, caves and hollow trees. They enter a state of torpor or hibernation, but will respond to sound, touch and movement. They will roost closely huddled together in the form of a larger body to help limit heat loss.

During the daytime, bats sleep in caves, crevices, tree cavities, human-made structures or exposed sites on trunks, limbs, and branches of trees. Nearly all bats roost, hanging by their hind feet; their weight causes the foot tendons to automatically grasp, firmly holding the animal in place. The thumb on the forearm acts as a hook for attachment as well.

ANATOMY

Bats are covered in fur, which is dense and has an unusual scale-like structure. The primary function of bat fur is for insulation; however, some hairs, such as those on the face, receive and transmit sensory impulses, much like cats' whiskers.

Bat wings are modified hand bones (phalanges) – the name of the bat order, *Chiroptera*, is Greek for 'hand-wing'.

The fingers are joined by a brown or black hairless, elastic membrane that attaches to the body sides and hind legs.

Each wing is made of a double layer of skin called the wing membrane or plagiopatagium (Fig. 8.2). The clawed thumb is free of the wing, and the bat uses this to cling to tree bark or the walls and ceiling of its roost.

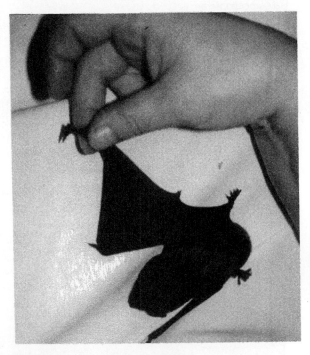

Fig. 8.2 Anatomy: stretched out wing.

Three pairs of flight muscles that attach to the bat's upper arms and chest produce the power for flight. Contractions of three other muscle pairs attached to the back cause the wing to raise in an upstroke, readying it for another downstroke.

The tail on the bat is almost as long as the body but is encased in the membrane and is curled under the body at rest. It is used for directional flight and as a storage place for insects.

The faces of bats also vary considerably in the shape and size of the ears, snout and fur cover. Many bats are able to turn their ears in the direction of faint noises.

Some bats have large, conspicuous eyes, while others may have small, beady eyes. This variation suggests that vision plays different roles in the lives of various species. Bats can see well in low light levels although they cannot see colour.

Like most mammals, bats have two sets of teeth. Depending upon the species, newborn bats are equipped with as many as 22 deciduous teeth. These teeth are replaced after a couple of weeks with 20–28 permanent teeth. The deciduous teeth are sharp and hooked; the permanent molars have ridged surfaces for grinding and slicing insects.

They have sharp and strong canine teeth for holding and catching prey during flight.

EXAMINATION

Firstly try to provide a sense of security and reduce stress by handling as little and as gently as possible. Bats are best examined by placing them across the inside of your fingers with the thumb resting on their dorsal surface to hold them in place. Wear thin gloves for protection against a bite.

Look for any blood or obvious signs of injury such as broken bones and holes in the wings. Then look for any external wounds including puncture wounds and abrasions. Bats often sustain injuries such as torn wings and cuts.

Consider if the bat is dehydrated, starving or suffering from poisoning and provide symptomatic treatment.

Begin supportive therapy to warm and rehydrate; in some cases this may be all the treatment required.

FIRST AID

The main reasons for bats requiring assistance include the following:

- Orphaned or injured young bats requiring hand rearing (British bats are very small and may be mistaken for young animals that have become separated from their mothers)
- Injured – wing damage or broken bones
- Dehydration or anorexia
- Injury from predation, such as cat attacks
- Hypothermia – from shock or possible problems following hibernation.

The most important initial care for the bat is to provide water and warmth. Shock and dehydration can be fatal to bats but following some guidelines will help a bat to survive.

> **Tip:** If willing to drink, offer Lectade or tepid water using a small, clean paintbrush or cotton bud and gently placing at the side of the mouth; the water will seep into the mouth and they will often begin sucking from the brush. This may be enough on its own to revive the bat.

Rehydrate using Hartmann's solution subcutaneously; approximately 0.3 ml for a pipistrelle or whiskered bat and 0.7 ml for the larger species such as serotines and noctules.

Grounded bats are likely to be injured or otherwise incapacitated. Do not put a grounded bat outside without proper assessment of the situation.

Use gloves, or a cloth, when handling, as frightened wild animals may try to bite. Handle the bat as little as possible initially, and keep it somewhere quiet. Avoid exposure to extremes of temperature, light or movement, which may increase the stress to the patient.

If the bat is injured and needs to be kept longer than a few hours, water should be offered regularly.

ACCOMMODATION

Place the bat in a small, secure container ensuring it is completely escape proof; bats can squeeze through the smallest of gaps.

Completely line the container with kitchen paper or toilet paper with a soft cloth hanging from the sides for the bat to hang on to. Then place tissues on the floor to allow hiding places.

Make sure there are adequate air holes for ventilation. Keep the bat in a warm place, where it can use all its energy for recovery. A dark, quiet area is ideal.

> **Tip:** A large food container or box with a lid is useful in an emergency. Drape a towel from the edges of the container hanging down inside the box, providing something for the bat to hang on to. Then replace the lid for security with air holes for ventilation.

DIET

Bats need to be warm before feeding; they may, therefore, need warming up. Mealworms (from pet shops) are the best food for bats but are often difficult to obtain; an adult pipistrelle will eat 10–15 mealworms a day.

Small chunks of meaty cat food are an alternative to feeding mealworms. If cat meat is being used it is important to use a vitamin and mineral supplement such as Vionate or Nutrabol to replace the valuable nutrients lost when not eating whole insects.

Bats usually need hand feeding at first to gain their interest.

> **Tip:** Use a very small, clean paintbrush for feeding cat food as it picks up the meat well, allowing the bat to take it off the brush.
> Tweezers can be used for mealworms (with heads removed), gently placing by the mouth (Fig. 8.3). Bats' sense of smell will enable them to locate the feed.

Other alternatives for feeding are waxworms. These are softer than the mealworms and often useful for very small, young or weak bats to get them on the road to recovery. There are also insectivore diets available in pet shops that contain dried grubs and beetles. These can be added to the cat food and fed again by brush to obtain a more balanced diet.

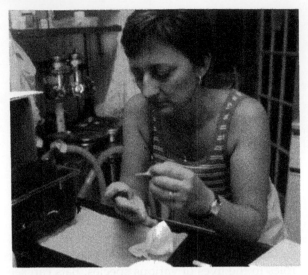

Fig. 8.3 Feeding using paintbrush and tweezers.

ORPHANS

Breeding places enormous strain on the female to produce milk and maintain condition and weight. In situations where there is poor food availability or bad weather the females may lose condition and be unable to feed the youngsters, resulting in underweight, poorly developed orphans.

Due to the size of British bats it is very difficult to tell if the bat is baby, juvenile or adult. If the bat has little or no fur it is only a few days old. If well furred then it can be difficult to tell the age. If the bat is very small, and its fur is very short then it is likely to be a young animal.

Babies are born between the months of May and July, depending on weather conditions and species. They take up to 6 weeks to become fully weaned and to reach adult size. They can fly from approximately 3–5 weeks.

YOUNG BATS: FEEDING AND CARE

The incubator must be at 32° – this is very important. If bats are not warm enough they will not digest the milk, and will become bloated and die.

If the bat is less than about 1 week old it will need toileting after every meal.

Baby bats are born with no fur and require intensive nursing. They need to be fed milk by pipette, dropper or paintbrush.

Feeding

Warm goat's milk or Esbilac milk should be given hourly from 6 am to midnight. Once they have been hand fed for 1 or 2 days (Fig. 8.4), put a few drops of milk in a very tiny, shallow dish with a small lip, and place in the incubator so they can help themselves. Change milk every 2 hours between about 8 am and 10 pm.

The bats can get very sticky so need their faces washing daily and occasional baths. Hold by the shoulders and gently lower into a small container of warm water (32°). They will spread their wings and the fur only needs a quick rinse with a finger to get clean. Remove from water, wrap in a soft facial tissue to dry, then replace in the warm incubator.

Once they are self feeding regularly, they get the hang of it and need less washing. Also the number of feeds can be gradually reduced.

Age 3 weeks

Give the middle of chopped mealworms as well as milk. Put a few bits of chopped mealworms in a shallow lid in the incubator so they can help themselves. Provide three to four meals per day. If the bat is thin, tapering away and falling away from the backbone, give as many feeds as possible.

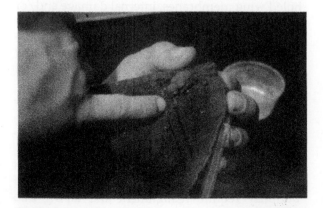

Fig. 8.4 Hand rearing babies.

Tip: Esbilac appears to be successful in hand rearing; using a paintbrush allows bats to suckle the brush ends containing the milk.

Tip: Hang a piece of furry material from the side of the cage. This will act as a mother substitute and provide privacy and warmth for the youngster to huddle into.

ANAESTHESIA

It is essential to use anaesthesia for any repair work on the wings or fracture repairs. Induce using an induction chamber or modified face mask. Isoflurane is suitable and effective for anaesthesia. Keep the animal on a heat source throughout the operation to minimise heat loss.

TORPOR AND HIBERNATION

Bats are warm-blooded animals, but unlike most other warm-blooded animals, they maintain their body temperature only when active. During the day, while resting in their roosts, bats let their body temperature drop to the temperature of their surroundings to conserve energy and, if cold, bats enter a sluggish state of suspended animation, known as torpor.

Torpor is a similar situation to hibernation but happens at higher temperatures and for shorter periods of time.

In colder times bats enter an extreme form of uninterrupted torpor, known as hibernation, that can last through the winter months.

During hibernation, a bat's metabolism drops, enabling the bat to conserve energy. The heart rate may slow to 25 beats a minute compared to 1000 in flight, and respiratory rate drops to less than five breaths a minute.

Hibernation permits bats, as well as other animals such as hedgehogs, to conserve energy, allowing them to survive in the leanest of seasons when food is scarce. However, bats hibernate to a greater degree than other animals.

During hibernation they are vulnerable, so may suffer dehydration if the hibernaculum

Table 8.2 Biological data of common species

| | Common name | | | |
	Pipistrelle	Brown long-eared	Natterer's	Serotine
Size	4 cm	4–5 cm	4–5 cm	6–8 cm
Weight	3–8 g	6–12 g	7–12 g	17–30 g
Colour	Brown, chocolate, black	Yellow buff on top, buff underneath	Grey brown, whitish underneath	Dark red/brown, pale underneath
Mating season	April–May	Autumn + spring	Autumn–spring	Autumn–winter
Gestation period	4–6 weeks	6–8 weeks	50–60 days	6–8 weeks
Litter size	1–2 born June	1	1	1
Development	Blind at birth, flight 21 days, adult size at 42 days	As for Pipistrelle	As for Pipistrelle	Blind at birth, flight 4–6 weeks, independent 2 months
Diet	Caddisflies and small moths	Moths and insects	Moths and insects	Large beetles and moths
Roost site	Buildings and trees	Buildings and trees	Trees, buildings, caves	Buildings and trees

(hibernation site) is not humid enough. They may also deplete their fat reserves to such an extent that the energy required to come out of hibernation puts too much stress on their body. Alternatively, they may starve.

If you receive a bat that appears to be in difficulty during or following hibernation you can assist by carrying out the following:

1. Allow the animal to warm up very gradually over a few hours to prevent shock from adverse temperature changes.
2. Rehydrate orally or by subcutaneous (SC) injection.
3. Provide feed and water until weight gain is observed and the bat reaches the recommended adult weight for the species (see Table 8.2).
4. Once recovered replace at site of rescue at dusk on a day with good weather conditions.

RELEASE

If there are no injuries, the bat should be released as soon as it is able to fly well enough. This must be close to where it was found, at the same spot if possible, and in mild weather at dusk. The sooner a fit bat is released the better its chance of survival.

Do not throw the bat into the air; ensure it is warm, place it in your open palm and hold it up, gently allowing your hands to drop away.

> **Tip:** For any bat maintained in captivity it is extremely important to have details of who found the bat, exactly where it was found and under what circumstances, to enable release back into the environment.

COMMON INJURIES AND DISEASES

Cat attacks

Damage from cat attacks often results in torn or holed wing membranes, internal damage and/or broken digits. With small tears the membrane may well repair itself without help. However, in some cases it will require suturing or glueing to assist repair. A bat with an injured wing will not fly and will ultimately die of starvation.

Puncture wounds may be present on the body and can be extremely small but may still require attention; clip away the hair from the wound site and treat with antiseptic gel.

Broken phalanges (fingers) are, to a certain extent, supported by the actual membrane itself but may require realignment and taping into position to allow healing in the correct position.

Matchsticks can be used as splints on the forearm to prevent damage whilst they move around on their limbs.

The wing should be firmly bound to the body and movement limited to prevent movement during healing. It may be necessary to place a small collar on the bat to prevent removal of the dressing with the teeth.

> **Tip:** For general antibiotic treatment following injury or infection treat with amoxycillin (oral drops) 40–50 mg/kg twice per day.

Wing repair

Torn wings are very common in bats and are usually caused by trauma of some form.

In some cases the wound, if small, may heal of its own accord; in others it may require surgical assistance.

Large tears will require suturing; use absorbable suture material to allow early release. Tissue glue is also useful for repair of smaller tears and again allows quick release.

Another useful method is debriding of the tear edges to allow the edges to be re-joined and heal correctly. This can be achieved using tissue glue and adhesive tape to keep the edges together. This, however, will mean a longer stay in captivity, as release will not be possible until the dressings have been removed.

Fracture repair

The wing bones of bats are fairly fragile and easily damaged through the membrane.

In most cases, especially the phalanges, the bones will require realignment and stabilisation to allow healing. The membrane itself offers a degree of support.

In the larger bones such as humerus, femur, etc., splinting may be required, especially as when bats are not able to fly they will crawl around on their limbs increasing the pressure and damage to a fracture.

Matchsticks taped to the wing will support smaller bones and padded aluminium finger splints can be attached to the large bones requiring additional support.

Bandaging the wing close to the body will minimise movement of the fracture site until healed.

> **Tip:** If the fracture is severe and requires amputation it should be taken into account that the animal will be committed to a life in captivity.

Poisoning

Bats may suffer secondary poisoning from eating insects that may have been treated with pesticides. Bats are extremely sensitive to poisoning. This will often result in fatality and only supportive and symptomatic treatment can be provided.

Parasites

Like all mammals, bats are prone to infestation by fleas, ticks and mites, which live in the fur. They are fastidious cleaners and groom themselves, assisting in parasite control.

> **Tip:** For ectoparasites, dust using a paintbrush with a pyrethrum-based powder, gently brushing through the coat.

Systemic treatment using ivermectin is possible at 0.02 ml/kg at a dilution of 1:99 propylene glycol.

Alopecia

If kept in captivity for a prolonged period partial alopecia may be observed. It is likely to be due to stress, dietary alterations or environmental changes. The pipistrelles are especially prone to this.

To avoid or treat, follow these basic principles:

- Handle as little as possible.
- Try to provide an appropriate diet with live insects.
- Try to reduce environmental stress.
- Release as soon as possible, avoid keeping bats unnecessarily.

Rabies

As warm-blooded mammals they have the ability to contract rabies and due to their ability for sustained flight, they are often transient through Europe and may be a source of infection. It is important to recognise signs of abnormal behaviour:

- overly aggressive
- attacking objects
- seizures.

In 2002 a Scottish rescue worker contracted rabies from a bat and became the first person to die from the disease in the UK for 100 years.

If you suspect rabies the best course is to euthanase the bat and send it to the Central Veterinary Laboratory for post-mortem examination.

CASE HISTORY

Patient

Adult long-eared bat that had been brought into the house following capture by the household cat.

Condition

The bat, initially thought to be a mouse, was found crawling around on the carpet with the cat watching. The house owners gently picked up the bat with a towel and placed it in a container; they were unsure of what to do and what may be wrong with the animal.

Capture

Bats on the whole are very placid animals and can be easily picked up using a towel for them to cling onto. They like to hold onto the material and travel better in darkness as they are nocturnal animals. Full household lighting can sometimes cause stress. However, they are well armed with teeth and so gloves or a towel should always be used. There also has been an isolated incident in the UK of a fatality from a rabies-infected bat bite. As mammals, they can carry rabies, so precautions should always be taken when handling bats.

Treatment

The bat was in shock and so initially was placed in a warm, dark environment to allow it to recover prior to any treatment. The bat was given fluids orally using a tiny pipette placed near the mouth. Other methods include using a small paintbrush that they can suck or even placing a drop of water onto the fur which they then lick during grooming; however, this is not a method that should be used until they are well and warm.

After a couple of hours when the bat was warmed through a thorough examination took place. All the actual bones in the wings were intact; however, the membrane had been punctured and torn in a couple of places. These could be stitched using fine suture material but now a more suitable option is a special bonding glue for skin – Vetbond – which acts like Superglue and immediately repairs the wound. For the next 2 days the bat was treated for shock, dehydration and fed on mealworms to help maintain condition.

Following this, the wound had sealed well and the bat was released back near the house to fly back to the original roost site. The release and flight were successful.

Chapter 9

Foxes

Sara Cowen

INTRODUCTION

The red fox (*Vulpes vulpes*) is a native canine species in Britain. The fox is at the head of the British food chain, being a top predator, feeding on small mammals and rodents (Table 9.1).

Table 9.1 Biological data of red fox	
Latin name	*Vulpes vulpes*
Life span	3–5 years
Description	Yellowish red-black, pointed ears, white chin, belly and tail tip, bushy tail
Average male weight	6 kg
Average female weight	5 kg
Average head and body length	70 cm
Average tail length	40 cm
Gestation period	53 days
Litter size	4–6 cubs
Breeding season	Jan–Feb
Average weight of neonates	120 g
Lactation period	4–8 weeks
Weaning age	4–6 weeks
Eyes and ears open	2 weeks
Hair erupts	Born furred, chocolate brown
Milk teeth incisors	2 weeks
Fully independent	4–5 months
Adult diet	Small mammals, birds, insects, carrion, berries, earthworms

The fox is commonly seen now in urban habitats, with populations thriving having adapted to the presence of humans and, as such, they are often referred to as pest species.

Foxes are sociable, living in family groups with usually related subordinate siblings. The dominant alpha male (dog) and female (vixen) will breed once a year and siblings will assist in rearing the cubs. The peak birth time for fox cubs is March, usually resulting in an increase in mortality rates from road traffic accidents in autumn, as youngsters naturally disperse and have to search further for food.

ANATOMY AND PHYSIOLOGY

In adaptation to nocturnal behaviour foxes have an additional layer behind the light sensitive cells in the eyes – the *tapetum lucidum*, passing the light back through the sensitive cells. This enables them to see better at low light levels as the sensitivity is increased. They also have an increased number of rods (photoreceptors in the eyes), which allows a better range of sensitivity to black, white and grey, perfect for low light conditions. The reduced numbers of cones, which pick up colour illumination, mean they are less likely to be able to distinguish colour.

They also have sensitive hearing with the ability to detect low-frequency noises allowing the location of the movements of prey.

HANDLING

Foxes are predators and as such are often aggressive when being handled or approached.

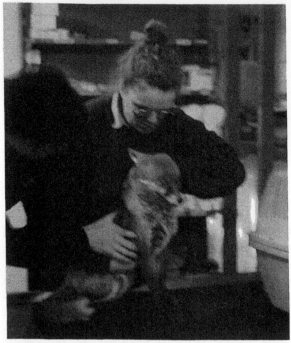

(a)

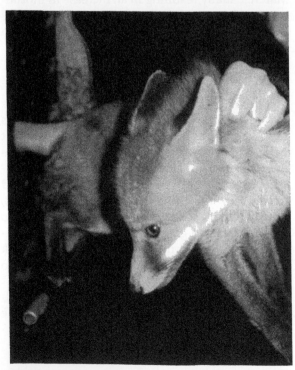

(b)

Fig. 9.1 (a, b, c) Fox handling.

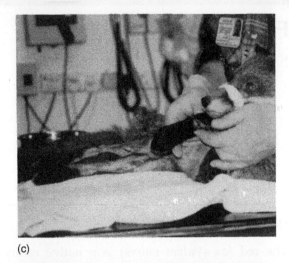

(c)

Fig. 9.1 *Continued*.

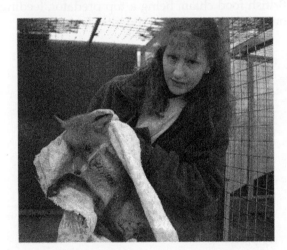

Fig. 9.2 Fox scruffed in towel.

For handling a frightened or injured fox the easiest method of capture and restraint is a dog-catcher (Fig. 9.1a,b,c). This enables the handler to restrain the animal securely at distance.

Once controlled, the fox can have a towel placed over its head to reduce stress and then be scruffed to allow closer examination to take place. Always support the body weight with the other hand. Once scruffed they are usually very calm and struggle little.

The towel assists in calming the animal during this procedure and offers an element of safety to the handler (Fig. 9.2). Always wear thick gloves, as they will bite!

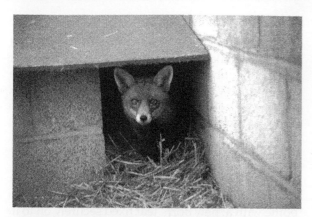

Fig. 9.3 Accommodation.

ACCOMMODATION

Foxes, like all wild animals, do not like being caged; however, for temporary periods of time this may be unavoidable.

Place them in dog kennels with metal bars to limit self-inflicted injury when trying to escape.

Place newspaper and straw bedding for warmth and absorption and place a box or upturned dog bed for them to climb under, providing security (Fig. 9.3).

Cover the front of the cage to avoid eye contact and minimise stress from passers-by and other animals, such as dogs, in the near vicinity.

If possible, during the day, darken the accommodation as they are nocturnal and will do better in the dark.

NUTRITION

In the wild, foxes will feed on small mammals and carcasses to gain a balanced diet.

If possible feed using kitchen scraps, day-old chicks, mice and such items as rabbits from the butchers, etc.

If none of these are available or they are in short supply, tinned dog food can be offered.

HAND REARING FOX CUBS

Cubs are usually presented in practice following the death or injury of the mother preventing her return to the den. The youngsters are usually found wandering around distressed, cold and hungry. They are usually 2–3 weeks old, as prior to this will remain underground, immobile, and will die of starvation.

Fox cubs can be reared along the same lines as puppies using a proprietary canine milk replacement such as Welpi or unpasteurised goat's milk. Add multivitamins such as Abidec to enhance levels.

Bottle-feeding may be necessary for the very young (1–2 weeks of age) (Fig. 9.4a,b). However, if they are mobile and active they will usually respond to warm milk in a bowl and lap it up.

During the first week they will require manual stimulation for defecation and urination using a damp piece of cotton wool wiped over the anogenital area before and after feeding.

If possible try to place with cubs of similar ages as they do much better and are likely to remain wilder if kept in pairs or groups.

If the cubs are less than 2 weeks old they will need a heat source of approximately 30°C to be provided as they are unable to thermoregulate.

Notes on feeding fox cubs (Tables 9.2 and 9.3)

Some quick reference points for fox cubs needing to be hand fed include:

- Fox cubs with their eyes closed are less than 2 weeks old.
- On arrival they should be weighed and all details entered onto their individual cards. They need to be weighed daily.
- An incubator is ideal for their sleeping quarters, and a cuddly toy helps them to settle in.

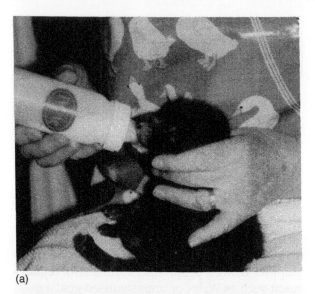

(a)

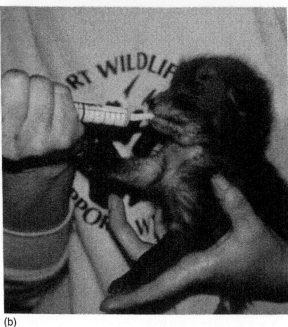

(b)

Fig. 9.4 (a, b) Fox cub feeding.

- Depending on how small the cubs are they can be fed 2–3 hourly.
- If they wake early or do not feed well adjust feeds accordingly, either times or quantities.
- Cubs need to be fed up until 12 midnight and then again at 6 am the next day.

1–2 weeks of age

If they are very tiny and have black fur, they should be fed on Esbilac as this contains the colostrum that these tiny cubs need. Feed using a 2 ml syringe with teat. Sew a thread to the teat in case they suck the tip off; you can then gently pull the string to remove from the mouth.

From 2 weeks of age

Cimicat or Esbilac milk are the best types of milk to feed the cubs, diluted 1:3. Feed using a baby's bottle with a 'new born' teat fixed securely on to it. Feed lying on their tummy so they can stretch out and suckle as they would from their mother. **Do not feed curled up in the hand as this is not a natural position.**

They may not stop for a rest or breath and if they push the teat out after taking an amount it means they have had enough or the milk has gone cold.

Care has to still be taken, to make sure that the milk does not come out of the teat too fast, as they will choke, but providing the teat used at first is a 'new born' all should go well.

You will need to support their head with your left hand (if you are right handed) and hold the bottle with your hand underneath it supporting the cub's front feet with the heel of that hand.

Cubs with their eyes shut will also need to be toileted before and after every feed. A piece of toilet tissue dampened with water is the most efficient way of stimulating their bladder and the bowel.

If a cub has an extremely hard tummy or finds difficulty in passing motions, boiled, cooled water or Lectade can be given for one or two feeds in place of milk. Glucose can be added if the cub refuses to take the plain water.

A healthy fox cub should gain about 15–20 g a day in the wild. If a cub loses weight for more than 2 days there is something very wrong.

Fox cubs with eyes shut weighing around 115–124 g take an average of about 10 ml of warm milk at each feed. They may find it difficult to accept the strange teat at first but if you persevere they usually get the hang of it, if not immediately.

When these cubs reach 250 g in weight they may need 'toddler' teats, as these give a better flow.

Table 9.2 Feeding guidelines

Age (weeks)	Identification	Frequency
0–1	Chocolate brown fur, blind, deaf, fully dependent, umbilical cord still present	2 hourly, Esbilac milk 6 am–12 pm
1–2	Eyes and ears still closed	2 hourly Esbilac 6 am–12 pm
2–3	Eyes and ears open, begin moving around, milk teeth begin to erupt	Cimicat 3 hourly 6 am–12 pm
3–4	Much more mobile and walking around, teeth develop	Cimicat 4 hourly 6 am–12 pm
4–5	Very mobile, well-developed teeth, interested in solids	Mashed puppy food mixed with Cimicat to milky consistency
5–6	Full set of teeth, very active, noisy and playful, red coat begins to appear	Puppy Chum and chopped chicks and meat
From 6 weeks	Miniature adults often develop aggressive behaviour at this stage	Solids only

Table 9.3 Comparison of milk

	Fox milk (%)	Goat's milk (%)
Protein	34.5	22
Fat	35	32
Carbohydrate	25	39
Solids	18.2	22

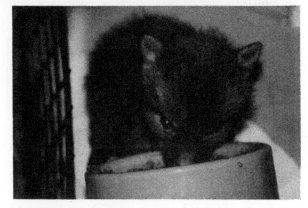

Fig. 9.5 Fox cub weaning.

When the cub sucks and sucks on the bottle and the milk is not going down the time is right to change to these types of teats.

Cubs that arrive with their eyes open can be more difficult to establish on a feeding pattern. They are more fearful and more aware of their surroundings. They are aware that the teat you are trying to push into their mouths does not belong to their mother.

If they weigh around 460 g they are about 3–4 weeks old, and may begin to take solids, if bottle feeding proves to be a problem. Solids should consist of a small amount of puppy/junior food finely mashed + Cimicat milk poured on top. Keep giving a bottle feed, if they are used to this, but lengthen the time between feeds until they are on solids totally (Fig. 9.5).

At 4 weeks old they can be introduced to finely chopped chick, but with beaks and legs removed, until older.

At 900 g they are 6 weeks old roughly and should be well established on the puppy/milk, feeding from a saucer. If a cub arrives at the centre weighing this amount it may not accept a bottle and, providing they can manage well feeding themselves and are getting enough to put on weight, the less they are handled the better, so no need to worry. Forget bottle feeding.

At 9 weeks old they can go up to an outside pen, and be housed five to six cubs together, mixed sex, given wood shavings on the floor, a wooden bed with straw for bedding, and an outside run. They should be fed twice a day with whole chicks, though still with no legs or beaks, thrown around at feed time so they squabble over them and learn

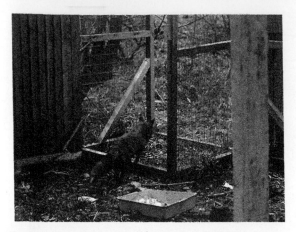

Fig. 9.6 Fox release.

to fight and fend for themselves. Puppy food can be put into one or two bowls as necessary, and clean water should always be made available.

> **Tip:** Try to vary the solid diet and reduce the amount of tinned meat – use road-kill carcasses, kitchen scraps, etc. Fur and bones are essential to the diet and lack of these will result in diarrhoea.

Fox cubs will imprint onto humans resulting in a tame individual if not prevented. Try to handle the youngster for feeding and examination purposes only. Other than that treat as a wild adult fox limiting human contact.

Hand-reared cubs cannot be released straight into the wild as they will not be shy of humans or have a natural hunting instinct and this may result in death through starvation. They have to go through a slow-release programme allowing adjustment to life in the wild. This should be carried out from 4–6 months of age when independent and should be via an experienced wildlife rehabilitator using a suitable programme, habitat and location (Fig. 9.6).

FIRST AID

Treatment

Initially the following should be provided:

- warmth
- darkness

- quiet
- oral fluids – Lectade
- intravenous fluids
- corticosteroids
- sedation if required – diazepam 1.0 mg/kg intravenously (IV) or intramuscularly (IM).

> **Tip:** For quantities of fluids and drug dose rates, give as for a dog of similar size.

ANAESTHESIA

Short-term effective sedation to allow examination and treatment can be achieved using diazepam at a dose rate of 1.0 mg/kg IM or IV.

Foxes can be treated as for dogs and cats. Induction may be gaseous, although this can cause stress to the animal so premedication or sedation is preferable.

They can then be intubated and maintained using halothane or isoflurane.

THERAPEUTICS

Treatment and administration of drugs to foxes is similar to dogs as a canine species and the correct dose rate can be calculated by weighing the fox on presentation.

Remember, they are likely to be very underweight, as if they were well and able they would not have been caught.

RELEASE

It is important that, if possible, the fox is released in the location where it was captured as foxes are territorial and have defined home ranges (Fig. 9.7).

However, this may not be possible due to the nature of the injury and safety of the area.

> **Tip:** Do not release a fox back into an area where the illness or injury will automatically reoccur, i.e. snares or deliberate poisoning.

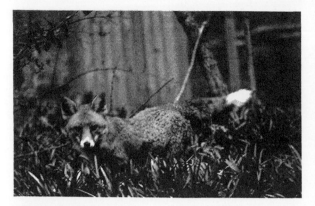

Fig. 9.7 Fox release.

COMMON ILLNESSES, INJURIES OR DISEASES

Parasites

Sarcoptic mange

Mange (*Sarcoptes scabiei*) is one of the most common conditions observed in foxes (Fig. 9.8a,b). The animals become debilitated from the condition, losing weight and coat condition. As sociable animals the disease is quickly spread through the group due to direct contact or indirect contact in the earth.

The mites live beneath the surface of the skin causing intense irritation and inflammation of the skin.

It is usually accompanied by hair loss, sores and weeping wounds. The fox will scratch the skin surface causing inflammation and sore patches to develop and the coat will appear to have a thick crusty surface where the wounds seep.

The most common places are on the base of the tail, abdomen and head resulting in conjunctivitis. The animal will lose condition and without treatment it can be fatal.

If actually caught the fox will usually be in poor condition requiring immediate fluid therapy and supportive treatment.

On presentation the fox should be treated with an injection of ivermectin 200 µg/kg (approx. 0.3 ml) subcutaneously (SC) or dectomax 300 µg/kg IM. With both treatments a course of three injections 2 weeks apart should be given.

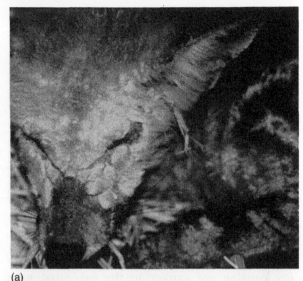

(a)

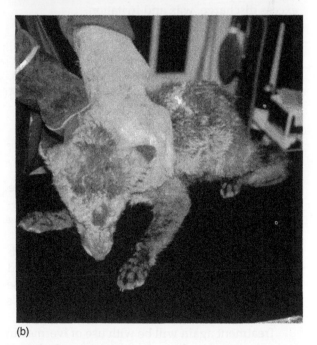

(b)

Fig. 9.8 (a, b) Mange.

It is advisable to treat with anti-inflammatories and antibiotics, e.g. amoxycillin LA.

Some baths and topical applicants, such as parasiticidal dips, may also assist in initial treatment to reduce symptoms and irritation; however, these will not be appreciated by the patient.

Remember to use barrier nursing to minimise cross contamination to domestic species, as the condition is zoonotic and highly infectious to other animals within the practice.

> **Tip:** If a client has a fox with mange but is unable to catch the animal, it can be treated orally with ivermectin in food that has been injected with the drug, such as meat. However, this can be toxic to some dogs and cats.
> An alternative is the use of arsenicum album and sulphur 30c, a homeopathic treatment that has no toxicity to other species. Place a few drops on food scraps daily until recovered.

Ear mites

Otodectes cyanotis is also an observed mite in the fox causing ear canker in the ear canal with excess discharge, wax and irritation.

Ticks and fleas

Foxes will often be infected with ticks, namely the hedgehog and dog tick species, and with dog and cat fleas. So treatment will follow the guidelines for dogs and cats.

Endoparasites

As with all wild animals they will normally be hosts to a number of parasites, including tapeworm (*Taenia serialis*) and roundworm (*Toxacara canis*), as in dogs.

They may also be hosts to lungworm or bladder worms due to the ingestion of insects and rodents that are often intermediate hosts for these species. It is only if debilitated that the animal's condition will be severely affected.

Treatment again will be with use of ivermectin injection or by the administration of droncit 5.5 mg/kg.

Infectious canine hepatitis

This disease is found in foxes and dogs, and rarely seen in the domestic situation, as the majority of people vaccinate their pets. It is a viral condition spread through urine, faeces and saliva. Again the fox is likely to be in very poor condition if it has been caught and brought into practice.

Symptoms

These include:

- poor condition
- lethargic
- jaundiced
- neurological symptoms
- corneal oedema (blue eye).

Treatment

This involves:

- fluid therapy
- antibiotics
- supportive treatment
- symptomatic treatment
- strict barrier nursing procedures to prevent cross contamination.

> **Tip:** A blood sample will confirm diagnosis; this should be considered as jaundiced individuals may be suffering from leptospirosis, which is zoonotic.

Canine leptospirosis

This bacterial disease (*Leptospira icterohaemorrhagiae*) is again rarely seen in practice in domesticated dogs. It was commonly referred to as lamp-post's disease as it was spread through the urine of infected dogs and picked up by others' sniffing of the lamp-post on exercise.

This disease is now commonly seen spread by rats', urine and is contractable by humans and known as Weil's disease.

Symptoms observed will be jaundiced mucous membranes and damage to the kidneys, and treatment will be the same as for infectious canine hepatitis.

Fractures

Unfortunately, the most common injuries to foxes are caused by man. Road traffic accidents are the most usual form of injury resulting in trauma, fractures and fatalities.

Foxes have a large home range and as such are often required to tackle roads and oncoming vehicles, especially during the winter months when they have to travel further and for longer periods of time to gain adequate nutrition.

The most common fractures observed will be fractured pelvis, femur, humerus or possibly, jaw.

In all cases the injuries can be fixed as for dogs and cats; however, the animal will be less tolerant of external fixations, stitches and casts.

> **Tip:** If amputation is a possibility, foxes will return adequately to the wild without a hind limb, but would be unable to cope without a forelimb and euthanasia or captivity should be considered.

Head injuries

These are commonly observed in foxes taking a minor blow or injury to the head and may cause temporary problems only.

Observed symptoms may include:

* concussion – head shaking, dilated pupils, nystagmus
* contusion – swelling from bruising or bleeding externally or internally
* compression – pressure on the brain resulting in disorientation, pain, unconsciousness (Fig. 9.9a,b)
* torticollis – head tilt.

Treatment should include the administration of a steroid to assist in reduction of swelling and reduction of pressure. Additional care will be required during this recovery period as the animal will be disorientated and may have adverse reactions to the presence of or handling by humans.

Keep the cage dark, quiet and covered. Animals may be hypersensitive to sound and movement causing further distress.

If unable to feed, gentle restraint will be required to administer fluids and liquid feeds.

Ensure the cage is safe and soft to prevent injury during disorientation and movement.

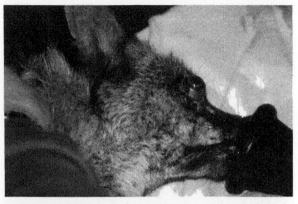
(a)

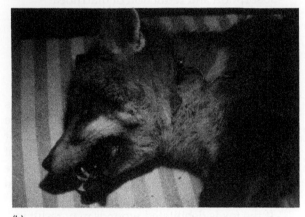
(b)

Fig. 9.9 (a) Head injury. (b) Snare injury.

Poisoning

Deliberate poisoning, although this practice is illegal, still takes place, as foxes are regarded as pest species. This may also occur due to accidental ingestion of parasiticides, insecticides used in the garden or the possible ingestion of rodent baits.

Animals are also poisoned by chemicals such as petrol, tar, etc., that may be lying around unprotected. Foxes may fall into pits with oil, and then try to clean themselves resulting in internal damage. In all cases the symptoms are similar to all poisoned animals:

* Collapsed and in shock
* Salivation
* Disorientation

- Nystagmus
- Diarrhoea – possibly with blood present
- Enteritis.

Treatment should be as for poisoning in general:

- Supportive and symptomatic
- Remove all residues of contamination if external
- Rehydrate the patient in the hope of diluting the effect of the poison
- Use kaolin and activated charcoal for absorption and reduction of diarrhoea
- Keep warm and quiet and treat symptomatically.

Wounds

Foxes will encounter conflict at various times and may be attacked by dogs or injury from wire fences or snares, etc., resulting in lacerated or puncture wounds (Fig. 9.10). The usual locality of these is the tail, limb and neck areas. If not severe the wound will be cleaned and will heal without intervention.

If the fox is debilitated wounds may result in:

- abscessation
- infection
- flystrike
- toxaemia and septicaemia if severe.

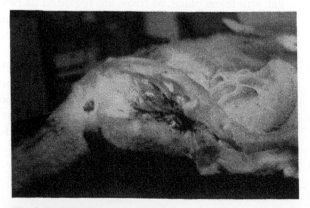

Fig. 9.10 Snared.

Treatment will involve:

- draining and cleaning of wounds
- debriding and suturing of wounds if appropriate
- fluid therapy
- broad-spectrum antibiotics – enrofloxacin 5 mg/kg SC daily.

CASE HISTORY 1

Patient

Female adult vixen of approximately 3 years of age.

Condition

Female found collapsed in the road, reluctant to move, disorientated and in obvious discomfort.

Her movement was restricted by a large abscess on her back resulting in infection, pain and swelling.

Capture

As she was collapsed the fox was approached slowly and a towel placed over her head. She was scruffed by the neck, the handler wearing thick gloves to prevent being bitten on moving. Her rump was supported as well as being scruffed and she was placed into a carry cage to secure during transport.

Treatment

On admission the fox was muzzled to allow a safe examination without aggravating the abscess. The abscess was then lanced and drained and flushed through with dilute hydrogen peroxide to assist in removing the pus and cleaning the wound. Once the wound was cleaned an antibiotic was placed into the abscess site. In addition, antibiotic and dexadresson were provided intravenously through a fluid replacement drip. The drip helps replace fluids lost through the injury and also assists in increasing body temperature and helps the blood circulate around the body.

She was then made comfortable in a heated enclosure to allow the drip to flow slowly over the next few hours. Food and water were placed nearby in case she was interested.

The following morning the fox still looked very ill but was no longer dehydrated; she had also eaten some of her food in the night. She slowly improved every day and began eating well over the next few days; she was given antibiotics every day for a week to help control the infection in the abscess site.

Over the next 3 weeks the wound healed and all the infection was cleared, she was very bright and lively, and showed her natural instincts and wild behaviour, and she was ready to go back. In the evening she was boxed and placed back where she came from to return to her earth.

CASE HISTORY 2

Patient

Male adult fox of approximately 2 years of age.

Condition

Adult male fox with sarcoptic mange, majority of fur was lost and scabs all over the body. The fox had crusty wounds and intense irritation over the body; he was very thin and a low weight for his age. He was also very dehydrated with pale gums and was anaemic. He was found collapsed in a barn on a farm and brought in by the property owner with a low temperature and very little sign of life.

Capture

As he was collapsed the fox was approached slowly and a towel placed over his head. He was scruffed by the neck with thick gloves to prevent the handler being bitten. His rump was supported as well as being scruffed and he was placed into a carry cage to secure during transport.

Treatment

On admission the fox was put on a drip to help encourage blood circulation and increase the body temperature. He was then given a general anaesthetic to allow the wound to be dressed and covered to prevent further injury to himself. While on the drip and following the wounds being cleaned the fox was given antibiotics, an antispasmodic and corticosteroids to help combat the shock. Multivitamins were also given to support the system and encourage eating.

At this point it was not possible to provide treatment for the mange as the fox was too ill and treatment can be toxic. He was placed in a warm enclosure and observed for 24 hours. By the next morning the fluids had made a huge difference and the fox was alert, interested in its surroundings and on his feet.

The fox continued to improve over the next week and the infections died down. He then began the treatment to control the mange with a course of three injections of ivomec 1 week apart. By the end of this period the hair had begun to regrow and the fox had gained weight, was healthy and appeared much more content. The man who had brought him in collected the fox 6 weeks after being admitted and released him back near the barn to return to his home territory.

Chapter 10

Hedgehogs

Sara Cowen

INTRODUCTION

The European hedgehog (*Erinaceus europaeus*) is one of the most commonly presenting wildlife casualties in the UK. Humans are usually the cause of injury and illness, and hedgehogs suffer frequently at the hand of man.

Hedgehogs have few natural predators, with badgers and foxes taking the occasional unsuspecting individual; however, domesticated dogs are often causes of injury.

They are well protected by a layer of tough spines (modified hair) running over their dorsal surface and have extensive powerful, circular muscles to enable them to curl into a ball when threatened, as a defence mechanism. An adult hedgehog has around 16 000 spines.

Having adapted to urban life, road casualties are common, usually resulting in death; however, the most commonly preferred habitat is the cultivated garden resulting in injuries from strimmers, poisoning due to pesticides, entanglement in netting and disturbance of nest sites resulting in abandonment.

Hedgehogs are unaggressive creatures that will tolerate human interaction within their habitat making monitoring and treatment of them fairly easy.

Hedgehogs are solitary in lifestyle coming together only to breed; they will have a large home range and will move freely within this area on daily foraging expeditions. They will have a number of nest sites within this home range where they rest during daylight hours.

Hedgehogs are nocturnal, being active and feeding at night.

In the wild, a hedgehog's life expectancy is 3–4 years increasing to up to 10 years in captivity.

> **Tip:** If a hedgehog is out during the day it will often mean that it is unwell or injured.

The hedgehog will present itself in surgery with a wide range of clinical problems usually categorised as:

- Injured or sick wild adults
- Over-wintered animals often underweight
- Tame/hand-reared orphans.

HEDGEHOG DEVELOPMENT

It is important to assess the age of your patient as it will indicate possible problems and likelihood of requirements (see Table 10.1).

INITIAL EXAMINATION

It is often difficult to assess their condition due to their inaccessibility.

Hedgehogs will often grunt or exhibit a jerky movement and will automatically roll into a ball when touched. However, a hedgehog that is unable to roll into a ball is one that is extremely ill and weak, and in need of immediate treatment.

Fully examine the dorsal surface for signs of trauma, puncture wounds or poor skin condition.

Many reported methods are described to assist in unrolling for examination. One that usually works is to allow the hedgehog to rest on the table and slowly unroll of its own accord then

Table 10.1 Biological data of hedgehog

Age	Weight	Appearance
Newborn	10–20 g	Born naked, white spines emerge in 1 hour, eyes and ears closed
2–3 days	20–25 g	Brown spines begin to emerge
1–2 weeks	50–60 g	Growth of hair on ventral surfaces, able to curl up at 11 days
3–4 weeks	100 g	Eyes open, deciduous teeth erupt, weight approx. 85–130 g
8–10 weeks	250–300 g	Permanent teeth develop
Adult	Up to 1500 g	Fully grown, covered in spines
Hibernation	Minimum 450 g	Often autumn young animals are underweight

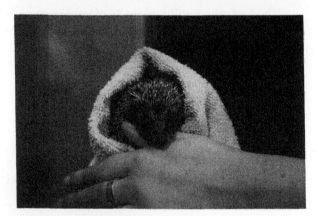

Fig. 10.1 Handling in towel.

gently stroke the dorsal surface along the back. The hedgehog will soon unroll completely allowing a better visual assessment. Once unrolled gently take hold of the hind legs leaving the front limbs touching the surface; this will then allow a closer examination to take place of the ventral surface.

Some hedgehogs may not be so co-operative (Fig. 10.1) and require sedation or anaesthesia to allow full examination.

Tip: Placing in a transparent plastic container will allow viewing of the ventral surface when unrolled.

FIRST AID

Provide a source of warmth immediately; many animals will be hypothermic on presentation as they may have been injured a while. Check all over the body, underneath, anogenital area, ears, eyes and mouth and around the face.

Flystrike is common and if this is the case it is vital to remove all maggots or eggs, using tweezers and flushing with saline.

If the animal is lively administer fluid orally (Lectade; approximately 10–20 ml). If in a collapsed state use Hartmann's or saline SC (approximately 20–40 ml).

Dress all wounds and control bleeding. Open wounds are likely to be infected so disinfect and dress. Administer antibiotics to control infection and disinfect all utensils and surfaces following contact.

If infective disease is suspected isolate the hedgehog from other animals.

Weigh the hedgehog to obtain initial weight on presentation especially during the winter months. Place in a warm, dark cage for the initial 12–24 hours to help treat stress, keep noise to a minimum and handle as little as possible.

Tip: When examining hedgehogs always wear gloves as many carry ringworm, which is zoonotic.

ACCOMMODATION

Provision of suitable housing and security whilst in practice can assist in minimising stress.

Hedgehogs are solitary animals and during treatment should be housed alone to prevent fighting.

Hedgehogs can be extremely dirty and produce large amounts of urine and faeces; therefore, place newspaper on the base of the cage for absorbency.

Place on hay bedding to allow the hedgehog to nestle underneath, but only if there are no external wounds or surgical sites.

The ideal material for a sick or post-operative hedgehog is a towel. This helps to prevent contamination of any wounds by bedding. Hedgehogs will sleep and rummage around underneath a towel.

Place an upturned cardboard box with a hole cut out for entry to allow them somewhere to hide away from daylight and artificial lighting.

NUTRITION

Providing the correct and adequate diet is highly important to assist the recovery process and prevent further problems.

Hedgehogs are insectivores and in the wild will feed primarily on invertebrates such as slugs, beetles, caterpillars, snails and earthworms, in addition to carrion such as young birds, mammals and eggs, when available. They will also feed on fruit, although this does not constitute a high proportion of their diet. They have a short digestive tract and the caecum is absent having little requirement or use for fibre in the diet.

Feeding adult hedgehogs in captivity is fairly easy (Fig. 10.2) and they will do well on a combination of meat flavoured moist and dry cat foods. The addition of invertebrates such as mealworms, worms, beetles, etc., can also be beneficial or proprietary insectivores' meals can be added to the meat. There are also specialised hedgehog diets now available on the market.

An adult hedgehog will eat approx 100 g of food per day.

> **Tip:** As they are nocturnal, hedgehogs have poor eyesight and rely heavily on their sense of smell to locate food and prey. Fruit such as bananas can be useful in stimulating feeding.

Many people supplement their diet these days in the garden with provision of artificial foods including bread and milk. On the whole it is ill advised to feed cow's milk and bread to hedgehogs as this can cause digestive upset due to their inability to digest lactose. However, a small amount of goat's milk may encourage a sick patient to eat.

Always ensure fresh water is available in a heavy weighted or untippable bowl. They are

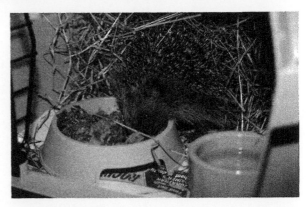

Fig. 10.2 Adult feeding.

unlikely to use a bottle as they would not drink in the wild using this method.

> **Tip:** For naturally nocturnal animals it is best to provide food supplies at night to stimulate natural behaviour.

PRE-OPERATIVE PROCEDURE

Once injury or illness is fully assessed it may be necessary to suspend surgical treatment until fully treated for shock or infection. Shock in itself will increase the anaesthetic risk and can kill on its own.

Many animals will have chronic infections, such as in severed limbs, and will require antibiotic treatment to prevent infection of the surgical site.

Providing premedication, e.g. domitor 0.2 ml intramuscularly (IM) for an adult, will allow unravelling of the animal to allow preparation of the surgical site and also access to the head in order to administer the gaseous anaesthesia.

Good site preparation is of the utmost importance as hedgehogs tend to roll in food and faecal material so the wound site can become heavily contaminated. If the injury is on the dorsal surface it will be necessary to remove the spines for access to the area. Cut them near the base and clear the whole area – they will regrow in time. If the injury is on the ventral surface then the area can be routinely clipped as this area is covered in hair not spines. Scrub the wound site with surgical scrub, although this may not result in a sterile wound site.

It is important to provide a heat source to prevent loss of body heat during surgery, as a drop in temperature due to heat loss via the surgical site can result in shock or a state similar to hibernation.

> **Tip:** Place on a heat mat through surgery and keep the surgical site to a minimum.

Pre-operative checks

Consideration should be given to the following:

- Minimise stress due to pre-operative handling by giving a sedative.
- Look for oculonasal discharge – this may indicate the presence of respiratory congestion.
- Listen to the lungs – impairment or damage may result in respiratory failure during surgery.
- If the animal has not been drinking, pre-operative fluids can be given subcutaneously.

ANAESTHESIA

A physical examination of every animal should be carried out prior to any form of anaesthesia as any health concerns may lead to complications and even death. In all small animals good surgical preparation and intensive post-operative nursing are essential, as they are generally not good candidates for anaesthesia.

Gaseous anaesthesia induced in a chamber is the most suitable method for induction, with isoflurane as the preferred agent. If not possible, halothane can be used.

Even rolled up hedgehogs can be induced with the use of a mask if turned over. Once induction begins they can be gently opened allowing a better seal on the mask preventing environmental contamination.

A good level of sedation can be created using domitor IM solely (or ketamine) or it can be used to assist in induction before administering gaseous anaesthesia.

> **Tip:** The advantage of domitor is that it has a reversant – antisedan.

If analgesia is incomplete, increasing the anaesthetic may result in overdose. Evaluation of depth of anaesthesia may be difficult – vital signs are often a poor indicator and heart rate may be immeasurable. Absence of pedal reflex and ear pinch are useful indicators of sufficient depth.

Response is extremely variable and recovery can be prolonged.

INTENSIVE POST-OPERATIVE NURSING

Place the animal on a heated mat. Removal of the heat source can result in rapid heat loss. Heat lamps can be used but avoid overheating and ensure that the animal can move away from the

Table 10.2 Biological and clinical data

Respiratory rate	50–100 r.p.m. (13 during hibernation)
Heart rate	120–170 b.p.m. (5–10 during hibernation)
Temperature	34–37°C (6°C during hibernation)
Urinary values	**Bayer diagnostics Multistix 10SG**
pH	6.0 – strongly acidic indicates starvation, dehydration or diabetes
Protein	0.30 – consider renal failure, urinary tract infection or congestive heart failure if high
Specific gravity	1.030 – if persistently low may indicate renal abnormality. If high may indicate dehydration
Leucocytes	Negative – if present indicates bladder or renal infection
Glucose	Negative – if present indicates elevated blood glucose levels, reduced renal absorption, stress
Blood sugar	125 mg/100 ml
Ketones	Negative – if present may be due to starvation or diabetes
Nitrite	Negative
Urobilinogen	0–3 – if elevated may indicate liver abnormalities or haemolytic anaemia
Blood	Negative – if present indicates renal disease or urinary tract infection
Bilirubin	Negative – if present may indicate hepatic or biliary disease

heat if it needs to – excessive heat can cause dehydration. Warm any fluids given to, or used upon, the animal to body temperature before use.

Administer oxygen and respiratory stimulants where necessary.

Keep the animal at a constant environmental temperature following recovery, i.e. approximately 28–30°C, and ensure all urine is cleaned up and the animal is dried to prevent hypothermia (see Tables 10.2 & 10.3 for relevant data).

COMMON CONDITIONS, INJURIES AND DISORDERS

Abandonment

This is fairly common resulting from nest disturbance or the mother being killed. The breeding season runs from May to September often resulting in late litters near to hibernation time and thus underweight juveniles. The young will stay with the mother until 8 weeks of age, when fully weaned and independent. The male takes no role in parental care and disappears after mating (Table 10.4).

Many autumn-born orphans are abandoned as the mother hibernates and they may not have reached weaning age.

Many nests are disturbed by accidental human intervention when gardens are tended to. Sheds and compost heaps are often favoured nest sites, and abandonment results from disturbance of them.

In this circumstance young will need to be hand reared and cared for.

Depending on the age of the youngster it will require a permanent, stable heat source for at least the first 3–4 weeks. An incubator or heat pad maintaining temperature at 30°C will be required for the first 2 weeks.

Use physical signs to determine the age of the youngest to enable assessment for feeding regime.

First, thoroughly check the hoglet for signs of flies, eggs or maggots. These will need to be removed and sites bathed with saline.

Young will need to be fed via syringe (Fig. 10.3a) regularly once their age has been assessed. Provide Lectade as the first initial feed to assist in rehydrating the patient.

The most suitable milk for hand rearing is fresh goat's milk containing colostrum or artificial milks, such as Esbilac, as this helps to provide the antibodies absent in powdered milk to assist in

Table 10.3 Normal blood values for hedgehogs	
PCV	36.0–38.5%
Haemoglobin	12.0–13.2 g/dl
Erythrocytes	7.03–7.64 10^3/µL
Leucocytes	6.6–9.6 10^3/µL
Neutrophils	1.6–2.8 10^3/µL
Eosinophils	0.36–2.4 10^3/µL
Basophils	0.096–0.45 10^3/µL
Monocytes	0–0.84 10^3/µL
Lymphocytes	3.72–6.14 10^3/µL
Thrombocytes	230–430 µL
Reticulocytes	8–14% of RBC
MCH	16.8–18.2 pg
MCHC	33.3–35.2 g/dl
MCV	49.1–53.2 fl
Serum protein conc	51–72 g/l
Urea	13.3–15.0 mmol/l
Sodium	132–138 mmol/l
Potassium	3.6–5.1 mmol/l
Calcium	2.0–2.3 mmol/l
Phosphorus	2.0–3.8 mmol/l
Blood glucose	7.6 mmol/l

Table 10.4 Breeding data	
Gestation period	35–40 days
Litter size	1–8
Weaning age	40 days
Leave nest	6–8 weeks
Hibernation weight	500 g minimum
Male	Hog
Female	Sow
Young	Hoglets

Table 10.5 Comparison of milk and available replacements

	Hedgehog (%)	Goat (%)	Cow (%)	Cat (%)	Esbilac (%)
Solids	21.6	12	12	27	97
Protein	33.3	22	26	40	33.2
Fat	46.3	32	26	28	43.0
Carbohydrates	9.3	39	39	27	15.8

Table 10.6 Feeding guidelines for hand rearing

Age	Feed amount	Frequency
1–3 days	1–2 ml	2 hourly, through the night
3–7 days	1–2 ml	3 hourly
8–14 days	2–3 ml	3 hourly
15–21 days	3–5 ml	4 hourly
22–27 days	5–6 ml	5 hourly and leave with youngster Begin weaning onto solid meat
28 days	Leave milk in bowl	Provide water, cat food and invertebrates
Up to 8 weeks	Phase out milk	Fully weaned

supporting the immune system. Hedgehog milk is rich in fat and protein but low in carbohydrates. Table 10.5 shows a comparison of the different milk types available.

Feed milk substitute warm, at body temperature (25°C), and via a syringe with a mothering teat on the end to stimulate suckling. Avoid frozen milk as essential vitamins are broken down during the freezing process. Thiamine deficiency has been observed in youngsters fed on frozen milk resulting in hind limb paralysis. The condition can be treated by the inclusion of thiamine (vitamin B_1) in the milk; there is no toxicity level with the addition.

Hedgehogs cannot digest cow's milk well and so it is unsuitable for hand rearing.

Following feeding, baby hedgehogs, up to 3 weeks of age, will require manual stimulation with damp cotton wool to encourage urination and defecation before and following feeding. Don't be alarmed at the presence of pale greenish blue stools following feeding of goat's milk as this is normal.

Keep in an incubator for the first 2–3 weeks or near to a reliable, constant heat source.

Place on a towel and vet bed to allow nestling.

Weigh them daily to ensure a steady weight gain.

Sterilise all feeding utensils following feeding and between individuals.

Tip: Identification of young will be required for individual weight and health assessment and different coloured correction fluid can be placed on the spines between the shoulders.

At around 4 weeks of age the hedgehog will begin to lap milk from the bowl reducing the frequency and amount required to be fed by hand (see Table 10.6 for feeding and weaning guidelines). Solid food can now be offered such as puppy meat. They will also feed on scrambled eggs, crushed rusks, cat biscuits, cereals, dried insect food and will attempt to eat small invertebrates. They will also show interest in mashed banana and soft fruits.

Provision of milk is still important until fully weaned at around 8 weeks (Fig. 10.3b). At this stage continue feeding with cat biscuits and/or cat meat with the addition of garden invertebrates such as snails and beetles.

Hibernation problems

Hibernation is a complex process that the body undergoes to preserve physical condition through periods of poor food supply. The animal's metabolic, cardiovascular and respiratory rates dramatically decrease and they rely on a sufficient fat reserve to maintain them through this period. In order to survive through this period they must have an adequate supply. Prior to hibernation the hedgehog should weigh **500 g minimum** to have a chance of surviving the winter.

Hedgehogs may give birth to hoglets later in the year, resulting in youngsters having only a

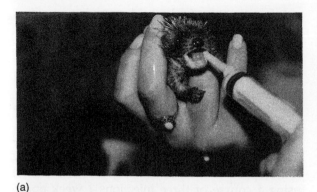

(a)

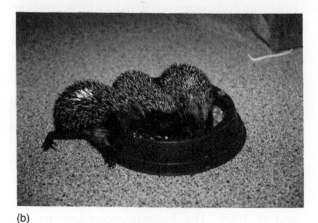

(b)

Fig. 10.3 (a) Syringe feeding. (b) Weaning.

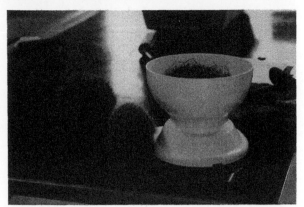

Fig. 10.4 Hedgehogs being weighed for hibernation.

short period to build up sufficient fat reserves to enable survival through hibernation.

During autumn months weigh any hedgehogs that present in the surgery, regardless of reason for presentation, to prevent hibernation whilst underweight (Fig. 10.4). It is possible to feed them up to weight and then allow the animal to go into hibernation at a later date than would happen in the wild.

Release on a suitable day such as a period of warm damp weather and place adequate nesting material to allow a nest for hibernation to be built. If in doubt hospitalise through the winter and release in April.

Hibernation usually begins in December lasting through until March, but is dependent on environmental conditions.

Hibernation usually occurs when the temperature falls below 9°C.

Periods of activity will be observed during this time for feeding excursions or change of nest site. Hedgehogs will slowly return to natural activity in spring.

Many animals may come out of hibernation in poor condition and require supplementary feeding or a temporary period of hospitalisation.

It is also important to check them for parasites and worm infestations during this time.

Bacterial respiratory illness

Infection of *Bordetella bronchiseptica* can cause pneumonia and rhinitis in hedgehogs. *Pasteurella multocida* is also often seen.

Hedgehogs will often tolerate chronic respiratory illness with little evidence of clinical symptoms.

Treatment with enrofloxacin and chloramphenicols should be considered.

Endoparasites

Due to the nature of the diet they ingest large numbers of invertebrates that are often temporary hosts for internal mammalian parasites. These further develop into adults within the hedgehogs' intestines or larvae may migrate to alternative organs in the body. Hedgehogs are susceptible to a large number of parasites including nematodes, cestodes and protozoa, exhibiting a range of symptoms from none to enteritis and respiratory disease.

Such endoparasites include threadworm, tapeworm and intestinal flukes.

Droppings with green gel-like appearance can indicate lung or intestinal worms.

Treatment includes:

- A single injection of praziquantel (Droncit) 5.5 mg/kg (approximately 0.1 ml/kg) or administration of ivermectin or fenbendazole.
- Coccidian can occasionally cause gastro-intestinal disturbance and will require treatment with sulphadimidine.

Lungworm

The most commonly found lungworm is *Crenosoma striatum*, a white segmented worm 0.3 mm in thickness and 10–20 mm in length. Infestation is transmitted across the placenta before birth. Segments are usually visible only in faeces following worming, although larvae can be identified in both faeces and saliva.

Threadworms, *Capillaria aerophila*, live in the trachea and lungs causing poor condition, laboured and noisy breathing, and oculonasal discharge. The adult worms are thin and 10–15 mm in length.

The larvae are coughed from the lungs and swallowed by the adult, and passed out through the faeces. The transport host then becomes an invertebrate species as they burrow into snails and slugs. Here they develop into third-stage larvae, which get back to the hedgehog through ingestion of the affected snails and slugs.

They then develop into adults in the hedgehog bronchi in approximately 3 weeks.

Symptoms of infestation are:

- chesty cough
- difficulty in breathing
- congestion during breathing
- discharge from nose
- weight loss
- poor condition
- bronchitis
- pneumonia
- death if untreated or if in hedgehogs that are old or young.

Infestation is fairly widespread and often reaches peaks during autumn and winter months.

To identify prepare a faecal or salival smear and examine via microscope; larvae often appear yellowish and are approximately 0.25 mm and mobile displaying thrashing movements.

Egg sacs may also be visible as yellow ovals measuring 0.07 mm.

Parasites can be successfully treated by administration of Lavamisol 20 mg/kg subcutaneously (SC) (approximately 0.5 ml/kg solution 1.25%) using a course of three injections 1 week apart. Treat with corticosteroids to reduce inflammation: methylprednisolone at 4 mg/kg in a single dose. Use antibiotics in case of secondary bacterial infection: amoxycillin LA 40 mg/kg SC (approximately 0.27 ml/kg).

> **Tip:** Dyspnoea during hospitalisation can be distressing; place hedgehogs on towel bedding to minimise dust and drop olbas or eucalyptus oil onto bedding to assist in relieving congestion.

Various *Capillaria* species inhabit the intestines and stomach. The hedgehog can lose weight, become weak and restless with a voracious appetite and is often seen foraging in the daytime.

Infestation can result in enteritis and diarrhoea.

Treat with anthelmintics such as Panacur granules.

> **Tip:** Place Panacur granules in the food; 1 sachet divided into three feeds will treat an adult hedgehog.

Fleas

Most hedgehogs will be infested with fleas (*Archaeopsylla erinacei*) on presentation as they are host specific. Always treat on presentation with Frontline spray or dusting with Pyrethrum powder.

Be wary of using any flea spray especially on juveniles of weight below 300 g, as this has been known to cause toxicity.

Mites

Mite infestations generally present themselves with skin in poor condition with a white flaky appearance and hair and spine loss.

Common species observed are *Caparinia tripilis* and *Sarcoptes, Notodres* spp, which often create severe mange problems (Fig. 10.5) and may be preliminary to ringworm infection.

Some may require identification under microscope following collection, possibly requiring skin scrapes for sub-surface mites.

They can be treated with ivermectin 400 μg/kg or acaricidal dips.

Ear mites are also common and appear as a sandy, dusty deposit around the ears. They can also be treated with ivermectin; however, often topical treatment is more successful such as with neomycin or permethrin drops.

> **Tip:** Hedgehogs will tolerate being bathed and this can be very soothing on the skin. Bathe weekly using a shower attachment in a sink with Seleen until condition improves. Always ensure they are dried and kept warm following bathing.

Ringworm

Symptoms on appearance are similar to mites; infestations can be due to a number of species, e.g. *Trichophyton erinacei* and *Microsporum* spp. *Trichophyton* spp. will not fluoresce like other species.

The appearance of the hedgehog will feature:

* flaky skin
* deposits around the base of spines
* possible missing spines.

Treat with griseofulvin placed in the food 25 mg/kg orally (PO) SID or a vial of program into food, or use of antifungal spray daily such as Imaverol at a 1:50 dilution.

Ticks

Usually *Ixodes hexagonus*, these are common and easily removed; however, heavy infestation may indicate an animal in poor condition and result in anaemia.

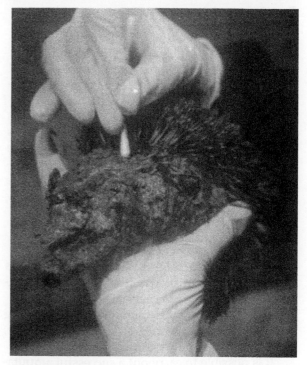

Fig. 10.5 Mange.

Myiasis – flystrike

This is a common condition seen in many species where blow fly eggs are laid on the animals. They hatch into larvae (maggots), which then feed on available faecal or wound material, or on the actual animal itself. This condition is fatal if not treated in time (Fig. 10.6).

In hedgehogs the eggs are often laid around the eyes, mouth and anogenital area. These will all require picking or brushing off, and flushing out of the mouth and eyes. If the maggots have hatched then again they will require removing or flushing out of wounds.

Also treat with an injection of ivermectin for any larvae that may have escaped or be internal, and a broad-spectrum antibiotic such as amoxycillin should be administered.

> **Tip:** A dental water jet is often useful for flushing out maggots from wounds.

Dental problems

Hedgehogs commonly suffer from dental problems including tartar build up, gingivitis and decay. Many adult hedgehogs presenting in surgery will be suffering from some form of dental decay resulting in hindered foraging and emaciation.

It is always important to check their mouths and treat with antibiotics to increase their chances of a successful release. Dental decay may have increased in incidence due to supplementary feeding of tinned meats provided by members of the public. Infected teeth may require removal as they will only cause the animals problems later in life.

Traumatic injuries

It is not uncommon to treat a hedgehog that has partial or fully amputated limbs following accidental damage by lawn mowers and strimmers.

They often survive for long periods following trauma as the site is lacerated and bleeds little; however, it is often seriously infected.

It is possible to carry out a successful amputation of hind limbs, but animals will be unsuitable for release if forelimbs have been removed as they may be unable to dig for food; however, semi-wild release is possible.

Provide first-aid treatment to allow assessment of the candidate for surgery.

In all case fluids, warmth and antibiotics should be provided to prevent death during anaesthesia.

Consider using long-term dissolvable sutures following surgery as this will prevent them having to be anaesthetised again for removal.

Skin wounds and lesions

These are common and may be due to attack from predators such as foxes, badgers or dogs. The spines are often damaged or broken and an infected open wound site visible (Fig. 10.7).

Remove all debris from the wound and try to clean as much as possible. If skin is missing then long-term wound management and hospitalisation will be required.

Wounds are often puncture wounds requiring flushing out and leaving open to allow any infection to track from the wound.

> **Tip:** Always check for other wounds opposite to the site to represent both top and bottom jaw entry sites.

Fractures

Fractures are common injuries and result from trauma such as road traffic accidents or injury from strimmers, etc.

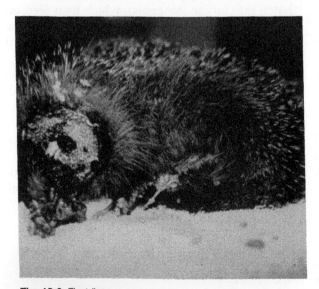

Fig. 10.6 Flystrike.

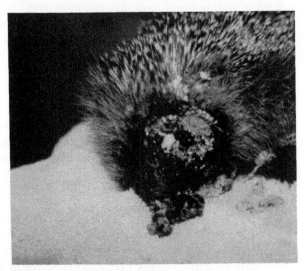

Fig. 10.7 Skin wounds/trauma.

It is possible to repair a limb but in some cases infection and injury may be so severe that it requires amputation. Hedgehogs cope well with three legs if a hind limb is being amputated but will not survive well in the wild if a forelimb is being removed.

For simple fractures a splint can be applied with the provision of adequate analgesia and an aluminium finger splint or a plaster of Paris cast to immobilise the limb. For compound or complicated fractures the areas will require surgery for internal (e.g. femur) or extracutaneous (e.g. radius and ulna) fixation prior to splinting.

There will usually be an infected and contaminated wound as many hedgehogs spend days with an injured limb before receiving treatment. Antibiotic treatment will assist in controlling infection with the use of Intrasite gel on the wound surrounding the fixators.

In some cases the animal may try to remove the dressing or splint and may require an adapted Elizabethan collar.

Prolapsed eyes

This condition is usually associated with some form of trauma and is often observed. It may heal and wither on its own; hedgehogs are often presented apparently with one eye.

Hedgehogs will cope well with only one eye but should not be directly released into the wild. Hedgehogs' eyesight is fairly poor but the loss of one eye will result in easier predation or injury. So once removed and healed a hedgehog-friendly garden should be sought for release.

Burns

Burns are common, usually resulting from injury from bonfires or fireworks. Bonfires make ideal nesting sites and many hedgehogs are going into hibernation at this time of year and are caught unsuspectingly. The area should be treated using a cold compress to reduce the heat and then thoroughly cleaned and ointment applied. It may be necessary to remove spines to allow adequate access to the site.

Poisoning

Methaldehyde poisoning from ingestion of slug pellets is still observed.

The animal will appear hypersensitive to sound and touch. Also observe for discoloration, pink or blue, of the faeces due to dyes present in the pellets.

Treatment is symptomatic as there is no actual antidote for methaldehyde. Rehydrate the patient using Hartmann's (approximately 10–20 ml) and also syringing or tubing activated charcoal into the gut to assist in absorbing some of the poison.

Many forms of poisoning can be seen from the usual chemicals kept in sheds, garages and used in gardens, and again treat as for shock and provide supportive treatment.

If the hedgehog is contaminated with oil or tar then wash in warm washing-up liquid or use Swarfega to remove all residues. Again, activated charcoal will also assist in case of accidental ingestion.

SELF-ANOINTING BEHAVIOUR

Without knowledge this unusual behaviour could be alarming. The hedgehogs roll on their side rapidly licking their spines producing frothy saliva (Fig. 10.8). It is often in response to the odour of certain materials, such as leather gloves during handling, or on the presentation of fruit to feed on, and is perfectly normal behaviour.

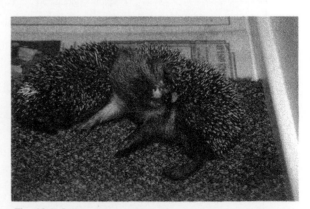

Fig. 10.8 Self-anointing behaviour.

DRUGS AND DOSE RATES

Subcutaneous injection can be administered in the back or sides and IM into hind legs. It is possible to use IP injection, but access to the ventral surface is often difficult (see Table 10.7 for drug dosage guidance).

RELEASE

Following successful treatment and care of wildlife the release back to the wild is the end result, and is highly rewarding.

Assessment is vital; the animal must be able to live a normal life.

> **Tip:** On consideration for release you must take into account the reason for the initial injury. It may not be a suitable site for release.

Prior to release, there are a number of things to consider as poor assessment may result in the animal having a poor quality of life or facing a life-threatening situation. However, keeping an animal too long in captivity can hinder its naturally wild behaviour and result in stereotypic

Table 10.7 Medical treatments

Condition	Medication	Dosage
Bacterial infection	Amoxycillin LA	20–40 mg/kg SC
	Clamoxyl	7 mg/kg SC
	Clamoxyl palatable drops	5–10 mg/kg PO, 0.25 ml/kg twice per day for 5 days
	Clamoxyl tablets	40 mg, 0.25 of tablet twice per day for 7 days
	Chloramphenicol	50 mg/kg twice per day SC, IM, PO
	Enrofloxacin 5%	5–10 mg/kg twice per day SC, IM, PO
	Oxytetracyclin	50 mg/kg twice per day PO
Parasites	Suphadimidine	1.5 ml/kg PO for 5 days
	Neo-sulphatrin suspension	1.2 ml/kg for 5 days
	Fendendazole	20–30 mg/kg 10 days PO
	Ivermectin	0.2–0.4 mg/kg SC
	Levamisole	20 mg/kg SC three injections 1 week apart
	Griseofulvin	25 mg/kg SID PO
Analgesia	Buprenorphine (Temgesic)	0.04–0.01 ml/kg IM every 6–8 hours
	Carprofen (Rimadyl)	0.05–0.01 ml/SC
	Flunixin (Finadyne)	0.05–0.01 ml/SC
Anaesthesia	Ketamin (Vetelar)	20 mg/kg IM
	Fentanyl/fluanisone (Hypnorm)	1–2 ml/kg IM
	Pentobarbitone sodium	25 mg/kg IP
	Halothane inhalation	2–4% + oxygen
Respiratory problems	Bisolven injection	0.25 ml/kg SC twice per day for 5–7 days
	Bisolven powder	One pinch daily for 14 days
Topical treatment	Alamycin aerosol	Spray over infected area
	Aureomycin powder 2%	Sprinkle over infected area
	Dermisol	Apply to infected area
	Sudocrem	Apply to infected area
	Betsolan	Apply to infected area
Ear infection/mites	Neomycin/Permethrin drops	One drop twice per day
Eye infections	Chloromycetin	5–6 times per day
	Orbenin	
Diarrhoea	Kaolin	
	Activated charcoal	
Microflora disruption	Avipro	Sprinkle one pinch on food daily
	Protexin	

SC: subcutaneous; PO: oral; IM: intramuscular; IP: intraperitoneal.

behaviour due to boredom. This may also lessen its instinct to be wary of humans thus putting it at risk once released.

Consider the following:

- The animal must be 100% fit.
- Consider the time of year for release; hedgehogs released in mid-winter may die.
- Consider the release habitat; it may be a different site to where the animal was captured and must be suitable.
- A hedgehog rescued from drowning in a garden pond would only face further danger if replaced in that locality.
- Hedgehogs are solitary and do not require replacing within a social group.
- A suitable release site is often indicated by the presence of other species in the area suggesting a suitable and viable food supply; however, beware of overcrowding.
- Hedgehogs are nocturnal and should be released early evening or at night to allow natural dispersal following release and assessment of their territory.

Some animals will be unsuitable for any wild release and may require a secure sheltered garden with provision of food until a later date or until old age. These animals include:

- Underweight animals during winter as they will not survive hibernation – release in spring.
- Hedgehogs who are unable to curl up and so have no protection and will not be able to hibernate.
- Completely blind or deaf hedgehogs, as they will be unable to avoid danger.
- Those with amputated front leg, as they are unable to dig or climb; animals with hind leg removals will do well.

> **Tip:** Assess whether the habitat is suitable for a hedgehog and will provide an adequate food supply naturally; if there are already hedgehogs there it can sustain them and is suitable.

CASE HISTORY 1
Patient

Adult male hedgehog, weighing 300 g.

Reason for hospitalisation

The hedgehog was seen in the client's garden during the day. The animal appeared in poor condition and reluctant to move. On moving the animal appeared to be circling around the lawn. The client offered it bread and milk but the animal was uninterested. It was left there most of the day and checked to see if it had moved off at any point but was still there at dusk. The client brought the hedgehog into the house in a box and was concerned about the animal's health as it appeared to be having difficulty in breathing. The client was also worried because the animal should have been in hibernation at that time of year. On presentation the animal was severely underweight and quite heavily infected with parasites, and internal lung parasites were suspected.

The hedgehog required anthelmintic treatment and increased weight gain prior to release and hibernation.

Type of accommodation and bedding material used

The hedgehog was placed in isolation due to parasitic burden for prevention of cross infection with domestic animals and to minimise stress from unfamiliar smells and noises. It was housed in a cat kennel, placed on newspaper for absorbency and hay for warmth and to allow nesting. A heat mat was placed under the newspaper to treat for possible hypothermia and to stimulate activity. The room was kept quiet and dimly lit, as hedgehogs are nocturnal.

Accommodation cleaning protocol

The hedgehog required daily cleaning due to the copious amounts of faeces and urine. The hedgehog was placed into a cat carrier during cleaning and was moved with leather gloves to prevent injury. All bedding material was removed and disposed of in bin liners. The cage was sprayed with Formula H disinfectant dilution 1:10 wearing rubber gloves. The spray was left for the recommended contact time of a couple of minutes and then thoroughly rinsed with warm water. The cage was allowed to dry and fresh newspaper and hay were placed back in the cage. Daily cleaning was continued as necessary to remove the parasite's eggs, larvae, etc., in excrement during treatment. The carrier was fully cleaned and disinfected following temporary use.

Feeding regime

The hedgehog was severely underweight and required feeding up to above 500 g before release could be considered. The bulk of the diet was from tinned cat food with the addition of a dried insectivore food mixed at the rate of approximately 1 teaspoon per feed. The hedgehog is nocturnal so feed was placed in the cage at early evening and early morning to follow natural feeding behaviour. Approximately one-third of a tin was provided for each meal. Fresh water was provided throughout the day in a shallow bowl.

Nursing care and monitoring of the animals

The hedgehog, being wild, required minimal handling and disturbance during its stay. Because of respiratory congestion the mouth and nose were cleaned daily with warm water to remove discharge and assist breathing. The animal was cleaned daily and wiped of any excrement obvious on the body and spines.

Eucalyptus oil was placed onto the bedding material (2–3 drops) to assist in clearing the airways. Weight was monitored weekly and a steady gain of 30–40 g was seen weekly.

Medication administered

On admission the hedgehog began a course of systemic antibiotics – baytril – initially given SC (0.1 ml) and then orally for the next 5 days during daily examination. This was to treat respiratory illness.

Anthelmintic drugs – Panacur granules – were placed in the food to treat internal parasites such as worms. A 20 g sachet was split into three and given daily for 3 days.

Date(s)

The hedgehog remained in the hospital for 5 weeks. Although treatment for respiratory

infection and parasites was complete in 1 week, the weight gain took 5 weeks to allow release at a hibernation weight for the winter.

CASE HISTORY 2

Patient

Male adult of approximately 1 year of age, weighing 455 g (underweight for age and time of year).

Condition

Adult male hedgehog found moving around in a garden with difficulty, limping and hind leg being dragged and not used. The hedgehog appeared to be coping but was unable to move properly and the client was very concerned. On admittance the hedgehog had obvious fly eggs around the hind limb and in the spines, he was very dehydrated and the dragging leg appeared to be swollen and infected.

Capture

Hedgehogs are easy to handle, especially if injured as they tend to curl up if startled. Pick up using garden gloves to prevent being harmed by the spines or any cross infection from disease, such as ringworm and place in a holding cage.

Treatment

On admission the hedgehog was obviously very dehydrated and the fly eggs suggested the animal had been ill, and infection was present in the leg requiring immediate treatment. The hedgehog had been mobile so an anaesthetic was given to allow a full observation and treatment. The hedgehog was placed under gaseous anaesthetic, isoflurane, to allow him to be uncurled. Under anaesthetic it was apparent that the left, hind leg was broken and the skin was torn. The fly eggs were present around the wound, and maggots had hatched and were present in the injured leg. The maggots and eggs were removed using a suction pump and tweezers ensuring every single one was removed. The wound was repeatedly flushed with saline to help the process, and was then cleaned and examined closely.

The leg was severely infected and would not be able to heal on its own and would require amputation. Hedgehogs cope well with rear limb amputations, but not front limbs, as they need these to dig for food. However, the infection and shock needed to be combated before this was possible. The hedgehog was given antibiotics and dexadresson to treat the shock and the wound was dusted with Negasunt powder to control any additional parasites. The antibiotics were continued for 3 days to reduce infection and at this stage the hedgehog was anaesthetised and the leg was removed.

The wound was checked 10 days later and had healed properly, so the stitches were removed. The hedgehog had improved dramatically and was bright, alert and eating well. The hedgehog was released 2 weeks later.

CASE HISTORY 3

Patient

Adult female hedgehog, approximately 3 years of age, plus four babies at 2 weeks of age.

Condition

Female hedgehog and four babies were found in a garden by the client having accidentally disturbed the nest during gardening. The client tried to restore the nest moving it to a quieter part of the garden but the mother ran away from the youngsters and the nest in fright. This would mean the babies were abandoned and would need hand rearing if the situation could not be resolved.

Capture

The babies and (having been found in the nearby bushes) the mother were captured together to try to prevent rejection. Hedgehogs are easy to handle especially if injured, as they tend to curl up if startled. Pick up using garden gloves and place in a holding cage. The gloves are used to prevent harm from the spines or any cross infection from diseases, such as ringworm, and also to prevent rejection of the babies by the mother due to human scent on the spines.

Treatment

On admission, the female hedgehog and babies were placed in a small enclosure with a heat lamp to assist in acceptance of the young and for the treatment of shock or hypothermia of the young.

Once warmed through, the babies were all given 1 ml of warm Lectade (fluid replacement). Following this they were replaced with the mother, and food and water were provided whilst a close observation was taken to see if she accepted the youngsters and began feeding. The mother and babies were left for a period of a week and the mother was active and feeding; however, it was impossible to check the babies for fear of further rejection. The following week the babies were seen coming out of the nest box and began weaning. The reintroduction had been successful and all five were doing well.

At 6 weeks following arrival all the family were placed in a holding cage and replaced in the garden where they were found. Hedgehogs are not gregarious and live solitary lives except when breeding. They naturally disperse to the surrounding neighbourhood to make a new territory for themselves.

Chapter 11

Squirrels

Sara Cowen

INTRODUCTION

In the UK there are two species of squirrel, the red squirrel (*Sciurus vulgaris*), which is native, and the introduced North American species, the grey squirrel (*Sciurus carolinensis*).

Although native, the red squirrel has been moved out of its foothold of distribution in the UK and is rarely seen. It is predominantly an inhabitant of pine forest being seen in Scotland, Wales and a population on the Isle of Wight where the grey squirrel has not taken over.

The grey squirrel is now referred to as the most common squirrel species of the UK, having been very successful in colonising deciduous woodland and urban areas over the red. Because of this, the grey squirrel is considered a pest species and there are legal restrictions to importations, release and the animal being held in captivity.

To keep grey squirrels a licence is required from the Ministry of Agriculture (now DEFRA). Red squirrels are also fully protected by the Wildlife and Countryside Act 1981 making it illegal to capture, disturb or harm them. These restrictions have obvious constraints over treatment and release of both species (see Table 11.1 for species data).

There are over 350 varieties of squirrels worldwide ranging from the African Pygmy squirrel to the Giant Asian. They fall into the categories of tree, flying and ground squirrels. The word squirrel is derived from the Greek words 'skia' meaning shadow and 'oura' meaning tail and translates roughly as 'the creature that sits in the shadow of its tail'.

Tip: Only grey squirrels can eat acorns as they have special digestive enzymes in their saliva, which protects them. Acorns contain polyphenols (tannic acid) and are poisonous to most species.

The main reasons for a squirrel ending up requiring veterinary assistance include:

- Abandonment or injury of young
- Injury due to falling or road traffic accidents
- Some form of poisoning.

ANATOMY AND PHYSIOLOGY

Squirrels, as typical rodents, have a large stomach and long intestine for handling and absorbing vegetable material.

Their physique is designed for an arboreal life and specialised for leaping and climbing. They have a well-developed spine, shoulders and pelvis for attachment of powerful muscles.

The coccygeal vertebrae form a long, flexible tail for balance.

Squirrels have short front limbs with four toes and long, powerful hind limbs with five toes. They have long, narrow paws and double jointed feet for climbing; during descent the hind feet rotate by 180°C to allow them to hang on.

Their skulls are flattened and they have rounded noses and sharp incisors. They have two upper and one lower premolar and three upper and lower molars with ridged grinding surfaces. The lack of canines allows the cheek to be drawn in creating two areas, one for chewing and one for

Table 11.1 Biological data of red and grey squirrels

	Red squirrel	Grey squirrel
Latin name	*Sciurus vulgaris*	*Sciurus carolinensis*
Life span	3–5 years	3–5 years
Average male weight (g)	280	515
Average head and body length (mm)	215	260
Average tail length (mm)	175	215
Average female weight (g)	260	500
Gestation period	38 days	44 days
Litter size	1–5	3–8
Breeding season	Spring – summer	Spring – summer
Average weight of neonates (g)	10–15	13–17
Lactation period	7–10 weeks	7–10 weeks
Weaning age	8–10 weeks	8–10 weeks
Eyes and ears open	28–32 days	28–35 days
Hair erupts	8 days	10 days
Lower incisors erupt	20–25 days	21–23 days
Upper incisors erupt	37–41 days	37–41 days
Adult diet	Seeds, nuts, berries, fungi, bark, foliage, insects, birds' eggs and nestlings	Seeds, nuts, berries, bark, foliage, acorns, hazelnuts, insects, birds' eggs and nestlings

biting. (In hamsters this is further developed into specialised pouches for food storage.)

They have continually growing incisors, which are covered in yellow enamel. This yellow colour indicates that the animal is in good condition.

The lower jaw is in two halves allowing them to slightly part the lower incisors enabling them to grab nuts. This is achieved due to specialised muscles around the jaw.

> **Tip:** If a squirrel appears very underweight and reluctant to eat check the incisors for overgrowth or malocclusion. They may require trimming; however, this may result in further overgrowth after release.

HANDLING

Handling of squirrels is always a tricky procedure, mainly because they are difficult to restrain, extremely lively, quick and are fiercely aggressive when provoked.

It is quite useful to consider similar handling techniques to restraining a ferret:

- Circle the neck using your thumb and forefinger.
- Gently circle the rest of the body behind the front legs allowing you to support the animal's weight.
- Your grip should be firm but do not squeeze the chest or abdomen.

Always wear gloves as their incisors are extremely sharp and if they bite will invariably hold on.

> **Tip:** Always wash your hands prior to handling as squirrels will become aggressive and bite in response to certain smells such as disinfectant and cigarette smoke.

Always be wary of squirrels; what may appear a shocked, sedate individual may rapidly change into an energetic patient once approached.

Use a towel to restrain the individual and cover the head, as this may have a calming influence. Once wrapped in the towel areas of the body can be revealed for examination whilst still providing a degree of protection and security for the animal. This is also useful if providing medication such as injections, as the animal may remain quieter during the procedures.

If full restraint is required, then clasp one hand around the shoulders and chest pushing the thumb gently under the chin to avoid being bitten.

ACCOMMODATION

Squirrels are housed suitably in cat carriers; however, in any situation it is vital that their accommodation is completely escape proof – a loose squirrel in a surgery is not a welcome distraction.

Try to keep them in an area that is warm (around 30°C), quiet and dark to reduce stress and anxiety. Darkness can be achieved by placing a towel over the front of the cage.

Placing a heat pad under the container can provide a suitable heat source.

> **Tip:** Do not place heat pads and hot water bottles directly in the cage, as squirrels naturally gnaw and will soon destroy such items, and this may result in burns if an electrical supply is chewed.

House adult squirrels separately as they may fight especially with unknown individuals.

Place suitable, soft and absorbent bedding materials in the cage. Newspaper should line the cage as it is absorbent for urine. Vet bed materials are useful for substrate, especially if the animal is in shock, as they retain warmth and are soft if traumatic injury has occurred.

Placing a towel on top of the bedding in the cage allows the squirrel to hide underneath and provides security and warmth. This is especially useful as it allows you to examine the cage, change water, etc., without disturbance of the patient.

Once in good health place some wooden twigs with bark for them to chew rather than the cage.

NUTRITION

This will depend on the age and condition of the patient. If it is a young animal requiring hand rearing, a substitute milk replacement will be required. If it is an adult and able to eat solids, then proprietary squirrel mixes are now available. Alternatively, the use of a hamster or gerbil mix will certainly be adequate. Use of muesli mixes and digestive biscuits can also assist in encouraging the patient to begin eating under stressful conditions.

It is important to provide them with logs and branches such as hazel, apple, willow, etc., for gnawing on in order to prevent overgrowth of teeth and subsequent malocclusion during hospitalisation.

HAND REARING

If a neonate arrives in surgery requiring hand rearing you may be well advised to contact a local rehabilitation centre. This is especially useful if only one baby is found; this way they can be placed with other youngsters making adjustment easier.

Young squirrels require hand rearing for numerous reasons such as the death of mother, nest disturbance, rejection or if they fall from the nest.

Initial treatment will include warming the baby, preferably by placing in an incubator (around 30°C). This will assist in providing a permanent stable heat source. Baby squirrels lose heat rapidly and can become hypothermic very quickly. Baby squirrels are unable to regulate their body temperature until fully furred, so a constant heat source will be required throughout the first few weeks.

Wrap the baby in a towel and place with the heat source, as this will provide and maintain warmth whilst giving the security of a nest.

Once warmed through, the young squirrel can be rehydrated by the provision of a warm fluid replacement such as Lectade. This will provide essential electrolytes, fluid, hydrate cells and will allow the gut to be rehydrated. This is vital if an animal is then to attempt to digest milk-replacement formulas. The baby can be rehydrated by syringing into the mouth or using a baby teat and feeder as for kittens or a 2 ml syringe.

At this stage do not attempt feeding, as the baby will be unresponsive and unwilling to suckle, and attempts may cause aspiration pneumonia.

There are a number of formulas and alternatives suggested for hand rearing, but the recommended ones are Esbilac and Cimicat. Cow's milk is not suitable and can cause serious nutritional problems as it does not provide adequate nutritional requirements (see Tables 11.2 & 11.3).

administration of the fluid. Babies will usually let you know how much they require and will stop suckling once full.

Following feeding it is necessary to stimulate defecation and urination. Failure to do so will result in constipation and bladder stress, as the babies will not release waste material until stimulated by the mother's licking. Use a damp piece of cotton wool and gently wipe over the anogenital region until defecation and urination are observed.

Tip:

Milk formula

Under 3 weeks of age
    Esbilac – one part powder to two parts water, boiled and cooled
    Cimicat – one part powder to three parts water, boiled and cooled

Over 3 weeks of age
    Powdered goat's milk – 15 ml measure
    Esbilac – 1 teaspoon
    Baby rice – Milupa – 2 teaspoons
    Cooled, boiled water – one-quarter pint

Mix well and refrigerate when not in use.

Tip: If the baby appears reluctant to feed and is refusing to suckle, test the temperature of the milk. Cool or cold milk is the most common cause for refusing to eat or stopping feeding half way through. Baby bottle warmers are extremely useful and ensure milk is kept at a constant temperature through feeding time.

Feeding should be carried out using a teat and a small syringe (Fig. 11.1). Gently placing the teat into the mouth of a youngster will soon initiate a suckling response and allow careful, slow

Table 11.3 Comparison of milk

	Grey squirrel milk (%)	Cow's milk (%)	Goat's milk (%)	Esbilac milk (%)
Protein	22	26	25	33
Fat	65	26	35	43
Carbohydrate	12	39	35	15
Solids	40	12	13	97

Table 11.2 Feeding guidelines

Age (weeks)	Identification	Frequency
0–1	Bald, blind, deaf, fully dependent, umbilical cord still present, approx. 25 g	2 hourly, Esbilac milk 6 am–12 pm, approx 0.5–1 ml
1–2	Slight fur covering body, eyes and ears still closed, approx. 55 g	2 hourly Esbilac 6 am–12 pm, approx. 1–2 ml
2–3	Eyes open, begin moving around, approx. 90 g	Cimicat 2.5 hourly 6 am–12 pm, approx. 2–3 ml
3–4	Much more mobile and walking around, teeth develop, approx. 120 g	Squirrel mix, 3 hourly 6 am–12 pm, approx. 3–4 ml
4–5	Fully furred and mobile, well developed tail and teeth, interested in solids, approx. 140 g	Squirrel mix 4 hourly, approx. 4–5 ml, proprietary squirrel dry food and chopped fruit such as apple, banana, grapes
5–6	Full coat, very active and climbing	Squirrel mix four times daily, approx 6–8 ml and solids available at all times
From 6 weeks	Miniature adults often develop aggressive behaviour at this stage	Solids only

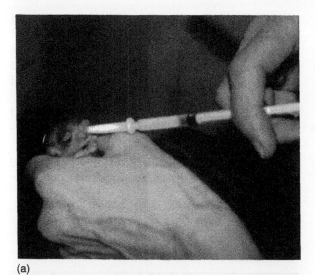

(a)

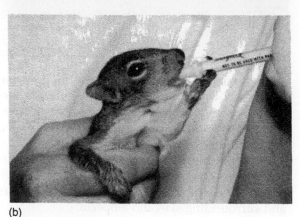

(b)

Fig. 11.1 Syringe feeding.

WEANING

Weaning can begin at around 6 weeks of age but it is important to remember that at this stage they will still require syringe feeding. The introduction of solids slowly is imperative and small amounts of varied feedstuff is important. Young squirrels will begin to accept soft feed from the time of the eruption of their incisors. A shallow bowl with bread soaked in the milk may evoke interest.

Youngsters can be introduced to small amounts of solids such as broccoli, apple, pear and corn, along with cereals such as sunflower seed, peanuts, rusks, digestives, etc. Each youngster will have preferences but it is important to provide a variety.

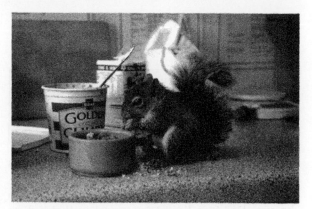

Fig. 11.2 Weaning.

To begin feeding, hand the solids to them as they prefer to hold the food in their hands and at this age they are a little awkward.

It is also useful to provide mineral supplementation, sprinkling a powdered version for additional source during the crucial developmental stages.

Rusk or digestive biscuits and baby formulas, such as Milupa, can be made into a moist mix and placed in a shallow lid or bowl. The youngster will start to lap up and swallow the mixture ensuring a gradual move to solids (Fig. 11.2).

The level of solids can be slowly increased up to the age of 10 weeks, where they will now show little or no interest in the milk. Provision of suitable proprietary pet mixes for hamsters, gerbils, rats, etc., can be used in addition to fresh food.

FIRST AID

The most important thing initially for squirrels is to treat for shock to allow them to survive the first few hours. Signs of shock include:

- shaking
- cold and motionless
- slow, shallow breathing
- hunched up appearance
- head tucked into chest
- eyes closed.

Treatment includes:

- warmth
- darkness
- quiet

- fluids, e.g Lectade – an adult dose would be 10–20 ml orally or 10 ml subcutaneously. This should be adjusted for young ones.

> **Tip:** It is always useful to keep some Bach's Flower Rescue Remedy in the practice. Wildlife casualties appear to respond well to a couple of drops in the mouth on arrival when suffering from shock.

Keep the patient clean and dry throughout this period to minimise stress.

If the animal is unable to eat, food will need to be supplied in a liquid form such as baby diets that are high in fibre and palatable. This may be required to be syringe fed or placed in a bowl to be lapped up. During this time the squirrel may have loose droppings but this will correct itself once back on solids.

To entice them to move onto solids use nuts such as peanuts, hazelnuts, almonds, etc.

ANAESTHESIA

As with all wild species there is little solid research evidence about drug dose rates and safety within these species.

Sedation and immobilisation in squirrels is useful for initial examination, allowing easy observation and reducing the stress of being handled.

Ketamin at 10–20 mg/kg intramuscularly will be effective, placing injection into the muscle whilst restrained in a towel.

Gaseous anaesthesia required for surgical procedures can be induced using a mask or more safely in an induction chamber using halothane or isoflurane.

THERAPEUTICS

Similar drug administration and dose rates are used as for large domestic rodents such as rats.

COMMON ILLNESSES, INJURIES OR DISEASES

Parasites

As wild animals they are prone to infestation by fleas and lice, which will be tolerated by the patient. It is unlikely these will be the cause of illness.

The species observed are *Orchopeas howardi* in the grey squirrel and *Monopsyllus sciurorum* in the red. They can be treated using a pyrethrum based powder or bird parasite sprays.

Capillaria infestations have been observed and are believed to be a reason for numerous grey-squirrel mortalities.

Also observed are coccidial (*Eimeria sciurorum*) infections, a gut parasite, causing enteritis. Symptoms include:

- wasting
- enteritis
- diarrhoea.

> **Tip:** Ivermectin can be used to treat parasites at a rate of 0.2 ml of a 10% solution for an adult. Adjust accordingly for youngsters.

A number of red squirrels examined were excreting oocysts without sign of illness; however, the presence can cause disease. Faecal parasitology will diagnose species and may be treated with sulphonamides.

Squirrels have also been observed with *Sarcoptes* mite and ringworm (*Microsporum cookei*). The animal will appear with crusty, flaking ears and surrounding skin and alopecia.

Internal parasites are common, such as intestinal parasites, ascarid worms, tapeworms and flukes.

Parapoxvirus

This condition observed in squirrels has similar symptoms to myxomatosis. It is believed that it may have been introduced by the grey squirrels and it has been documented in red squirrels. The virus is found in the eyelids of the animal and is thought to be stress related. It is debilitating and highly contagious.

Observed symptoms are:

- lethargy
- oculonasal discharge
- conjunctivitis
- swollen eyelids
- blindness

- disorientation
- pneumonia
- stomatitis
- alopecia.

Euthanasia should be considered rather than treatment.

Squirrel fibroma

It viral condition is considered to be spread by the vector of biting insects.

It appears as raised flattened nodules over the body areas such as limbs, tail, head and abdomen. Pathogenesis occurs as with other pox viruses with multiplication in the lymph nodes spreading to the blood. Lesions appear as fibromas spreading to multiple nodules over a period of 2–3 weeks. It is possible for the nodules to become ulcerated and infected with secondary bacterial infections or fungal infestation.

Accompanying symptoms may also be inappetence and anorexia, dyspnoea and general lethargic behaviour.

Histopathological examination of the nodules will confirm diagnosis.

Treatment includes antibiotics (amoxycillin) to control secondary infections 0.1–0.2 ml. The use of vitamin injections or Echinacea orally (a couple of drops directly into the mouth) may assist in boosting the immune response to the condition.

Cat attack

This is a frequent reason for presentation in surgery, especially of young, with lacerations or puncture wounds. Cats carry *Pasteurella* bacteria in their saliva and infection may affect the central nervous system.

In all cases of cat attacks a broad-spectrum antibiotic should be administered to control infection at the site of the wound.

Puncture wounds should be flushed and then left to heal to prevent abscesses forming inside the wound.

Head injuries

These are commonly observed in youngsters that have fallen from the nest or in adults who have been involved in road traffic accidents. Observed symptoms may include:

- concussion – head shaking, dilated pupils, nystagmus
- contusion – swelling from bruising or bleeding externally or internally
- compression – pressure on the brain resulting in disorientation, pain, unconsciousness
- torticollis – head tilt with circling behaviour.

Treatment includes the administration of a steroid, e.g. dexamethasone 0.1–0.2 ml to assist in reduction of swelling and reduction of pressure. Additional care will be required during this recovery period as the animal will be disorientated and may have adverse reactions to the presence of or handling by humans. Keep the cage dark, quiet and covered – animals may be hypersensitive to sound and movement causing further distress. If unable to feed, gentle restraint will be required to administer fluids and liquid feeds. Ensure the cage is safe and soft to prevent injury during the period of disorientation. Place solid food on the floor of the cage and water in a bottle; don't place bowls in the cage until the animal is calm again to prevent injury or soaking. Keep the squirrel as clean as possible from urine or faecal spoiling, as these are fastidiously clean animals and soiling causes further stress and discomfort.

Poisoning

This may occur due to accidental ingestion of parasiticides, insecticides used in the garden or the possible ingestion of rodent baits. In all cases the symptoms are similar to all poisoned animals:

- collapsed and in shock
- salivation
- disorientation
- nystagmus
- diarrhoea – possibly with blood present
- enteritis.

Treat as for poisoning in general and rehydrate the patient in the hope of diluting the effect of the poison. Feed high fibre liquid feeds to assist in gut movement forcing the poison through the gut. Use kaolin and activated charcoal for absorption and reduction of diarrhoea. Keep warm and quiet, and treat symptomatically.

Metabolic bone disease

This is a condition observed in youngsters that are reared on a diet deficient in vitamin D, and thus have inadequate absorption of calcium and phosphorus.

Calcium and phosphorus are major mineral constituents of the body and are associated with growth and development of the skeleton. Calcium also assists in blood clotting, nerve and muscle excitability and contraction. Phosphorus is involved in metabolism such as nutrient metabolism, e.g. of fats, carbohydrates and amino acids. Metabolic bone disease (MBD) occurs when the dietary phosphorus content is too high. The appropriate ratio is 2:1 calcium to phosphorus.

It is for this reason that it is vitally important to provide a varied diet supplying all the vitamins and minerals required for growth and development.

It has been observed that diets high in peanuts and sunflower seeds predispose to MBD.

The condition will appear within 5 days of the deficiency and often at around 2–3 months where seizures may be observed that can progress to paralysis and death.

Initial symptoms are:

- excessive sleeping
- lethargy
- reluctance to move
- pain
- swollen joints
- splayed legs
- loss of weight
- curvature of the spine.

To treat, administer direct supplementation of calcium by injection and continuation through the diet. Improvement of the animal should be observed in a few days. However, in all cases prevention is better than cure.

RELEASE

This is a problematic area as it is illegal to release a grey squirrel back into the wild. Schedule 9 of the Wildlife and Countryside Act 1981 makes it an offence to release or allow them to escape, so it is important to consider that a life of captivity is the alternative. Although hand-reared animals will often live well in captivity, do not be under the illusion that they will remain tame; they are still wild animals.

For assistance and rehoming contact your local wildlife rehabilitator for their support network.

CASE HISTORY
Patient

Adult male squirrel involved in a collision with a car at low speed.

The driver checked the animal and observed that it was still moving and picked it up from the roadside.

Condition

The squirrel was in obvious shock and appeared fairly sedate and calm. There was blood present from the mouth possibly inferring internal injuries or a fractured jaw due to direct trauma. There was a swelling to the head and pupils were fixed and dilated. The animal was breathing but this was shallow.

Capture

The car owner covered the animal in a jumper, as it appeared not to be moving and placed it in the car footwell. In this situation there was no problem with this procedure; however, squirrels often appear immobile until handled and then can become ferocious causing severe bites and injury. They may also be in initial shock and then recover during transportation. Squirrels should always be restrained using thick leather gloves and be placed in some form of confinement.

Treatment

Initial treatment involved injections of dexadresson and rimadyl, and being placed in darkness with a heat mat to assist in controlling the shock. At this stage it did not receive fluids as the accident had just taken place. The squirrel was left in confinement overnight to assess status the following day.

There appeared to be little improvement the following day and the swelling to the head had increased. A thorough examination indicated the animal was suffering from concussion and had a fractured jaw. The squirrel was unresponsive and would require surgical intervention to try to repair the jaw.

At this stage a decision was taken to euthanase the animal as no improvement had been observed, and a fractured jaw may cause problems in the wild due to the nature of their diet if repair is not satisfactory.

It also has to be considered in every case with squirrels that it is illegal to release grey squirrels back into the wild, as they are non-endemic species, so if a suitable captive environment cannot be found euthanasia must be fully considered.

Chapter 12

Deer

Sara Cowen

INTRODUCTION

There are currently six species of deer living wild in the UK; however, not all are native – only the roe and red deer are. A number of the species are escapees from deer parks that have colonised successfully. The main three likely to require treatment in practice are fallow, roe and muntjac deer (see Table 12.1).

ANATOMY AND PHYSIOLOGY

As deer are ruminants they have four distinct regions of the stomach. The first stage, the rumen, is the largest and leads directly off the oesophagus. This then enters the reticulum, with raised surfaces, the omasum with a folded lining and finally the abomasum, with a smooth lining that is similar to normal mammalian stomachs.

Table 12.1 Biological data of fallow, roe and muntjac deer

	Fallow deer	Roe deer	Muntjac deer
Latin name	*Dama dama*	*Capreolus capreolus*	*Muntiacus reevesi*
Description	Red brown coat with spots, white around rump, palmate antler in males	Red brown coat, white rump patch, tail barely visible, tubular with pointed ends antlers in male	Very small, brown, white underneath tail but not rump, small single pointed antlers
Average male weight (kg)	75	25	14
Average female weight (kg)	45	24	12
Average head and body length (m)	1.3–1.7	1–1.4	0.9–1
Average tail length (cm)	15–24	2–3	15
Gestation period	32 weeks	7 months	7 months
Breeding season	Oct–Nov	Aug–Oct (delayed implantation)	Throughout the year
Litter size	1	1–2	1
Fawns born	June–Oct	April–July	All year
Average weight of fawn (kg)	4.5	2	1
Weaning age	7–8 months	2–4 months	3–5 months
Lie up until	2–3 weeks	2 weeks	1–3 weeks
Fully independent	1 year	1 year	1 year
Adult diet	Grasses, herbs, fruit, bark	Leaves, buds, herbs, fruits	Leaves, shrubs, brambles, hawthorn, ivy

Deer have no upper incisors and, therefore, following partial chewing food is passed into the rumen. At a later stage the bolus of food is regurgitated (the cud) into the mouth. The rumen and reticulum are full of beneficial bacteria to aid digestion of cellulose material. Once the bolus has been chewed by the molars it then travels through the rest of the stomach chambers where absorption of nutrients takes place.

HANDLING

Deer can be extremely difficult to handle, but if they allow you to approach they are invariably in poor condition.

The most important factor in handling is to cover the head. This has a calming influence over the deer. A hood can be made by cutting the corner off a pillowcase and placing it over the head with the nose protruding through the corner that has been removed allowing the animal to breathe.

Wrapping deer in blankets and placing onto stretcher helps to restrain them and protect you from the damage of flaying limbs.

For male deer with antlers it is wise to consider sedation (diazepam 1 mg/kg intramuscularly (IM)) as severe wounds can be inflicted from these.

When transporting they should be placed either on their keel bone or on their side to prevent distress and accumulation of fluid in the lungs.

Smaller deer, such as muntjacs, can be transported safely in large pet carriers.

ACCOMMODATION

Deer, by their sheer nature, are difficult animals to capture, restrain and not least accommodate in practice. It is highly unlikely that there will be any specific housing for the animal but until it is stable and can be moved to a specialised rehabilitation centre, you will have to adapt.

The most important consideration is safety for both you and the animal. They are extremely nervous animals and are naturally wary of predators, fleeing from noises such as dogs, etc. You will have to keep the deer somewhere as quiet as possible and away from the sound and smell of dogs.

An isolation room or walk-in kennel may be appropriate but will have to have solid fronted

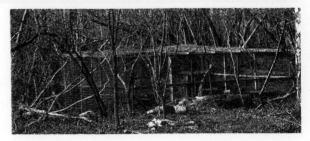

Fig. 12.1 Release pens.

doors and walls so no injury can be caused if the animal panics. A metal barred cage would be the perfect death trap for a deer in fright resulting in fractured legs and concussion.

If necessary, pad the walls and door from any protrusions or possible dangers.

Darken the room to low illumination or red light allowing you to view and check the animal without the stress of bright lights; remember they are dawn and dusk animals and on the whole prefer this light intensity.

Always enter the room very quietly and carefully and preferably with an outer safety door in case the deer bolts.

The practice may well have a shed that could be temporarily converted. However, again, ensure safety, covering any protrusions such as nails, etc., and making sure all windows are boarded up.

Use newspaper, straw and hay for bedding as this is more natural and creates a slightly more natural smell in the otherwise sterile conditions. If the deer is likely to be lying down try to place a highly absorbent surface under the bedding. This will prevent the deer having to be moved or cleaned out daily thus reducing stress from handling.

Once initial treatment has been provided and the animal is stable or well enough to be moved, place in the care of a wildlife centre that has facilities and accommodation for deer during the recovery period (Fig. 12.1).

NUTRITION

In captivity it is important to remember that you can sustain deer on proprietary mixes such as goat mix or deer or sheep pellets; however, they may refuse this type of feed as it is unfamiliar. The best

Table 12.2 Comparison of milk

	Deer milk (%)	Lamlac (%)
Protein	39	24
Fat	34	24
Carbohydrate	19	–
Solids	19	60

Table 12.3 Feeding guidelines

Age (weeks)	Frequency
0–1	2 hourly
1–2	2–3 hourly
2–3	3–4 hourly
3–4	4 hourly
4–7	4–5 feeds daily
7–12	3–4 feeds daily; begin weaning
Up to 7 months	1 feed daily

These are rough guidelines and will depend on the strength and feeding interest of the fawn. Once suckling they will monitor their intake, usually being a fairly frenzied rapid suckling. Deer wean very late and it is important to remember they will still take a bowl of milk daily in some breeds, such as fallow, up to 7 months of age.

form of feed to provide is browsing food such as branches of shrubs and bushes, etc. They may take hay but fresh leaves and bark are preferable, e.g. brambles and apple (not evergreens).

HAND REARING

Fawns are often brought in mistakenly thought to have been abandoned. The fawns will lie up in the wild while the mother forages a distance away. Dogs may discover or disturb them. It is vital not to undertake hand rearing unless the fawn is actually abandoned or the mother has been hit by a car and the fawn has been left lying up nearby.

Once hand-reared, it is highly unlikely that they can be released as they become tame and could endanger themselves in the wild.

Lamlac or Ovilac has been very successful in hand rearing deer. If the fawn is still in the early stages where meconium is still being produced, it is advisable to add sheep colostrum to the milk for the first few days (Table 12.2).

Fawns will feed from the bottle; however, aspiration pneumonia can be a problem. On initial feed from a bottle only provide Lectade to allow the fawn to get used to suckling from the bottle.

Tip: Deer feed underneath their mother whilst she licks around the hind end. Standing over a fawn like a mother can often make the feeding technique easier for the youngsters. Whilst suckling rub the coat, especially around the hind end to stimulate suckling and toileting.

If the youngster does not take to the bottle try getting it to suckle your finger and then gently lower your finger into a shallow bowl. In my experience they will suckle from a bowl at a very early age making feeding easy from there on.

Gradually solids can be introduced such as goat's mix and leaves; alfalfa and hay are also taken well (Table 12.3).

Tip: Placing browse in a large plant pot upright assists in encouraging natural foraging behaviour. Provide fresh twigs and leaves daily.

During the period of hand rearing they will need daily exercise. If an enclosure is not available it should be considered to walk them with a dog harness and lead around the chest. However, ensure the area is safe and secure from dogs, etc.

Whilst hand-reared deer cannot be released, it may be possible to place them in a managed deer park where they have a secured area; otherwise keeping in captivity will be necessary.

FIRST AID

Initial treatment includes the provision of:

- warmth
- darkness
- quiet
- oral fluids – Lectade
- intravenous fluids, e.g. 1 l of glucose/saline or Hartmann's, as appropriate

- corticosteroids for post capture myopathy
- sedation if required – diazepam 1.0 mg/kg intravenously (IV) or IM.

COMMON ILLNESSES, INJURIES OR DISEASES

Natural death of deer is invariably due to starvation, parasite, disease or old age and, in some cases, extreme weather conditions can affect mortality.

Starvation may be due to the inability to eat in older individuals with dental problems or worn-down teeth. Often it is due to overcrowding, as the habitat just does not have enough vegetation to support all the deer.

Males often sustain injuries during the rutting season, when they are sorting out their dominance hierarchy and fighting to breed.

Parasites

Deer are hosts to a number of parasites and on the whole these should not cause a problem, although heavy infestation will weaken a deer in the long term.

Ticks (*Ixodes ricinus*) are very common as with all wild animals; however, they are also the carrier for Lyme's disease, a zoonotic debilitating and crippling disease in humans. The symptoms in humans may be:

- inflammation at site of bite
- headaches
- stiff neck
- flu-like symptoms
- malaise
- arthritis
- meningitis
- possible paralysis.

Treatment is with antibiotics and is usually effective, and the condition is rarely fatal.

Other such parasites are lice and flat flies, which scuttle around in the coat of the deer causing minor irritation.

Internal parasites comprise lungworms and liver fluke and again will not normally pose a problem. Treatment with ivermectin is effective at a dose of approximately 0.6 ml (not diluted).

Post capture myopathy

Although not a cause of injury requiring treatment on presentation, this is often the condition that deer will die from following capture.

Essentially the flight and fright response causes the body to actually shut down resulting in paralysis and necrosis of muscle tissue. The condition is almost always fatal and can occur from 3 days to 2 weeks following capture.

On initial capture it is extremely important to administer corticosteroids such as dexamethasone IV or IM at a dose of approximately 3–4 ml to help minimise the risk of the onset of this condition.

Symptoms of onset are:

- lethargy
- depression
- head tilt
- rigidity of muscles
- convulsion
- death.

Fractures

Following a road traffic accident it is highly likely the deer will have fractures of the limbs or pelvis. They have a solid body but have extremely fragile legs with little protection.

It is possible to splint and fixate limbs in the normal manner; however, thought has to be given to whether it is practical and possible to provide after care. It is unfair to try and keep deer in surgery, and specialised wildlife units should be approached to provide long-term care up to release.

With a fractured pelvis it must be considered that if repair is possible a female must not be released unless spayed, as pregnancy following a fractured pelvis will invariably result in death of the deer and fawn due to malformation of the pelvic girdle.

Wounds

The most commonly observed are open wounds from a fracture or bites from dogs (Fig. 12.2a). The wounds usually involve the rump with tissue and muscle damage, and extremely deep lacerations, often with loss of skin.

The wounds will require thorough cleaning and management to prevent infection. Treat with systemic and topical antibiotics to control bacterial infections.

Wounds may require to be left open to allow any infection to drain away.

Other wounds may be from wire fencing (Fig. 12.2b) and these may present as tears in the neck or appear as an actual ligation around limbs as a snare would around the neck of an animal.

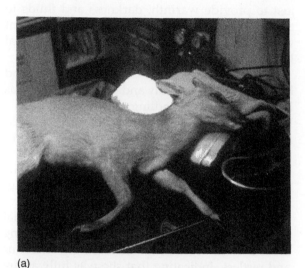

(a)

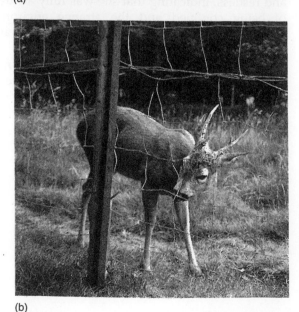

(b)

Fig. 12.2 (a) Dog attack. (b) Caught on wire.

If the limb has been affected there may be damage to tendons, ligaments and blood vessels. Immediately place the limbs on a heat source, preferably wrapped around the foot to encourage blood supply.

Open wounds and lacerations from fencing can be debrided and sutured in the usual manner.

> **Tip:** If treating with antibiotics you will need to administer probiotics in the food as the antibiotics will kill beneficial bacteria in the gut. Probiotics will help stabilise the bacteria and prevent gut dysbiosis.

CASE HISTORY 1

Patient

Adult, female roe deer.

Condition

The deer was victim of a dog attack. She was set upon by two German shepherd dogs that were out of control, and had tear and puncture wounds to her rump and hind legs. She was in a severe state of shock and was very stressed.

Capture

The deer was wrapped in a blanket to include all the legs and the head covered to reduce stress. Deer will usually not struggle if they are hooded and legs enclosed. She was then placed on a stretcher to be moved to the hospital. The wounds were extensive but fairly superficial but would require surgery to treat.

Treatment

The deer was injected with dexadresson to treat the shock and placed on a drip to combat the shock and fluids lost through the injuries. The wounds were dressed and bandaged and an antibiotic injection given.

She was then placed in a warm, dark shed with a heat lamp overnight. Surgery at this point and a general anaesthetic would be dangerous, as the shock would kill the deer. The wounds were covered and the antibiotics would assist in keeping any infection at bay prior to further treatment.

The following day the deer was alert and appeared to be coping with the stress of the attack and captivity. Later that day the deer was given an anaesthetic to allow the wounds to be stitched back together. The wounds were cleaned and were able to be stitched back together well. She was given further antibiotics and pain relief to help in the post-operative period. She was placed back in the shed under a heat lamp and given browse foods, rabbit mix, and fresh fruit and vegetables. She began eating and drinking approximately 6 hours after the operation, which was a good sign.

Over the next few days the wounds were healing well and there was no infection present; the deer was eating and drinking well.

The stitches were removed 10 days later and the deer was returned back to the area where she was found.

CASE HISTORY 2

Patient

Female roe deer, 8–9 months old.

Condition

The deer was a victim of a road traffic accident, was concussed and very unsteady, disorientated and unable to stand. No other physical damage or injuries were obvious.

Capture

The deer was wrapped in a blanket to include all the legs and the head covered to reduce stress. She was then placed on a stretcher to be moved to the hospital.

Treatment

The deer was injected with dexadresson to treat the shock and placed in a warm, dark shed with a heat lamp overnight. Deer do not tolerate high levels of stress as this can cause the immune system to turn on the animal. It is always advisable just to provide warmth, darkness and fluids to allow the adrenaline release to stop as treatment would be ineffective and may harm the animal long term.

The following day the deer was able to stand but the legs were wobbly and weak. The deer was left with minimal handling and provided with a bowl of milk replacement, Lamlac, a cereal-based rabbit mix, a variety of browse foods (leaves and buds from trees), chopped apple, carrot and Lectade to assist in preventing dehydration. She was then left in a heated shed with closed-circuit television for observation.

Over the next 11 days there was gradual improvement, with her walking and moving around and becoming increasingly nervous and restless, indicating that she was fully aware of being confined and the strange environment she was in, thus the wild instinct was returning.

She began feeding well and required no further treatment or observation and was returned to the wild, being placed back near her place of capture.

Chapter 13

Badgers

Sara Cowen

INTRODUCTION

Badgers are a native species to the UK and are fully protected under the Wildlife and Countryside Act 1981 and the Badgers Act 1973.

It is illegal to remove, handle, kill or injure a badger unless it requires emergency help due to injury or illness. Badgers' setts are also fully protected against disturbance.

They are sociable individuals living in setts with a dominant male (boar) and female (sow) (see Table 13.1 for biological data).

> **Tip:** Approximately 10 000 badgers a year are killed in road traffic accidents so the majority of injuries will be fractures, wounds and trauma.

HANDLING

Badgers are extremely powerful animals and are aggressive, especially if injured and in pain. No attempt should be made to handle a badger without protective equipment, leather gloves and a dog grasper (Fig. 13.1).

> **Tip:** If believed to be unconscious prod with a broom first before attempting direct handling. If no response the animal can be scruffed by the neck and the rump to support the weight. Use the broom to restrain the head until securely scruffed. Always place into secure transport as the animal may well come round quicker than expected.

Table 13.1 Biological data

	European badger
Latin name	*Meles meles*
Life span	3–5 years
Description	Black and white haired coat, black stripe across the eyes and under chin, white either side of face
Average male weight	11 kg
Average female weight	10 kg
Average head and body length (cm)	70–80
Average tail length (cm)	15
Gestation period	60–65 days, delayed implantation
Breeding season	Feb–Mar, implant Dec
Litter size	1–4 cubs
Cubs born	Jan–Mar
Average weight of neonates (g)	100
Lactation period	1–12 weeks
Weaning age	12–16 weeks
Eyes and ears open	30 days
Hair erupts	Slightly furred on birth
Milk teeth incisors	4 weeks
Deciduous teeth	4 months
Fully independent	At least 6 months
Adult diet	Omnivorous – earthworms, small rodents, hedgehogs, vegetable matter, insects, birds, eggs, cereals, berries

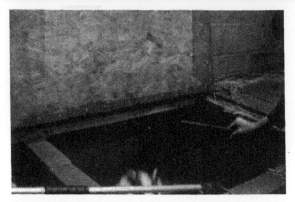

Fig. 13.1 Handling and restraint: scruff and graspers.

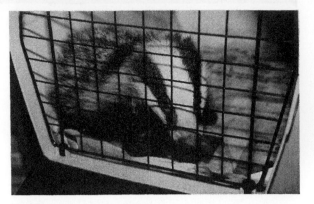

Fig. 13.2 After-rescue housing.

> **Tip:** Badgers can be muzzled, as with dogs, assisting handling; however, be sure the animal has no injury to the face and jaw, which is common with road traffic accidents, or is likely to vomit causing asphyxiation, such as with poisoning.

ACCOMMODATION

Badgers should be kept in metal barred cages, as they are so powerful both their and your safety must be ensured.

If possible, a double enclosure is ideal allowing the animal to be moved from one side to the other whilst the cage is cleaned out. This will prevent the additional stress of being handled repeatedly.

Place newspaper and hay and straw in the cage for warmth.

Badgers keep their beds/nests very clean and tend to defecate in latrines, so it is likely that a formed nest under an upturned dog bed will not require cleaning out. You may find they remove dirty bedding and will replace on their own if left with a fresh pile of straw.

As badgers are a nocturnal species, they should be kept in low light conditions and have the cage covered at all times to reduce fear from captivity (Fig. 13.2).

NUTRITION

Badgers are omnivores and will feed on a wide variety of available vegetable material, such as

Table 13.2 Comparison of milk

	Badger milk (%)	Esbilac (%)	Lamlac (%)
Protein	39	33	24
Fat	34	43	24
Carbohydrate	19	16	–
Solids	19	97	60

Table 13.3 Feeding guidelines

Age (weeks)	Frequency
0–1	2 hourly
1–2	2–3 hourly
2–3	3–4 hourly
3–4	4 hourly
4–7	4–5 feeds daily
7–12	3–4 feeds daily; begin weaning

carrots, peas, potato, etc., and on dog meat, dog biscuits, day-old chicks and peanuts.

If they appear to be reluctant to eat, peanut butter or honey spread onto bread may stimulate feeding, and cheese is often relished.

They will also feed on cereals, so rodent or dog mixes will provide variety. In addition, fresh fruit and berries will also be taken.

HAND REARING

Badgers can be hand reared using a puppy milk substitute, e.g. Welpi or Esbilac. Some have been given ewe replacement effectively such as Lamlac and will initially feed from a teated syringe moving up to a puppy or baby's bottle when larger (Tables 13.2 & 13.3).

> **Tip:** Lactol has been observed to cause baldness in some cubs hand reared on this replacement.

During the first 2 weeks they will require manual stimulation for defecation and urination. Using a damp piece of cotton wool, wipe over the anogenital area before and after feeding (Fig. 13.3a,b,c).

If possible try to place young with cubs of similar ages as they do much better and are likely to remain wilder if kept in pairs or groups.

If the cubs are less than 2 weeks old they will need a heat source of 30°C to be provided as they are unable to thermoregulate, and will continue to require some heat up to 4–6 weeks.

Cubs can be weaned onto dog meat, initially as a milky slop increasing the solid content over time.

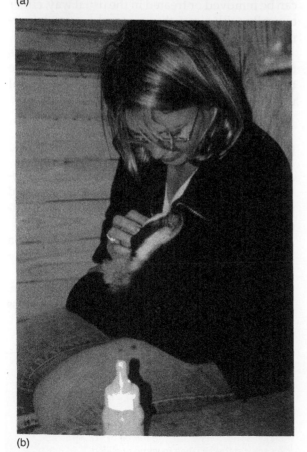

(a)

(b)

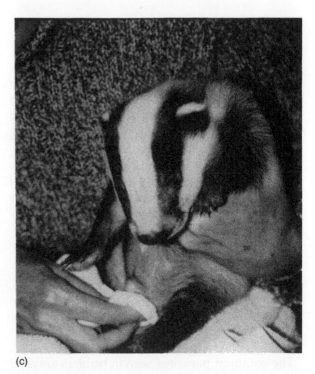

(c)

Fig. 13.3 (a) Bottle feeding. (b) Young cub. (c) Manual stimulation of cub.

At a later stage they will also take small chicks and rodents, eating the whole carcass. They also relish peanuts and honey sandwiches, which can often be used to tempt a reluctant feeder.

Hand-reared badgers cannot be placed in a sett or area where other badgers are present; a completely new location and an artificial or disused sett will be required. Always rehabilitate over a long period of time and integrate with other youngsters setting up a new colony.

FIRST AID

Initial treatment includes the provision of:

- warmth
- darkness
- quiet
- oral fluids – Lectade
- intravenous fluids – approximately 500 ml of an appropriate solution
- corticosteroids
- sedation if required – diazepam 1.0 mg/kg intravenously (IV) or intramuscularly (IM).

ANAESTHESIA

Anaesthesia can be effective, administering a ketamine injection of 20 mg/kg IM. This is useful, as it is unlikely that you will be able or willing to anaesthetise gaseously or intravenously due to the aggressive nature of the animal. Intramuscular injections can be administered in the hind leg during restraint with a dogcatcher.

Combination anaesthesia of domitor 100 μg/kg and ketamine 5 mg/kg IV can be used, and revival can be effected with antisedan. This shortens anaesthetic time and lessens the risk of respiratory depression.

Sedation can be achieved using diazepam 1 mg/kg and can be administered IM (Fig. 13.4).

COMMON ILLNESSES, INJURIES OR DISEASES

Parasites

The common parasites seen in badgers are similar to all wildlife.

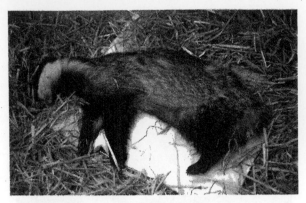

Fig. 13.4 Badger post-operatively.

Badgers are invariably infested with fleas (*Paracerus melis*), ticks (*Ixodes hexagonus*, *Ixodes canisuga*) and lice (*Trichodectes melis*), and these can be removed or treated in the usual way, either topically with a pyrethrum powder or with ivermectin injection.

The nematode *Skrjabingylus nasicola* often affects the nasal passages of badgers and, again, can be treated with ivermectin (adult dose: 0.4–0.5 ml undiluted) or Dectomax.

FRACTURES

As robust animals they have an element of protection from injury; however, hind limbs and pelvic fractures are common in road traffic accidents, as are skull and jaw fractures.

They should be treated in the same way as a small dog and receive internal fixation as casting will be less well tolerated.

Analgesia should be administered (carprofen, buprenorphine) to control pain and reduce stress from injury and captivity.

> **Tip:** Badgers requiring amputations are unsuitable for release into the wild. Forelimbs are used for scratching, foraging and digging for food and for managing the nest site. They would be unable to carry out normal activity. Hind limb removal may lead to attack from dominant badgers without the ability to retreat fast or fight back. A semi-captive situation must be provided.

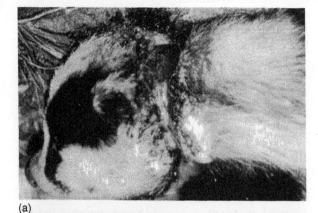

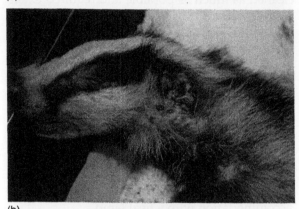

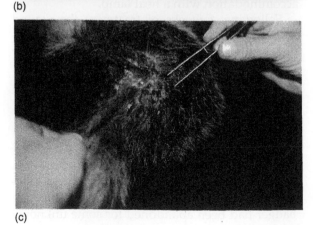

Fig. 13.5 (a) Snare injury. (b) Neck injury. (c) Rump injury.

WOUNDS

Many badgers are found following fights within the group or snare injuries (Fig. 13.5a,b,c). Badgers can lose their dominant position within the group

and be ousted. They often present with severe bite wounds to the rump and neck regions. On arrival the injury may well be septic and infested with maggots.

The wounds will need cleaning thoroughly and debriding prior to suturing. Puncture wounds should be left open to drain and heal.

Flystrike is a killer in these animals and all maggots must be picked or flushed out of the wounds. The wounds can be dusted with Negasunt powder to kill any remaining or hatching larvae. A useful method for syringing maggots is using the dental suction pipe.

Following treatment the badger will need IV fluids to rehydrate and should be placed in a warm, dark environment to recover.

If badgers have been ousted from the colony they cannot be returned and advice must be sought for a suitable release site from your local badger group.

Canine distemper

Both canine distemper and parvovirus are believed to be diseases that badgers are susceptible to, as are foxes. Symptomatic and supportive treatment should be provided.

Bovine tuberculosis

There are ongoing and controversial claims that badgers are a possible source of bovine TB with culling programmes in place to remove badgers from areas of infection. The issue was raised when various dead animals were tested and were found to be positive.

Some observed symptoms are:

- arthritis
- enlarged lymph nodes
- pneumonia
- nephritis
- pericarditis
- hepatitis
- osteomyelitis.

Tip: Following treatment and potential release, badgers, especially cubs, should be vaccinated against TB.

RELEASE

Contact your local badger group for assistance on release.

It is important that they are released where they were found as long as it is safe to return to the original sett. As they will not mix with others, introducing them to areas where there are unfamiliar badgers can result in fighting and potential further injury.

Your badger group will know where the setts in the area are and will advise on the procedure to adopt. Alternatively they will have access to artificial setts that have been set up to colonise with a new group, such as hand-reared cubs, and will allow full observation and protection during this time.

CASE HISTORY 1

Patient

Male badger, 1 year old, identifiable by the animal's size and teeth: presence of first set of deciduous teeth, clean with no calculi present and weight was approximately 6 kg, which is the size of a young adult.

Condition

The badger was immobile and found near collapse and unresponsive in undergrowth.

Capture

The badger was restrained by means of a dog grasper and placed into temporary accommodation for transport. On initial examination the badger was aggressive despite obvious circulatory collapse and extensive visual rump injuries. The badger was sedated for examination to assess the extent of the rump injuries as a result of rejection from the sett and aggression from mature sett individuals. The injuries sustained were extensive bite wounds to the rump region with subsequent infection. Badgers will tolerate fight injuries to the head, ears and rump regardless of impediment, infection and disability, and carry on without too many problems. Wild animals have the ability to mask pain, regardless of severity of injury, and sustain a quality of life that would be comparable to a domestic species suffering from a mild infection.

Treatment

The badger was sedated with domitor and torbugesic, and then placed on isoflurane to allow full examination and treatment. The wound was cleaned as much as possible and required extensive debriding. The wound was repaired with sutures and a drain was put in place for 3 days to allow seepage as the wound was very dirty and infected. The wound was packed with Intrasite gel and antirobe.

The badger was injected with dexadresson and duphamox. Pain relief and antibiotics were continued for 2 weeks as the infection was difficult to control, and the wound was cleaned regularly under general anaesthetic.

The badger was placed on a drip to support the circulatory system and housed in suitable accommodation with a heat lamp.

Following 4 weeks of treatment the wound healed and any breakdown healed with granulation. The badger was released in the evening near the area where it was found to relocate to its sett.

CASE HISTORY 2

Patient

Male badger, 4 weeks old, found on the roadside. The animal was distressed but appeared uninjured. It was assumed at this stage that either the badger had been abandoned for some unknown reason or it was lost.

Condition

The badger was in good condition, although dehydrated. The members of public had kept it overnight but had fed it nothing. The badger was crying but lively.

Capture

The badger was easily restrained and was not aggressive. It was just a cub, small and in need of contact. The badger was placed on a hot water bottle to increase its body temperature as it was fairly cold from lack of food and had been kept overnight in a cat basket outdoors.

Treatment

The badger was given a couple of hours to settle from the rescue and being kept captive, and to increase body temperature. The badger appeared hungry and was very active. At this stage a baby bottle feed of warm Lectade was given rather than milk. This would assist in rehydrating the cub but also enable assessment of the suckling ability of the animal. It is always safer to feed Lectade for the first feed, rather than milk, in case of aspiration pneumonia. Water in the cub's lungs is more easily rectified than milk substitute.

The badger took approximately 20 ml of Lectade and no problems were encountered on feeding.

A bottle feed of warm Esbilac milk was fed 1 hour later at a concentration of two parts water to one part Esbilac powder.

The badger was very enthusiastic over feeding and took to the teat well, taking 50 ml of milk. Over the next couple of weeks, following 3 hourly feeds between 8 am and 10 pm, the badger steadily gained weight and condition, and at this stage was taking 200 ml each bottle feed. At this point puppy Chum and Esbilac were mixed together and fed to initiate weaning. The bottle feeds were gradually reduced to 4 hourly and to four feeds a day. The badger was supplementing the diet by eating solid food of Chum and milk.

By 8 weeks of age only two bottle feeds a day were being given and the badger was placed into an outside enclosure with two other cubs of similar ages. Bottle feeds were removed to encourage solid feeding and a mixture of chopped day-old chicks and fresh and dried fruit was provided. The badger weaned onto the feed and no milk substitute was given from 10 weeks of age.

At this point all human contact was removed in order to begin rehabilitation to the wild. The badgers were relocated with two others to establish a new group. Badgers cannot be relocated into an existing group as they are aggressive in nature, and there would be the risk of fatal injury to the new individuals. An artificial sett in a safe environment or a suitable disused sett has to be used. The badgers were relocated to the sett in September once fully independent and rehabilitated to a wild group. Feeding was supplemented following relocation and they were observed until they were foraging and feeding independently.

Appendix 1

RABBITS

Normal body temperature	38.5–40°C
Normal respiratory rate	30–60 breaths/minute
Normal heart rate	180–300 beats/minute

RABBITS

Appendix 2

DRUG DOSAGES

Analgesia IM, SC or IV. Premedication IM, SC or IV		
	Concentration	
	10 mg/ml	10 mg/ml
Cat (weight in kg)	Torbugesic (dose IM) 0.4 mg/kg	Torbugesic (dose IV) 0.1 mg/kg
2.0	0.08 ml	0.02 ml
3.0	0.12 ml	0.03 ml
4.0	0.16 ml	0.04 ml
5.0	0.20 ml	0.05 ml

Sedation: double combination IM or SC		
	Concentration	
	10 mg/ml	1 mg/ml	5 mg/ml
Cat (weight in kg)	Torbugesic (dose IM, SC)	Domitor (dose IM, SC)	Antisedan (dose IM, SC)
1.5	0.06 ml	0.08 ml	0.04 ml
2.0	0.08 ml	0.10 ml	0.05 ml
2.5	0.10 ml	0.13 ml	0.06 ml
3.0	0.12 ml	0.15 ml	0.08 ml
3.5	0.14 ml	0.18 ml	0.09 ml
4.0	0.16 ml	0.20 ml	0.10 ml
4.5	0.18 ml	0.23 ml	0.11 ml
5.0	0.20 ml	0.25 ml	0.13 ml

Trauma/post-operative analgesia IM, SC or IV

Dog (weight in kg)	Concentration (10 mg/ml)
	Torbugesic (dose IM, SC or IV) 0.25 mg/ml
5	0.10 ml
10	0.30 ml
20	0.50 ml
30	0.80 ml
40	1.00 ml

Premedication IM or IV

Dog (weight in kg)	Concentration	
	10 mg/ml	1 mg/ml
	Torbugesic (dose IM)	Domitor (dose IM)
5	0.05 ml	0.05 ml
10	0.10 ml	0.10 ml
20	0.20 ml	0.20 ml
30	0.30 ml	0.30 ml
40	0.40 ml	0.40 ml

Sedation: double combination IM or IV

Dog (weight in kg)	Concentration		
	10 mg/ml	1 mg/ml	5 mg/ml
	Torbugesic (dose IM or IV)	Domitor (dose IM or IV)	Antisedan (dose IM)
2.5	0.03 ml	0.06 ml	0.06 ml
5	0.05 ml	0.13 ml	0.13 ml
10	0.10 ml	0.25 ml	0.25 ml
15	0.15 ml	0.38 ml	0.38 ml
20	0.20 ml	0.50 ml	0.50 ml
25	0.25 ml	0.63 ml	0.63 ml
30	0.30 ml	0.75 ml	0.75 ml
40	0.40 ml	1.00 ml	1.00 ml

Anaesthesia: triple combination IM

Cat (weight in kg)	Torbugesic	Domitor	Vetalar	45 mins post-induction
	Concentration			
	10 mg/ml	1 mg/ml	100 mg/ml	5 mg/ml
	Torbugesic (dose IM)	Medetomidine (dose IM)	Ketaset (dose IM)	Atipamezole (dose IM)
1.5	0.06 ml	0.12 ml	0.08 ml	0.06 ml
2.0	0.08 ml	0.16 ml	0.10 ml	0.08 ml
2.5	0.10 ml	0.20 ml	0.13 ml	0.10 ml
3.0	0.12 ml	0.24 ml	0.15 ml	0.12 ml
3.5	0.14 ml	0.28 ml	0.18 ml	0.14 ml
4.0	0.16 ml	0.32 ml	0.20 ml	0.16 ml
4.5	0.18 ml	0.36 ml	0.23 ml	0.18 ml
5.0	0.20 ml	0.40 ml	0.25 ml	0.20 ml

New anaesthesia: triple combination IM

	Concentration			
	10 mg/ml	1 mg/ml		100 mg/ml
Dog (weight in kg)	Torbugesic (dose IM)	Domitor (dose IM)		Ketaset (dose IM)
2.5	0.03 ml	0.06 ml		0.13 ml
5	0.05 ml	0.13 ml		0.25 ml
10	0.10 ml	0.25 ml		0.50 ml
15	0.15 ml	0.38 ml	Wait 15 minutes	0.75 ml
20	0.20 ml	0.50 ml		1.00 ml
25	0.25 ml	0.63 ml		1.25 ml
30	0.30 ml	0.75 ml		1.50 ml
40	0.40 ml	1.00 ml		2.00 ml

Anaesthesia: triple combination IV – any stage

	Concentration			
	10 mg/ml	1 mg/ml	100 mg/ml	5 mg/ml
Cat (weight in kg)	Torbugesic (dose IV)	Domitor (dose IV)	Ketaset (dose IV)	Antisedan (dose IM)
1.5	0.02 ml	0.06 ml	0.04 ml	0.03 ml
2.0	0.02 ml	0.08 ml	0.05 ml	0.04 ml
2.5	0.03 ml	0.10 ml	0.06 ml	0.05 ml
3.0	0.03 ml	0.12 ml	0.08 ml	0.06 ml
3.5	0.04 ml	0.14 ml	0.09 ml	0.07 ml
4.0	0.04 ml	0.16 ml	0.10 ml	0.08 ml
4.5	0.05 ml	0.18 ml	0.11 ml	0.09 ml
5.0	0.05 ml	0.20 ml	0.12 ml	0.10 ml

For badgers and foxes use dose rates for dog (of equivalent size).

For all other species use dose rates for cat (of equivalent size).

These dose rates *do not* apply for deer.

Appendix 3

GENERAL INFORMATION ON HAND REARING MAMMALS

On arrival all baby mammals should be weighed, toileted and given a first feed of dilute Lectade before any milk feeds.

Esbilac milk

- In a clean, sterilised jug, mix:
  —One measure of powder
  —Two measures hot water (previously boiled and cooled)
- Stir thoroughly, using a small whisk
- Use clean, sterilised teats and syringes or bottles and teats
- Store excess in a sterilised, **labelled** bottle.

  This type of milk is fed to:

- Baby badgers
- Tiny fox cubs (black fur)
- Baby hedgehogs
- Dormice
- Mice.

Squirrel mix

- In a clean, sterilised jug, mix:
  —3 tbsps of dried goat's milk
  —1 tsp Esbilac
  —2 tsp baby rice
  —¼ pint hot water (previously boiled and cooled)
- Stir with small whisk until all lumps have gone

- Use clean and sterilised syringes and teats
- Store excess in a sterilised, **labelled** bottle.

  This type of milk is fed to baby squirrels over 3 weeks of age.

Cimicat milk

- In a clean, sterilised jug, mix:
  —One measure of Cimicat powder
  —Three measures hot water (previously boiled and cooled)
- Stir thoroughly using a small whisk
- Use clean and sterilised syringes and teats for feeding
- Store excess in a sterilised, **labelled** bottle.

  This type of milk can be fed to:

- Baby squirrels, birth–2 weeks
- Baby rabbits plus Abidec multivitamins plus probiotic – Avipro
- Fox cubs
- Weaning older hedgehogs.

FEEDING AND CARING FOR BABY MAMMALS

1. Weigh and record weight and sex on patient card.
2. Toilet. It may have lost its mother hours before and have a very full bladder!
3. Place in an incubator. Use a small piece of wool blanket on top of soft towels for bedding. A soft toy can be added as a surrogate mother. Do not attempt to feed until the animal feels warm.

4.   First feed should consist of warm Lectade or similar given diluted as per directions on the packet and fed via 1 ml syringe plus teat. (Always use boiled, cooled water and sterilised teats and syringes.) Subsequent feeds should consist of the appropriate milk feed for the type of animal. **Feed very slowly and carefully**.

When caring and feeding for these little creatures throughout the day and into the evening, special attention should be paid to:

1.   Feeding and toileting at regular intervals.
2.   Using a previously sterilised 1 ml syringe and teat (squirrels, rabbits and hedgehogs) or baby bottle and large teat (fox cubs, badgers and fawns) or 1 ml syringe and cannula (mice, dormice and other tinies).
3.   Sterilising feeding utensils successfully. They should be filled with sterilising solution to *cover* the contents. There should be one clean feeding utensil in the pot for each baby in the incubator at every feed. After use they must be taken apart and thoroughly washed in hot soapy water, rinsed and placed back into the sterilising pot.
4.   Toileting. Always use a soft piece of toilet paper dampened with water. The urinary area should be gently stroked or tickled and the movement continued until all urination and defecation has ceased. They do not always defecate but they should pass water every time they are toileted.
5.   Being patient when feeding these helpless babies. Concentrate on the job in hand, watch their mouths carefully and stop feeding them immediately they stop sucking, otherwise they will choke, milk will go down their noses, into their lungs, and they will become sick and die.
6.   Use clean woollen gloves when feeding bald babies as their temperature drops quickly if your hands are cold. Concentrate on holding them safely; baby rabbits can jump out of your hands in an instant!!
7.   If the milk is already made up, give the container a good shake every feed as it can settle in the fridge and the last babies to be fed get a thick, sludgy mix!

WHICH MILK FEED FOR WHICH BABY?

Baby badgers

- Are fed Esbilac milk, mixed one part Esbilac powder to two parts boiled water using a sterilised baby bottle with a large teat.
- They can be weaned on puppy food and Milupa baby food – they love the fruit puddings best. They also like chopped chicks with beaks and legs removed at first.

Fox cubs

- Are fed on Cimicat milk mixed one part Cimicat powder to three parts boiled water using a sterilised baby bottle and large teat.
- If they are really tiny Esbilac milk, mixed one part Esbilac powder to two parts boiled water, is best at this early stage.
- Fox cubs are weaned on puppy food and Cimicat milk mixed together; chopped chicks are very popular, but need the beaks and legs removed at first.

Squirrels

- 1–3 weeks Cimicat only, one part Cimicat to three parts water.
- After 3 weeks give 'Squirrel mix', which has to be measured and mixed daily.
- To feed them use a 1 ml sterilised syringe and small teat.
- They are weaned on brown bread, rabbit/squirrel mix and chopped fruit, e.g. apple.

Baby rabbits

- Are also fed on Cimicat plus Avipro and Abidec.
- Use a 1 ml syringe and small teat attached, that has been previously sterilised.
- Feed 2 hourly from 6 am–12 pm and they will need one feed in the night.
- They are weaned on dry plain rabbit mix, brown bread and chopped apple. No fresh green food at first.

Dormice

- If their eyes are shut they need feeding 2 hourly with Esbilac milk, mixed one part Esbilac powder to two parts boiled water; use a cannula fixed onto a 1 ml syringe (sterilised) to administer the milk. They need to be toileted and kept warm and dry.
- When the eyes open they need to be weaned in the usual way; offer them grated apple, Milupa baby food (fruit variety) and jars of fruit puree can be used. Grain and blackberries can also be given; a very shallow dish with water on a tissue will be fine for drinking.

Woodmice

- Same milk feed and toileting as for dormice.
- They are weaned on brown bread, apple, grain, sluis and water on a tissue.

All these animals in the process of being weaned need a **small** shallow bowl of water in their cage. Mice need a small lid with a tissue soaked in water.

Appendix 4

FEEDING AND CARING FOR BABY BIRDS

1. Weigh and record result on the patient card.
2. Place in an incubator. Make sure it is switched on! Not too hot and not too cool. If they are bald make a nest for them using a plastic dish (nest shape) and line with paper towelling.
3. For ducklings a cotton mophead can be hung from the top of the cage as a surrogate mother.
4. Water birds will also need an incubator but with a towel covering the newspaper.
5. First feed should not commence until the bird feels warm, and looks reasonably alert. **For birds that gape** use a pair of plastic tweezers or if very tiny a paintbrush and offer the food in **tiny** amounts.
6. Offer water too with a 1 ml syringe before and after feeding.
7. If very small, they may need feeding hourly, but remember too little is safer than too much food. **Water birds are self feeding**, so once they are warm, they will need the appropriate food and water in their incubator at all times.

When caring and feeding these little creatures throughout the day and into the evening, special attention should be paid to:

1. Feeding at regular intervals.
2. Using a clean, previously sterilised pair of tweezers for birds that gape. After using the tweezers they must be washed and stored in a pot of sterilising solution. The solution must completely cover the contents.
3. Picking up only tiny pieces of food to pop into their open beaks each time. Do not scoop up a large amount and try and feed each baby off this one tweezer full. They will try and force down too much in one go and often end up choking!
4. Squabs (baby pigeons) are tube fed.
5. All swifts are tube fed.
6. Make sure, as far as possible, that they produce a dropping each time you feed them.
7. Remember as far as possible to weigh each bird daily when cleaning the cage. When they have fledged and begin to fly, procedure will become impractical, and it should be discontinued.

WHICH FOOD FOR WHICH BABY BIRD?

Blackbirds, thrushes, sparrows, robins, starlings and finches

All are fed cat food finely mashed, with sluis and chopped maggots and a few drops of water offered on plastic tweezers; usually 1–2 hourly feeds, depending on age of bird (first feed of the day should have a pinch of Vitracel ZM or SA 37 added).

When ready to feed themselves they are given a small dish of cat food, sluis and live maggots in their cage. They show interest in the wiggly maggots and it encourages them to peck. A small bowl of water should also be available at this stage.

Finches and sparrows eventually like to eat mixed seeds, including millet, sunflower seeds and sluis.

Crows, jays, jackdaws and magpies

Are fed mashed cat food with a drop of water added and finely chopped up dead, day-old chicks. This is fed to them with plastic tweezers. 2–3 hourly depending on age (first feed of the day should have a pinch of Vitracel ZM or SA 37 added).

When ready to begin to feed themselves they should be given a small bowl of cat food and chopped chick plus a bowl of water in their cage. Do not give the crow family low, shallow dishes to feed from; they stand in them and get foot problems.

Food dishes should also be placed to the side of the cage, as if they are at the front the birds will stand in them.

Housemartins, swallows, wrens and other small-beaked birds

Are fed finely chopped maggots or mealworms. Feed 1–2 hourly depending on age, and offer with tweezers (first feed of the day should have a pinch of Vitracel ZM or SA37 added).

When ready to begin to feed themselves, they should be given a small bowl of sluis and live maggots, plus a small bowl of water in their cage.

Tits

Need the same treatment as above, but will need to be hand fed with tweezers for much longer than other garden birds. Even when they are outside in an aviary and seem to be feeding themselves, they need to be hand fed at least four times a day. They spend quite a long period of time after they have left the nest, following their parents around and being fed in the trees.

Swifts

Soak meaty cat biscuits in water until soggy, add some sluis plus a pinch of Nutrobal and a pinch of Avipro, all liquidised and sieved. This should be the consistency of soft ice cream.

Suck it up into a 5 ml syringe and attach to this a small soft tube about 3″ long. Wrap the bird up in a small piece of towelling to confine the wings, or get someone to hold it for you. Pass the tube down the bird's throat to the crop (avoiding the air passage at the base of the tongue) and ease about 2–4 ml into its crop. Do this four times a day.

Watch the bird's beak at all times to make sure the mixture does not come back up its throat. Babies and adults are all fed in this way.

Woodpeckers

If young enough they will gape and can be fed mashed cat food and chopped maggots. If they are older and refuse to eat they should be fed as for swifts. Once ready place cat meat, honey and sluis packed into the holes in an upstanding log. They will peck the food out of the log and it is a natural way for them to eat.

Kestrels, owls and sparrowhawks

If fluffy yellow feathers are present, feed tiny pieces of chopped chick (no beak, legs or egg sac until older); add a vitamin and calcium supplement daily, Nutrobal plus ACE vitamins and SA 37 are both suitable. Feed 2–3 hourly to begin with and adjust accordingly as the bird gets older.

Coots, lapwings and moorhens

Hand feed chopped maggots to begin with, and also tiny pieces of whitebait. Later when they are beginning to self feed, give them a small bowl of sluis and live maggots, and whitebait in a small bowl of pond water.

Cygnets, ducklings and goslings

Feed with chick crumbs and bread soaked in pond water. Place this in small bowls, too small for them to sit in. If they get wet at this early, fluffy stage they cannot keep themselves warm. They do not naturally have oil on their feathers and rely on their mother for this, by nestling under her wings; the feathers are also not water repellent. They will need a towel covering the newspaper and a mophead can be hung from the top of the cage to act as a surrogate mother.

Baby pigeon (squab) feeding

Baby pigeons with yellow feathers are fed Kaytee Exact. The babies are tube fed Kaytee in just the same way as the other birds mentioned above, taking care not to force the tube down too far, as they are very small. They need to be fed 2 hourly if very young.

All must have warmth, peace and quiet, and food regularly supplied, whether by hand or placed in the cage for them to help themselves.

PIGEON MIX RECIPE FOR FORCE FEEDING

- 150 g dry chick crumbs
- 420 ml hot water (previously boiled and slightly cooled)
- Or if to be used immediately, 300 ml hot water and after soaking, cool with 120 ml cold water (all previously boiled).

1. Soak chick crumbs in hot water for at least 15 minutes. If using hot and cold water add cold water after soaking in hot.
2. Mix well and spoon into liquidiser, replace lid, switch on. Liquidise for at least 30 seconds, spoon into a suitable sieve.
3. Push mixture through the sieve using a large spoon.
4. Keep sieving until the mixture has virtually all disappeared into the bowl below. It takes time, but if this is not done thoroughly, all the pigeons get to eat is thin coloured water, instead of a thick even mix of chick crumb and water.
5. **The finished product should be thick and creamy**, and will easily draw up into a tube and syringe. If it doesn't, then the mixture has not been sieved correctly and it will need to be re-sieved. **Store in the refrigerator.**
6. When feeding the pigeons, the mixture must be warmed to blood heat. **Do not heat up the whole basin of mix.** Remove an estimated amount from the bowl (depending on how many birds there are to feed) and heat this up separately. It can then be discarded and not re-heated every feed time.

KAYTEE EXACT

1. This powder must be mixed up freshly every feed.
2. A very small amount can be made up each feed (half a scoop is enough for two 50 g squabs).

Category	Hospital foods	No. of feeds/routine
Blackbird, bunting, finch, robin, sparrow, starling, thrush	Maggots and/or cat food (mashed finely) Fine strips of raw ox heart with scrambled egg and a dusting of vitamin powder SA 37. Alternatively hard boiled egg	Every hour 6 am–10 pm
Coot, lapwing, moorhen	Maggots and sluis with plenty of water	Ad lib
Crow, jackdaw, jay, magpie	Catfood mashed with a dash of water	Every hour 6 am–10 pm
Cygnet, duckling, gosling	Chick crumbs with plenty of water	Ad lib
Housemartin, swallow, swift, tit, wren	Maggots and mealworms (chopped) and sluis with a pinch of SA 37	Swift does not gape – open beak very carefully, put food beyond tongue
Kestrel, owl, sparrowhawk	Chopped chick (small pieces or strips)	No water to be given
Pigeon	Pigeon mix	Does not gape – open beak carefully, insert syringe beyond tongue

3. Use hot water to mix (previously boiled).
4. Let the mixture stand for a few minutes to thicken and cool to blood heat.
5. It should be a creamy consistency.
6. If the squabs' crops do not empty between feeds the Kaytee mix is too thick and should be made thinner, for one or two feeds.

7. Use the designated syringe, tube and small plastic tub for mixing, which should be kept in a pot of sterilising fluid, and labelled with hourly feeds.
8. When the feeding has finished, wash the tube and syringe well in hot, soapy water, rinse and return to the sterilising pot.
9. Throw away any Kaytee that is left over.

Index

A

Acts of Parliament
  Protection of Animals Act (1911)
      (live prey) 69
  Wildlife and Countryside Act (1981)
      (protected species) 69, 207
Aeromonas infections, reptiles 60
allergies, rats and mice, case history
      42–3
alopecia
  birds 156
  rodents 33
anaesthesia
  badgers 225
  bats 175
  birds 129–31, **132**, 138, 154–6
  chelonians 100
  dogs and cats, weight tables **233–5**
  emergencies **133**
  hedgehogs 202
  inhalation **132**
  lizards and snakes 78–9
  rabbits 13–14
  reptiles 78–9
  rodents 29
analgesia
  birds 130
  dose rates 202, **233–5**
  rabbits 10, 15
  wildlife 169
anorexia
  birds 126–7
  chelonians 102, 109–13
  lizards and snakes 73–5
  rabbits 9–11, 15, 20–3
anthelminthics 17, 106, 203
antibiotics, dose rates 202
antidiuretic hormone (ADH) 36–7
antiparasitics, dose rates 202
antisedan, dose rates **233–5**

appendixes
  baby bird care and feeding 241–4
  baby mammal care and feeding
      237–40
  drug dosage rates 233–6
  milk formulas **237**
  rabbit data 231
Archaeopsylla erinacei, hedgehog flea
      198
aspergillosis, birds 145, 156
atipamezole, dose rates **235**
atropine, dose rate, birds 133, 134
avian pox 157

B

baby birds, care and feeding 241–4
baby mammals
  hand rearing 237–9
  see also named species
badgers 223–9
  accommodation 224
  anaesthesia 226
    table (dog weights) **234–5**
  analgesia, table (dog weights) **233**
  biological data **223**
  bovine tuberculosis 227
  case histories 228–9
  common conditions/diseases
      226–7
    parasites 226
    trauma 226–7
  first aid 226
  food and feeding 224
  hand rearing 225–6, 228–9, 238
    milk formula 238
  handling/restraint 223
  release 226, 228
  and tuberculosis 227
barbarism, rodents 39

bats 171–8
  accommodation 173
  anaesthesia 175
  anatomy 172–3
  assessment and first aid 173–4
  behaviour 172
  case history 178
  common conditions/diseases 176–8
  fluid therapy 173–4
  food and feeding 174–5
  hand rearing orphans 174
  rabies 178
  species
    biological data **176**
    conservation status **171**
  torpor and hibernation 175–6
betamethasone, rodents 37
biological data
  badgers **223**
  bats **176**
  deer **217**
  foxes **179**
  hedgehogs **192**
  rabbits 231
  rodents **25**
  squirrels **208**
birds *(incl.* cage and wild birds)
      119–63
  accommodation 125–6, 150
  anatomy 119–22, 141–2
  assessment 122–4
    Lansdown Hospital form 127
  average weights **130**
  baby bird care and feeding 241–4
  case histories 137–41, 161–3
  classification 119
  common conditions/diseases
      135–7, 156–61
    alopecia 156
    anorexia 126–8
    aspergillosis 145, 156
    avian pox 157

birds (*continued*)
  botulism 157
  feather plucking 136
  fish hooks/lines 160, 162
  lead poisoning 160
  metabolic bone disease 161
  oiling 159–60
  paramyxovirus 157
  parasites 144–5, 156
  psittacine beak and feather
    disease (PBFD) 136–7
  psittacocis/ornithosis 136
  respiratory disease 135–6
  salmonellosis 136
  trauma/fractures 135, 137–8,
    145–8, 158, 160, 161–2
  wing and feather damage 157–8
emergencies 134–5
  cardiopulmonary arrest 134–5
  dehydration 134
  hypocalcaemia syndrome 134
  hypothermia 134
equipment list **123**
first aid 132–4, 143–4, 153–6
fluid therapy 129–30, 138, 154
food and feeding 128–9, 150–1, **152**
  gavaging 154
hand rearing 151–3, 241–4
handling/restraint 122–3, 149
hospitalisation 123–6
hypocalcaemia syndrome 134
hypothermia 133, 153, 155
medication 124–5, 138, 161
  anaesthesia 130–2, 138–41
  emergencies **133**
monitoring 124, 126
pre/postoperative care 154–6
  anaesthesia 130–2, 138, 154–6
  emergencies 132
skeletal system 119, 120
vital signs 131–2
see also birds of prey
birds of prey 141–8
  anatomy 119–21, 141–2
  baby bird care and feeding 241–4
  case histories 147–8
  common conditions/diseases 144–7
    aspergillosis 145
    bumblefoot 146
    fractures/trauma 146, 147–8
    parasites 144–5
    respiratory infections 145
    starvation 146–7
    trichomoniasis 145
  first aid 143–4
  food and feeding 142, **143**
  hand rearing 142–3, 242

handling/restraint 142
  see also birds (*incl.* cage and wild
    birds)
bone disease *see* metabolic bone
  disease
Bordetella bronchoseptica infections 197
Borrelia, Lyme disease, reptiles 60
botulism, birds 157
bovine tuberculosis 227
bumblefoot, birds of prey 146
burns, lizards and snakes 62

C

caecotrophs 8
cage and wild birds *see* birds
cages *see named species*:
    accommodation
calcium: phosphorus ratios,
    fruits/vegetables 70, 71
calcium
  hypocalcaemia 37–8
  metabolism in reptiles **58**
  metastatic calcification in rodents 38
calcium borogluconate 76
calcium gluconate
  dose rate
    birds 133
    reptiles 76
calcium stones *see* urolithiasis
Campylobacter infections, reptiles 60
canine distemper, badgers 227
canine leptospirosis, foxes 186
Capillaria infestations
  birds 144–5
  hedgehogs 198
cardiopulmonary arrest, birds 134–5
carnidazol, trichomoniasis 145, 156
cat, analgesia, dose rates **233–5**
chelonians 87–113
  accommodation 51, 55–9, 87–93
    cleaning and hygiene 92–3
    lighting 91–2
    water 92
  anatomy and physiology **89**
    airways 99
    carapace and plastron 90
    thermoregulation 90–1
  assessment/monitoring 67
  case histories 102, 109–13
  common conditions/diseases 47,
    62–6, 103–8
    anorexia, post-hibernation 102,
      109–13
    dystocia 108
    ear abscess 106–7

    hypocalcaemia 103–4
    hypovitaminosis A 104
    metabolic bone disease 98–9, 103
    parasites 106
    penile prolapse 107, 110–13
    runny nose syndrome 105
    shell rot 105–6
    stomatitis **105**
  dehydration 61
  examination 48–9
  food and feeding
    problems 98–9
    stomach tubing **110**
    tortoise 95–7
    tortoise hatchling 96–7
    turtle/terrapin 97–8
    water provision 96
  handling/restraint 94
  hibernation (brumation) 89, **111–12**
  monitoring 93–4
    assessment of weight ratio **109**
    records 93
  pre/postoperative care 76–80,
    99–101
    induction of anaesthesia 100
    injection sites **77**, 99
  species, lists **89**
Cheyletiella infestation, rabbits 18
chinchillas 24
  biological data **25**
  clinical data **30**
  handling 26
chlamydiosis 135
Cimicat milk 237
cisapride 20
CITES protection, chelonians **88**
Citrobacter infections, reptiles 60
classification of small mammals **24**
clinical data
  hedgehogs **194**
  rodents **30**
Clostridium botulinum, botulism in
  birds 157
coccidiostats, poisoning 40
corticosteroids *see* dexamethasone
cranberry juice 41–2
Crenosoma striatum (lungworm),
  hedgehogs 198
cystostomy, urolithiasis, rodents 34–5

D

deer 217–22
  accommodation 218
  anatomy and physiology 217–18
  case history 222

common conditions/diseases
    parasites 220
    post capture myopathy 220
    trauma 220–1
  first aid 219
  food and feeding 218–19
  hand rearing 219
  species, biological data **217**
degu 24, 36
dental disease, rabbits 4, 15–16, 20–3,
    32
dexamethasone
  deer 220
  rodents 37
  squirrels 213
dextrose, emergency use, birds 133
diabetes insipidus, rodents 36–7
diabetes mellitus, rodents 36
diazepam 130
  dose rate, birds 133, 155
diuresis, in urolithiasis 42
dog, analgesia, dose rates **234–5**
domitor, dose rates **233–5**
dormice, hand rearing 239
doxepram, dose rate, birds 133, 134
drug administration, parenteral routes,
    reptiles **77**
dysecdysis, lizards and snakes 62
dystocia (egg-binding)
  chelonians 108
  lizards and snakes 63, 80–3

E

ear abscess, chelonians 106–7
ear infections 202
ecdysis, lizards and snakes 62
eclampsia, rodents 37–8
ectoparasites
  badgers 225
  bats 177–8
  birds 144–5, 156
  chelonians 106
  deer 220
  foxes 185–6
  hedgehogs 198–9
  lizards and snakes **64**
  squirrels 212
egg-binding, lizards and snakes 63,
    80–3
Encephalitozoon cuniculi
  rabbits 17
  in rabbits 17
endoparasites
  badgers 225
  birds of prey 144–5

chelonians 106
foxes 186
hedgehogs 197–8
lizards and snakes **64**
reptiles 60
squirrels 212
enrofloxacin 20
enteritis/diarrhoea, rodents 29–30
Enterobacter infections, reptiles 60
enterotoxaemia 29, 31
epinephrine, emergency use, birds
    133, 134
Esbilac milk 237
eye infections 202

F

feet, pododermatitis in rodents 38–9
fibroma, squirrels 213
fleas
  badgers 225
  hedgehogs 198
  rabbits 17
fluid therapy
  bats 173–4
  birds 129–30, 138, 154
  lizards and snakes 61, 78, 82–3, 85
fly strike (myiasis) 18–19, 199, 204, 226
foxes 179–89
  accommodation 181
  assessment and first aid 184, 188–9
  biological data **179**
  case histories 188–9
  common conditions/diseases
    endoparasites 186
    mange 185–6, 189
    mites 186
    poisoning 187–8
    trauma 186–8
  food and feeding 181–4
  hand rearing 181, 238
    milk formula 238
  handling/restraint 179–81
fractures
  birds 146, 147–8, 158
  lizards and snakes 62–3
frounce 145, 156
fruits, calcium : phosphorus ratios **70**,
    71

G

gapeworm, birds of prey 145
gastrointestinal disease
  enterotoxaemia 29, 31

rodents 29–31, 35–6
  clinical signs 31
  enteritis/diarrhoea 29–30
  enterotoxaemia 29, 31
  scurvy 31–2
  trichobezoars 31
  wet tail (proliferative ileitis)
    35–6
gerbils 23, **24**, **25**
  biological data **25**
  clinical data **30**
  handling 26
  see also rodents
glucose deficiency, pregnancy
    toxaemia, rodents 37
guinea pigs 23, **24**, **25**
  biological data **25**
  clinical data **30**
  eclampsia/hypocalcaemia
    37–8
  handling 25
  pregnancy toxaemia/ketosis 37

H

haematological data
  hedgehogs **195**
  rodents **30**
halothane 131
hamsters 23
  biological data **25**
  clinical data **30**
  handling 26
  see also rodents
hand rearing
  baby mammals 237–9
  badgers 225–6, 238
  bats 174–5
  birds 151–3
  birds of prey 142–3
  deer 219
  dormice 239
  foxes 181, 238
  hedgehogs 195–6
  milk formulas **210**, **237**
  rabbits 238
  rodents 239
  squirrels 209–10, 238
  wood mice 239
handling/restraint
  badgers 223
  birds 121–2, 149
  chelonians 94
  hedgehogs 191–2
  lizards and snakes **81–2**
  squirrels 208–9

hedgehogs 191–205
 accommodation 192–3, 203–4
 anaesthesia 202
 anatomy 191
 assessment and first aid 191–2
 biological data **192**
  breeding data **195**
 case history 203–5
 clinical data **194**
  blood values **195**
 common conditions/diseases
   195–202
  abandonment 195–6
  burns 201
  dental disease 200
  endoparasites 197–8
  flystrike 199, 204
  hibernation problems 196–7, 203
  mange 199
  mites 199
  poisoning 201
  prolapsed eye 201
  respiratory infections 197
  ringworm 199
  trauma 200–1
 food and feeding 193
 hand rearing 195–6, 205
 handling/restraint 191–2
 medication 202, **202**
 pre/postoperative care 193–5
  anaesthesia 194
 release considerations 202–3
 self-anointing behaviour 201
herbivores, vegetable/fruit
    calcium : phosphorus ratios 70,
    71
hibernation
 bats 175–6
 chelonians 89, **111–12**
 hedgehogs 196–7
 lizards and snakes 69, 74
housing *see named species*:
    accommodation
hypocalcaemia
 birds 134
 chelonians **103–4**
 rodents 37–8
hypothermia 29
 birds 133, 153, 155
hypovitaminosis A, chelonians **104**

I

ileitis, proliferative (rodents (wet tail))
   35–6
isoflurane 131

ivermectin
 bird 145
 fox 185, 186

J

jird 24

K

ketamine 130
 dose rate, birds 155
ketaset, dose rates **233–5**
Klebsiella infections, reptiles 60

L

lagomorphs *see* hares; rabbits
Lansdown Hospital form 127
lead poisoning, birds 160
leptospirosis, foxes 186
lice
 badgers 225
 birds 156
lighting *see* accommodation *under*
    named groups/species
lizards and snakes 47–86
 accommodation 51, 55–9
  lighting and vitamin D3 58–9, 71
 anatomy and physiology **52–3**, 77–8
 assessment and first aid 60–7
 case histories 80–5
 common conditions/diseases 47,
   62–6
  anorexia 73–5
  burns 62
  dehydration 61, 82–3
  dysecdysis 62
  dystocia (egg-binding) 63, 80–3
  fractures 62–3
  metabolic bone disease 75–6
  necrotic dermatitis 62
  parasites **64**
  respiratory disease 65, 83–5
  stomatitis 62
  tail autotomy 66
  thiamine deficiency 65
 dehydration 61, 82–3
 ecdysis **53**, 62
 examination 48–9
 fluid therapy 61, 78, 82–3, 85
 food and feeding **54**, 68–75
  anorexia 73–5
  by species **54**

carnivores 71–2
herbivores 70–1
omnivores 72
prey items compared **68**, 69
vitamin D3 58, 71
water 72–3
 handling/restraint **81–2**
 hibernation (brumation) 69, 74
 pre/postoperative care 76–80
  drug administration **77**
  ECG 79
  induction of anaesthesia 78–9
  pulse oximetry 79
 species
  food requirements 70–3
  lists 47–8, **54**
 temperature regulation 57–8
 water and humidity 72–3
 zoonoses **60**
lungworm
 deer 220
 hedgehogs 198
Lyme disease
 deer 220
 reptiles 60

M

mange
 foxes 185–6
 hedgehogs 199
medetomidine, dose rates 130, **235**
meloxicam 20
metabolic bone disease
 birds 161
 chelonians 98–9, **103**
 lizards and snakes 75–6
 squirrels 214
metronidazole, trichomoniasis 145,
   156
microflora, disruption 202
Microsporum infections, hedgehogs 199
midazolam 130
milk formulas **210, 237**
  see also hand rearing; *specific animals*
    under food and feeding
mites
 birds 156
 ear mites 202
 hedgehogs 199, 202
 rabbits 18
 reptiles 60, 64
 rodents 33–4
 zoonoses 60
muscle diseases, myodystrophy in
   rodents 39

myiasis (fly strike) 18–19, 199, 204, 226
myodystrophy, rodents 39
myopathy, post capture, deer 220
myxomatosis 17–18

N

necrotic dermatitis, lizards and snakes
    62
nitrous oxide 131

O

obesity, rodents 32–3

P

paramyxovirus, wild birds 157
paraphimosis, penile prolapse,
    chelonians 107, 111–13
parapoxvirus, squirrels 212–13
parasites *see* ectoparasites (skin);
    endoparasites (internal)
Pasteurella multocida infections
    birds of prey 145
    hedgehogs 197
penile prolapse, chelonians 107, 111–13
pineapple juice, trichobezoars 31
pododermatitis, rodents 38–9
poisoning, rodents 40
poisonous plants 40
praziquantel, hedgehogs 198
pregnancy toxaemia/ketosis, rodents
    37
probiotics 29
propofol 130
Protection of Animals Act (1911), live
    prey 69
Proteus infections, reptiles 60
psittacine beak and feather disease
    (PBFD) 136
psittacosis/ornithosis 136
Psoroptes cuniculi (ear mite), rabbits 18
pulse oximetry
    birds 132
    reptiles 79, 101

R

rabbits 3–23
    accommodation 7–8
    analgesics 10, 15

assessment 6–7
biological data 231
caecotrophs 8
case histories 19–23
common conditions/diseases 5,
    15–19
    anorexia 9–11, 15, 20–3
    dental disease 4, 15–16, 32
    Encephalitozoon cuniculi 17
    infections/parasites 17–19
    overgrown incisors 20–3
    respiratory disease 16–17
    spaying 23
first aid situations 5, 7
food and feeding 8–9
gut motility stimulants 10–11
hand rearing 238
    milk formula 11, 238
operation
    anaesthesia 13–14
    pre-anaesthesia care 9, 11–13
    postoperative care 14–15
    reversal of anaesthesia 14
rabies, bats 178
rats and mice
    biological data **25**
    clinical data **30**
    food and feeding 27, 42–3
    handling 25
    reproductive data **25**
    see also rodents
reproductive data, rodents **25**
reptiles 45–113
    accommodation 51, 55–9, 87–93
    common conditions/diseases **62–6**
    dehydration 61, 82–3
    drug administration, parenteral
        routes **77**
    examination 48–9
    food and feeding, vitamin D3 58, 71
    handling/restraint **81–2**
    zoonoses **60**
    see also chelonians; lizards and snakes
respiratory infections
    birds 145
    birds of prey 145
    hedgehogs 197, 202
    lizards and snakes 65, 83–5
    rabbits 16–17
restraint *see* handling/restraint
Rickettsia, Siberian tick typhus, reptiles
    60
ringworm, hedgehogs 199
rodents 23–43
    accommodation 26
    biological data **25**
    case histories 41–3

classification **24**
clinical data **30**
common conditions/diseases 29–41
    alopecia 33
    barbarism 39
    calcification 38
    dental overgrowth 32
    diabetes 36–7
    eclampsia/hypocalcaemia 37–8
    gastrointestinal 29–31, 35–6
    mites 33–4
    myodystrophy 39
    obesity 32–3
    pododermatitis 38–9
    poisoning 40
    pregnancy toxaemia/ketosis 37
    scurvy 31–2
    torticollis 35
    urolithiasis 34–5
    vitamin C deficiency 31–2
food and feeding 27, 42–3
hand rearing 239
operation
    anaesthesia 29
    pre/postoperative care 28
see also rabbits; *named rodents*
runny nose syndrome, chelonians 105

S

salmonellosis
    birds 136
    reptiles 60
scurvy, rodents 31–2
sedation, table (dog weights) **234–5**
shell rot, chelonians 105–6
Siberian tick typhus, reptiles 60
skin sloughing (ecdysis), lizards and
    snakes 62
Skrjabingylus nasicola (nematode),
    badgers 225
small mammals
    biological data **25**
    classification **24**
    hand rearing 237–9
    see also rodents; *named species*
spaying, rabbits 23
squirrels 207–15
    accommodation 209
    anaesthesia 212
    anatomy and physiology 207–8
    biological data **208**
    case history 214–15
    common conditions/diseases 212–14
        fibroma 213
        metabolic bone disease 214

parapoxvirus 212–13
parasites 212
poisoning 213–14
trauma 213, 215
first aid 211–12
food and feeding 209–11
hand rearing 209–10, 238
milk formula 237
weaning 211
handling/restraint 208–9
release 214
Staphylococcus aureus pododermatitis 38–9
starvation, birds of prey 146–7
stomatitis
chelonians **105**
lizards and snakes 62
Syngamus tracheae (gapeworm), birds of prey 145

T

tail autotomy, lizards and snakes 66
thiamine deficiency, lizards and snakes 65
threadworms *see Capillaria* infestations
ticks
badgers 225
deer 220
foxes 186
reptiles 60, 64

torbugesic, dose rates **233–5**
torticollis, rodents 35
tortoises/turtles *see* chelonians
trichobezoars 31
trichomoniasis, birds 145, 156
Trichophyton erinacei, hedgehogs 199
tuberculosis 227

U

urolithiasis
rodents 34–5
case history 40–2

V

vegetables, calcium : phosphorus ratios 70, 71
viral haemorrhagic disease, rabbits 18
vitamin A, hypovitaminosis A, chelonians **104**
vitamin B1, deficiency, reptiles **65**
vitamin C, deficiency, rodents 31–2
vitamin D3
reptiles
calcium metabolism 58
supplementation issues 71
vivaria 51–9
substrates/materials **55**

W

Weil's disease 186
wet tail (proliferative ileitis), rodents 35–6
wildlife 149–229
assessment and receiving casualty 168–9
pain 169
procedure flowchart 167
see also birds; *named species*
Wildlife and Countryside Act (1981), protected species 69, 207
wood mice, hand rearing 239

X

xylazine, dose rate, birds 130, 155

Z

zoonoses
leptospirosis in foxes 186
Lyme disease 60, 220
mites 60
psittacocis/ornithosis 136
rabies in bats 178
reptiles **60**

Printed and bound by CPI Group (UK) Ltd, Croydon, CR0 4YY

03/10/2024

01040345-0007